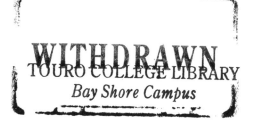

Musculoskeletal Aspects of Haemophilia

To my wife (Hortensia) and the rest of my family
for their constant and patient support.
E.C. Rodriguez-Merchan

To my family for their continued forebearance,
love and encouragement.
N.J. Goddard

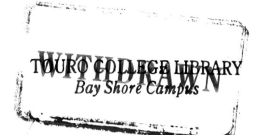
Musculoskeletal Aspects of Haemophilia

E.C. RODRIGUEZ-MERCHAN
MD, PhD
Consultant Orthopaedic Surgeon
Service of Traumatology and Orthopaedic Surgery
Haemophilia Centre
La Paz University Hospital
Madrid, Spain

N.J. GODDARD
MB, FRCS
Consultant Orthopaedic Surgeon
Department of Orthopaedics
Royal Free Hospital, London, UK

C.A. LEE
MA, MD, DSc(Med), FRCP, FRCPath
Professor of Haemophilia
Haemophilia Centre and Haemostasis Unit
Royal Free Hospital, London, UK

**Blackwell
Science**

© 2000 by
Blackwell Science Ltd

Editorial Offices:
Osney Mead, Oxford OX2 0EL
25 John Street, London WC1N 2BL
23 Ainslie Place, Edinburgh EH3 6AJ
350 Main Street, Malden
  MA 02148-5018, USA
54 University Street, Carlton,
  Victoria 3053, Australia
10, rue Casimir Delavigne
  75006 Paris, France

Other Editorial Offices:
Blackwell Wissenschafts-Verlag GmbH
Kurfürstendamm 57
10707 Berlin, Germany

Blackwell Science KK
MG Kodenmacho Building
7–10 Kodenmacho Nihombashi
Chuo-ku, Tokyo 104, Japan

First published 2000

Set by Sparks Computer Solutions Ltd,
Oxford, UK
Printed and bound in the United Kingdom
at the University Press, Cambridge.

DISTRIBUTORS

Marston Book Services Ltd
PO Box 269
Abingdon, Oxon OX14 4YN
(*Orders*: Tel: 01235 465500
          Fax: 01235 465555)
USA
Blackwell Science, Inc
Commerce Place
350 Main Street
Malden, MA 02148-5018
(*Orders*: Tel: 800 759 6102
              781 388 8250
      Fax: 781 388 8255)
Canada
Login Brothers Book Company
324 Saulteaux Crescent
Winnipeg, Manitoba r3j 3t2
(*Orders*: Tel: 204 837 2987)
Australia
Blackwell Science Pty Ltd
54 University Street
Carlton, Victoria 3053
(*Orders*: Tel: 3 9347 0300
      Fax: 3 9347 5001)

A catalogue record for this title
is available from the British Library

ISBN 0-632-05671-1

Library of Congress
Cataloging-in-Publication Data
Musculoskeletal aspects of haemophilia/
  [edited by] E.C. Rodriguez-Merchan, C.A.
  Lee, N.J. Goddard.
    p. ; cm
  Includes bibliographical references and index.
  ISBN 0-632-05671-1
  1. Hemphilia—Complications. 2. Hemarthro-
    sis. 3. Musculoskeletal system—Diseases. 4.
    Orthopedic surgery. I. Rodriguez-Merchan,
    E.C. II. Lee, Christine A. III. Goddard, N.J.
  [DNLM: 1. Hemphilia A—complications. 2.
    Musculoskeletal Diseases—etiology. 3.
    Musculoskeletal System—physiopathology.
    WH 325 M985 2000]
616.1′572—dc21   00-023044

For further information on
Blackwell Science, visit our website:
www.blackwell-science.com

Contents

Rehabilitation and Physiotherapy

Miscellaneous

Contributors

G. Alonso-Carro MD, PhD, Head, Service of Traumatology and Orthopaedic Surgery, La Paz University Hospital, Madrid, Spain

Y. Amit MD, Israel National Hemophilia Centre, Tel Hashomer Hospital, Israel

P. Arranz PhD, Consultant Psychologist, Haemophilia Centre, La Paz University Hospital, Madrid, Spain

J.A. Aznar-Lucea MD, Director, Haemophilia Centre, La Fe University Hospital, Valencia, Spain

K. Beeton, Senior Lecturer, Department of Physiotherapy, University of Hertforshire, Hatfield, UK; Honorary Lecturer, Royal Free and University College Medical School, University College, London, UK

J.W.J. Bijlsma MD, PhD, Professor, Department of Rheumatology and Clinical Immunology, University Medical Centre Utrecht, Utrecht, Holland

M. Blanco MD, Orthopaedic Surgeon, Service of Traumatology and Orthopaedic Surgery, La Paz University Hospital, Madrid, Spain

H.H. Brackmann MD, Director, Haemophilia Care Unit, and Institute for Experimental Haematology and Transfusion Medicine, University Hospital, Bonn, Germany

B.M. Buzzard MSc, Post Grad Dip, MCSP, Superintendent Physiotherapist, Haemophilia Reference Centre, Royal Victoria Infirmary, Newcastle upon Tyne, UK

H.A. Caviglia MD, Consultant Orthopaedic Surgeon, Department of Orthopaedics, Hospital Juan A Fernandez; Argentinian Haemophilia Foundation, Buenos Aires, Argentina

H. de la Corte MD, PhD, Consultant Specialist in Rehabilitation, Doce de Octubre University Hospital, Madrid, Spain

W. Effenberger, Haemophilia Care Unit and Institute for Experimental Haematology and Transfusion Medicine, University of Bonn, Bonn, Germany

H.H. Eickhoff MD, Consultant Orthopaedic Surgeon, Orthopaedic Hospital St. Josef, Troisdorf, Germany

F. Fernandez-Palazzi MD, Head, Orthopaedic Unit, National Haemophilia Treatment Centre, Municipal Blood Bank; Head, Pediatric Orthopaedic Unit, Hospital Vargas, Caracas, Venezuela

J. Gago MD, Consultant Haematologist, Haemophilia Centre, La Paz University Hospital, Madrid, Spain

G. Galatro MD, Consultant Orthopaedic Surgeon, Argentinian Haemophilia Foundation, Buenos Aires, Argentina

M.S. Gilbert MD, Consultant Orthopaedic Surgeon, Manhattan Orthopaedic and Sports Medicine Group, New York, USA

N.J. Goddard BSc, MB, FRCS, Consultant Orthopaedic Surgeon, Department of Orthopaedics, Royal Free Hospital, London, UK

L. Heijnen MD, PhD, Director, Rehabilitation Centre De Trappenberg, Crailoseweg, Huizen, Holland

M. Heim MD, Consultant Specialist in Rehabilitation, Department of Orthopaedic Rehabilitation, Israel National Haemophilia Centre, Tel Hashomer Hospital, Israel

F. Hernandez-Navarro MD, Head, Service of Haematology; Director of the Haemophilia Centre, La Paz University Hospital, Madrid, Spain

L. Hess, Haemophilia Care Unit and Institute for Experimental Haematology and Transfusion Medicine, University of Bonn, Germany

J.L. Hicks MA, MB, BCh, FRCS, Department of Orthopaedics, Northampton General Hospital, Northampton, UK

V. Jimenez-Yuste MD, Haematologist, haemophilia Centre, La Paz University Hospital, Madrid, Spain

F.P.J.G. Lafeber, PhD, Professor, Department of Rheumatology and Clinical Inmunology, University Medical Centre Utrecht, Utrecht, Holland

C.A. Lee MA, MD, DSc(Med), FRCP, FRCPath, Director, Haemophilia Centre and Haemostasis Unit, Royal Free Hospital, London, UK

C. Lopez-Cabarcos MD, Consultant Specialist in Rehabilitation, Haemophilia Centre, La Paz University Hospital, Madrid, Spain

J. Luboshitz MD, Israel National Hemophilia Center, Tel Hashomer Hospital, Israel

A. Martinez-Lloreda MD, Orthopaedic Surgeon, Service of Traumatology and Orthopaedic Surgery, La Paz University Hospital, Madrid, Spain

U. Martinowitz MD, Director, Israel National Hemophilia Center, Tel Hashomer Hospital, Israel

R. Miller, Social Worker/Family Therapist and Honorary Senior Lecturer, Haemophilia Centre and Haemostasis Unit, Royal Free Hospital and Royal Free and University College Medical School, London, UK

M. Ortega-Andreu MD, Consultant Orthopaedic Surgeon, Service of Traumatology and Orthopaedic Surgery, La Paz University Hospital, Madrid, Spain

R. Perez-Bianco MD, Consultant Haematologist, Argentinian Haemophilia Foundation, Buenos Aires, Argentina

L. Perlick, Department of Orthopaedics, University Hospital, Bonn, Germany

F. Querol-Fuentes MD, Consultant Specialist in Rehabilitation, Haemophilia Centre, La Fe University Hospital; Lecturer, Department of Physiotherapy, Valencia University, Valencia, Spain

M. Quintana Sr MD, Consultant Haematologist, Haemophilia Centre, La Paz University Hospital, Madrid, Spain

M. Quintana Jr MD, PhD, Fellow, Haemophilia Centre, La Paz University Hospital, Madrid, Spain

W.J. Ribbans BSc, MCh Orth, FRCS Orth, Consultant Orthopaedic Surgeon, Department of Orthopaedics, Northampton General Hospital, Northampton, UK

E.C. Rodriguez-Merchan MD, PhD, Consultant Orthopaedic Surgeon, Service of Traumatology and Orthopaedic Surgery; Haemophilia Centre, La Paz University Hospital, Madrid, Spain

G. Roosendaal MD, PhD, Van Creveld Clinic, National Haemophilia Centre, Division of Internal Medicine, University Medical Centre Utrecht, Utrecht, Holland

M.J. Sanjurjo MD, Haematologist, Haemophilia Centre, La Paz University Hospital, Madrid, Spain

G. Schumpe MD, Department of Biomechanics, Orthopaedic University Hospital, Bonn, Germany

H. Semper, Department of Orthopaedics, University Hospital, Bonn, Germany

A. Seuser MD, Kirotherapy, Kaiser-Karl Clinic, Bonn, Germany

M.T. Sohail MD, Professor of Orthopaedics, Postgraduate Medical Institute, Lahore General Hospital, Lahore, Pakistan

H.M. Van den Berg MD, PhD, Van Creveld Clinic, National Haemophilia Centre, Division of Internal Medicine, University Medical Centre, Utrecht, Holland

A. Villar MD, Consultant Haematologist, Haemophilia Centre, La Paz University Hospital, Madrid, Spain

T. Wallny MD, Department of Orthopaedics, University Hospital, Bonn, Germany

B. White MB, MsC Path, MRCPI, Senior Research Fellow, Haemophilia Centre, Royal Free Hospital, UK

J.D. Wiedel MD, Professor and Chairman, UCHSC Department of Orthopaedics, Denver, Colorado, USA

J. York MD, FRACP, FRCP, Professor, Department of Rheumatology, The Rachel Forster Hospital, Sydney, Australia

Preface

Haemophilia is a lifelong inherited bleeding disorder characterized by severe, spontaneous bleeding resulting in chronic, painful joint deformities. Without treatment, individuals with haemophilia will die in childhood or early adulthood. Thus, in a monograph from the US by Carroll Birch in 1937, the life expectancy of a haemophilic patient was approximately 20 years, and it was rare for the patient to survive to the age of 40. This is in vivid contrast to a patient in London who died recently at the age of 85 years, having received a shoulder replacement several years earlier which had substantially improved his quality of life.

The development of safe and effective clotting factor concentrate has enabled the orthopaedic surgeon to approach the patient with haemophilia with almost the same security as a patient without a bleeding disorder. Large pool clotting factor concentrates manufactured from human plasma became available in the developed world in the 1970s, and from 1986 this has become relatively 'safe' from viral transmission; in particular there has been no transmission of HIV following treatment with virucidally treated factor replacement since 1986 anywhere in the world. More recently, the development of high-purity concentrates has enabled perioperative delivery of clotting factor by continuous infusion, giving added safety during the period of surgery and the possibility of more intensive physiotherapy postoperatively. The newer recombinant clotting factor concentrates are particularly easy to deliver by continuous infusion.

The large epidemics of transfusion-transmitted disease resulting from the widespread use of large pool plasma derived clotting factor occurred during 1961–86 for the hepatitis C virus (HCV) and 1978–86 for human immunodeficiency virus (HIV). Thus, the generation of haemophilic patients who had poor treatment in their childhood and consequently are now needing orthopaedic procedures such as joint replacement are the patients most likely to be infected with HCV and HIV. This has presented problems for the orthopaedic surgeon and his team – destroyed joints can bleed extensively! Nevertheless, there are no reported transmissions of HIV or HCV to the operating team from a haemophilic patient. There have been many needle-stick accidents requiring an intervention with anti-retroviral therapy for HIV which has caused much physical and psychological morbidity. Clearly, there need to be rigorous operating procedures in place, and continuing vigilance. The advent of anti-retroviral therapy for HIV has the added concern of 'bleeding' in association with protease inhibitors reported in the haemophilic patient.

In parallel with the development of safe and effective clotting factor concentrates, the management of newly diagnosed children with haemophilia involves prophylaxis, or regular injections with clotting factor to stop bleeds, particularly joint bleeds. In well-resourced parts of the world this is performed using recombinant clotting factor for reasons of viral safety. This has enormous resource implications, and the cost–benefit analysis has to take into account that such individuals will grow up to expect a normal life and will not require expensive orthopaedic procedures. Although the use of continuous infusion can reduce by one-third the clotting factor concentrate used to cover a joint replacement, it still equates to about the average yearly use for an adult, that is 70 000 units, at a cost of approximately $20 000.

It has been suggested that worldwide 80% of those with haemophilia do not have access to adequate medical care. Many of those individuals are undiagnosed and untreated, and therefore suffer enormously. Often, expert orthopaedic care cannot be provided to the haemophilic patient because of the constraint of lack of clotting factor provision for economic reasons. There have been initiatives supported by the World Federation of Haemophilia and the fractionating industry to enable orthopaedic surgery to take place, and there are studies using continuous infusion with the maintenance of lower levels of clotting factor. Of course, orthopaedic care is dependent on first-class support from the physiotherapist. Fortunately, in less resourced parts of the world the provision of skilled personnel is sometimes better than in the so-called 'developed' world because of the relatively lower salaries paid. As a consequence, as a generation of children grow up on prophylaxis, healthcare professionals will have much to learn from their more experienced counterparts in less resourced countries.

The patient with haemophilia presents a particular challenge for those providing musculoskeletal care: quality of life can be transformed by such care. We all hope that there is a generation of children with haemophilia growing up who will not have musculoskeletal problems – but until then, this wide-ranging book will provide a useful reference for the comprehensive care team.

E.C. Rodriguez-Merchan
N.J. Goddard
C.A. Lee
Editors

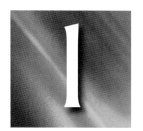

Haemostasis

CHAPTER I

The Diagnosis and Management of Inherited Bleeding Disorders

B WHITE AND C A LEE

INTRODUCTION

The haemostatic response to vessel injury involves vasoconstriction, the generation of a platelet plug, activation of the coagulation cascade resulting in fibrin clot formation and clot lysis (fibrinolysis). Platelets adhere to the site of vessel injury by interactions between platelet membrane glycoproteins and components of the subendothelium such as collagen and adhesive proteins including von Willebrand factor (VWF) and fibronectin. Platelets are then activated by a variety of agonists at the site of vessel injury resulting in shape change, aggregation, release of secretory granules and the expression of a procoagulant phospholipid surface which provides an ideal bed on which the coagulation cascade is activated. Tissue factor (TF) is expressed at the site of vessel injury and binds to and activates factor VII (FVII) leading to the generation of TF:FVIIa. This complex is critical in the initiation of the coagulation cascade *in vivo* and activates FX either directly or via FIX activation. Activated FX (FXa) converts prothrombin to thrombin, which in turn cleaves fibrinogen to fibrin. Factor XIII cross-links fibrin to produce an insoluble fibrin clot. Factors V and VIII are essential cofactors in the activation of FX and prothrombin, respectively. The final component of the haemostatic response involves clot lysis which is mediated by the fibrinolytic system. Plasmin is produced by the action of urokinase or tissue plasminogen activator on plasminogen and cleaves fibrin, leading to the dissolution of the clot (Fig. 1.1).

Inherited disorders have been described in all aspects of the haemostatic response and these abnormalities can be detected by appropriate laboratory investigations (Table 1.1). Severe deficiency of factors VIII, IX and X are frequently associated with recurrent spontaneous musculoskeletal bleeding which may lead to severe haemophilic arthropathy. FVIII (haemophilia A) and FIX (haemophilia B) deficiency are by far the commonest of these bleeding disorders, and therefore these patients are most likely to attend for orthopaedic review either at the time of diagnosis or for the management of chronic joint disease. Qualitative or quantitative defects in platelets or VWF result in primary mucocutaneous bleeding including epistaxis, gum bleeding and menorrhagia,

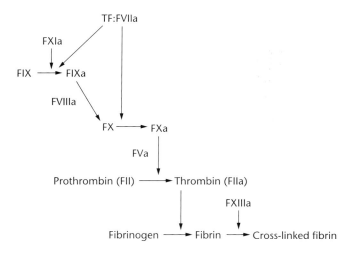

Fig. 1.1 Simplified overview of the coagulation cascade. The key events in the coagulation cascade that lead to fibrin clot formation are illustrated in this diagram. The generation of thrombin plays a critical role in this process and activates platelets, FV, FVIII, FXIII and FXI in addition to cleaving fibrinogen to fibrin. The activated form of each clotting factor is denoted by the letter 'a' (TF = tissue factor).

Table 1.1 Appropriate laboratory investigations to detect inherited bleeding disorders and their common clinical features and haemostatic support.

	Laboratory investigations	Common clinical features	Haemostatic support
Factor VIII or IX deficiency	Prolonged APTT	Musculoskeletal, genitourinary, gastrointestinal bleeding	FVIII or FIX concentrate DDAVP (mild FVIII deficiency) Tranexamic acid
Quantitative platelet defect	Full blood count	Epistaxis, mouth bleeding, skin bleeding, menorrhagia	Platelet transfusion
Qualitative platelet defect	Prolonged skin bleeding time Abnormal PFA-100™ Abnormal platelet function tests	Epistaxis, mouth bleeding, skin bleeding, menorrhagia, gastrointestinal bleeding	DDAVP, platelet transfusion Tranexamic acid
von Willebrand's disease	Prolonged skin bleeding time Abnormal PFA-100™ Reduced VWF (functional and antigen assay) Reduced FVIII	Epistaxis, mouth bleeding, skin bleeding, menorrhagia, gastrointestinal bleeding	DDAVP Tranexamic acid VWF containing concentrate Purified VWF concentrate

PFA-100™ = platelet function analyser. This commercially available machine assesses platelet and VWF function. APTT = activated partial prothrombin time. DDAVP = desmopressin. VWF = von Willebrand factor.

however, with the exception of a severe variant of von Willebrand's disease (VWD), these bleeding disorders do not result in spontaneous musculoskeletal bleeding. In this chapter, we will review the principles of management of inherited bleeding disorders with particular reference to the management of patients with severe haemophilia A and B who require surgery.

TREATMENT OPTIONS FOR INHERITED BLEEDING DISORDERS

The treatment of inherited bleeding disorders requires the correction of the coagulation defect. Treatment options include factor concentrates, plasma, platelets or desmopressin (DDAVP). In addition, systemic or topical tranexamic acid (which promotes clot stability by inhibiting fibrinolysis) may be used alone or in combination with other treatments.

Factor concentrate

The provision of factor VIII or IX replacement for haemophilia has evolved since the late 1960s from the use of cryoprecipitate and plasma to the development of recombinant FVIII and FIX concentrates. Factor concentrates are prepared from plasma which has been collected from several thousand donors, separated into different fractions and purified using a variety of techniques, including chromatography. The availability of factor concentrate had a major beneficial impact on the morbidity and mortality of haemophilia. However, the enthusiasm associated with the advent of highly effective therapy was soon tempered by the catastrophic outbreak of HIV and hepatitis C infection in the haemophilia population due to the contamination of factor concentrates [1–6]. Appropriate safeguards are now in place to prevent infection, including polymerase chain reaction (PCR) testing of donor plasma and the incorporation of validated viral inactivation steps in the purification process. Current plasma derived factor concentrate is safe, however, the risk of viral infection remains due to the failure of the viral inactivation process to destroy non-enveloped viruses such as hepatitis A and parvovirus B19 and the risk from as yet unidentified infectious agents [7,8].

Recent concerns have focused on the possibility of infection from plasma derived concentrates contaminated with new variant Creutzfeldt–Jakob disease (nvCJD). It is likely that this disease represents the human form of bovine sclerosing encephalitis (BSE) which infected a large number of cattle, especially in the United Kingdom, in the 1980s and early 1990s. There are insufficient data to accurately assess the risk to the haemophilic population. The risk is likely to be low since nvCJD has never been shown to develop as a result of transfusion of blood products either in clinical practice or in animal models [9]. However, nvCJD has been demonstrated in the plasma of infected patients and is unlikely to be destroyed by current viral inactivation processes. Furthermore, there is no effective screening test. As a result, plasma collected from donors in Britain is not currently used for the production of factor concentrates.

The risk of infection from plasma products provided the impetus for the development of recombinant factor concentrates. These products are produced by transfecting animal cells *in vitro* with FVIII or FIX cDNA. Some FVIII products are formulated with human albumin. Despite the potential for viral infection of animal cells and the risks associated with the addition of human albumin, recombinant products are recognized as being the safest available treatment option for patients who require factor replacement therapy. When the use of recombinant products is restricted by local financial constraints, children, women of child-bearing age and previously untreated adults usually receive priority.

Clotting factor concentrates may be administered on demand (that is, at time of bleeding episode) or as prophylaxis (that is, to prevent bleeding episodes). The dose of coagulation factor is determined by the following equation:

$$\text{Dose of factor concentrate} = \frac{\text{Desired rise} \times \text{weight in kg}}{K}$$

The K value is assigned to each factor concentrate and reflects the half-life and recovery of the product. The site and severity of bleeding determine the desired rise and frequency of administration.

Primary prophylaxis refers to the treatment of young children with the aim of preventing spontaneous musculoskeletal bleeding and ultimately chronic haemophilic arthropathy. This usually involves the administration of 25–35 IU/kg of FVIII (thrice weekly) or FIX (twice weekly). The less frequent administration of FIX reflects its longer half-life. The aim of this treatment strategy is to maintain the patient's coagulation factor above levels sufficient to prevent spontaneous bleeding. There is considerable clinical evidence that primary prophylaxis results in a dramatic decrease in the spontaneous haemarthrosis and subsequent arthropathy [10]. Secondary prophylaxis refers to the prevention of bleeding episodes in patients with established joint disease. This approach is also appropriate for the prevention of bleeding during the rehabilitation period following joint replacement.

Factor concentrate is usually reconstituted and administered as a bolus dose. However, the use of continuous infusion may be more appropriate for patients who require high-intensity factor replacement at the time of surgery or for severe bleeding complications. This method of administration avoids the peaks and troughs of bolus dosing, allows an accurate measurement of steady levels and is associated with a significant reduction in product requirement [11,12].

A specific problem arises in the treatment of haemophilic patients who have developed inhibitors to FVIII or FIX. These inhibitors are immunoglobulin-G (IgG) antibodies and bind to endogenous or exogenous FVIII or FIX and neutralize its procoagulant function. Approximately 20% of patients with severe FVIII deficiency develop inhibitors, although this complication is rare in FIX deficiency [13,14]. Patients with low responding FVIII inhibitors can be treated with large doses of factor replacement therapy or porcine FVIII, however patients with high responding inhibitors need specific inhibitory bypassing agents such as recombinant factor VIIa or prothrombin complexes [15]. Recombinant VIIa is highly effective in the presence of FVIII or FIX inhibitors. However, adequate levels are not achieved in a small percentage of patients who have a suboptimal clinical response [16].

Desmopressin (DDAVP) is a synthetic analogue of the pituitary hormone antidiuretic hormone. It can be administered by subcutaneous, intravenous or intranasal routes and results in the release of endogenous FVIII and VWF and may also correct a variety of platelet defects. It is used in responsive patients with mild FVIII deficiency, VWD and platelet function defects [17]. The response to DDAVP is not predictable, and therefore patients should undergo a DDAVP trial at diagnosis or prior to surgical procedures [17]. It is contraindicated in children less than one year old because of the risk of hyponatraemia, and in adults with ischaemic heart disease because of the risk of arterial thrombosis.

While DDAVP is a useful alternative to factor concentrate, it is not effective in FIX deficiency or severe FVIII deficiency. In addition DDAVP is not universally accepted as an effective treatment for responsive patients who require major surgery. As a result DDAVP is rarely used as haemostatic cover for major orthopaedic procedures.

There is no specific concentrate available for patients with FV or FX deficiency. A factor concentrate which contains a combination of clotting factors including FX is used for patients with FX deficiency, while fresh frozen plasma is used for the management of patients with FV deficiency. Platelet transfusions may be used for patients with platelet function defects and may occasionally be used as a source of platelet VWF in VWD. Platelet transfusions should be used sparingly in Bernard–Soulier syndrome and Glanzmann's thrombasthenia because of the risk of platelet antibody formation which would render the patient refractory to subsequent platelet transfusions.

SURGICAL MANAGEMENT

Preoperative assessment

Surgery should only be undertaken in centres which can provide continuous access to medical, nursing and laboratory coagulation expertise throughout the patient's hospital stay. The preoperative assessment of patients by the haemophilia service should include the following.
• *Definition of the nature and severity of the bleeding disorder.*
• *Investigation for the presence of an inhibitor and documentation of prior inhibitor formation.* Surgery in patients with inhibitors to FVIII or FIX is hazardous and those patients with high responding inhibitors should only undergo surgery as a matter of absolute necessity. The decision to proceed with surgery should only be made when the surgeon and patient are fully aware that, despite current treatment options with inhibitor bypassing agents, adequate haemostasis may not be achieved in a small number of patients.
• *Confirmation of the immunity to hepatitis A and B.* The immune status of patients is usually assessed on a yearly basis and vaccinations administered accordingly. The purpose of vaccination is to protect patients from viral infection secondary to contaminated red cell transfusions or plasma derived concentrates [18].
• *Documentation as to whether patients are infected with HIV, hepatitis B or hepatitis C.* Surgical, anaesthetic and nursing staff should be aware of the viral status of patients. It is important to identify additional risk factors for bleeding associated with infection (for example, thrombocytopenia or liver dysfunction) or antiviral therapy (protease inhibitors). Protease inhibitors are an integral component of current anti-retroviral treatment strategies. These agents are associated with an increased risk of spontaneous and surgery-related bleeding complications [19]. As a result, we discontinue protease inhibitors for 48 hours prior to major orthopaedic surgery and for approximately 1 week post-operatively. A treatment strategy to correct all other additional risk factors for bleeding complications should be formulated prior to surgery.

- *Liaison with surgical, anaesthetic and nursing staff regarding postoperative analgesia.* Intramuscular injections are contraindicated because of the risk of intramuscular bleeding. In addition, nonsteroidal anti-inflammatory agents should be avoided because of the risk of gastric erosion and platelet dysfunction. Spinal or epidural analgesia can be undertaken provided the postinfusion factor levels are within the required therapeutic range and there are no additional risk factors for bleeding such as inhibitors, thrombocytopenia or concomitant protease inhibitor use.
- *Documentation of management plan.* A treatment strategy should be selected for each patient and should be available to the medical and nursing personnel who will be responsible for patient care. Adequate stocks of factor concentrate should be available to cover surgery and the postoperative period.

Operative care

Patients are usually admitted the day prior to major surgery or on the day of surgery in a similar manner to patients without haemophilia. Blood is crossmatched according to the normal surgical blood-ordering policy of the hospital. Additional units may need to be crossmatched for patients with additional risk factors for bleeding.

A bolus of factor concentrate is administered 1 hour prior to surgery. If it has been decided to administer factor concentrate by a continuous infusion, then this should be commenced preoperatively. It is important to confirm that the postinfusion factor level is within the required therapeutic range *prior* to commencing surgery.

Postoperative care

The postoperative management of patients varies depending on the type of surgery and the practice of each haemophilia centre. We use a continuous infusion for 7 days after major surgery and aim to maintain factor levels at 100 IU/dL during this period.

Thereafter, we treat daily and then on alternate days until day 14 postoperatively [20]. However, there is considerable variation among haemophilia centres in the surgical management of these patients. Some authors recommend a continuous infusion with the aim of maintaining FVIII or FIX levels of 50 IU/dL on the day of surgery, reducing to 30 IU/dL thereafter [21]. There is currently insufficient evidence to justify one approach over the other and current practice reflects the experience of individual centres. Factor concentrate should be administered prior to physiotherapy and removal of stitches, in order to provide optimal haemostasis at the time of greatest risk of bleeding. Furthermore, the administration of prophylactic FVIII (thrice weekly) or FIX (twice weekly) after joint replacement allows the patient to undergo similar rehabilitation programmes to non-haemophilic patients without additional bleeding complications.

ORTHOPAEDIC SURGERY AND UNDIAGNOSED HAEMOPHILIA

Orthopaedic surgeons may be asked to review patients with undiagnosed haemophilia who present with unexplained joint swelling or pain due to haemarthrosis. In this situation, an invasive procedure without coagulation support will result in further joint bleeding and morbidity. Therefore, surgeons should be alert to the possibility of haemophilia in children who present for orthopaedic review and should always perform a basic coagulation screen of activated partial prothrombin time (APPT) and prothrombin time (PT) prior to surgery. This screen should detect the vast majority of bleeding disorders associated with spontaneous haemarthrosis. Orthopaedic patients with a bleeding history should be referred to a haematology or specialist coagulation unit. While many of these patients will not have a defect associated with spontaneous musculoskeletal bleeding, haemostatic support may be required at the time of surgery.

SUMMARY

Severe FVIII and FIX deficiency are the commonest bleeding disorders associated with spontaneous haemarthrosis and subsequent joint disease. The vast majority of other inherited bleeding states are not associated with spontaneous musculoskeletal bleeding but will require coagulation review prior to orthopaedic procedures.

Surgery can be safely performed in patients with severe inherited coagulation disorders provided the coagulation defect can be corrected with replacement therapy. The presence of high responding inhibitors to FVIII or FIX poses a considerable therapeutic challenge and requires the use of inhibitor-bypassing agents such as recombinant FVIIa. While these therapies are usually highly effective, adequate haemostasis cannot always be guaranteed, and invasive procedures should only be performed as a matter of absolute necessity.

It is imperative that surgery is only performed on patients with inherited bleeding disorders in centres that can provide comprehensive coagulation support. Unfortunately, this cannot always be achieved in poorly resourced countries, and this is likely to lead to an increased risk of surgical morbidity and mortality. Thus, the major challenge of the twenty-first century in haemophilia is to provide the resources and training so that these basic principles of haemophilia care can be applied to all patients worldwide.

REFERENCES

1 Ragni MV, Tegtmeier GE, Levy JA *et al*. AIDS retrovirus antibodies in hemophiliacs treated with factor VIII or factor IX concentrates, cryoprecipitate, or fresh frozen plasma: prevalence, seroconversion rate, and clinical correlations. *Blood* 1986; **67**: 592–5.

2 Lee CA, Kernoff PB, Karayiannis P, Thomas HC. Acute fulminant non-A, non-B hepatitis leading to chronic active hepatitis after treatment with cryoprecipitate. *Gut* 1985; **26**: 639–41.

3 Rickard KA, Batey RG, Dority P, Johnson S, Campbell J, Hodgson J. Hepatitis and haemophilia therapy in Australia. *Lancet* 1982; **2**: 146–8.

4 Colombo M, Mannucci PM, Carnelli V, Savidge GF, Gazengel C, Schimpf K. Transmission of non-A, non-B hepatitis by heat-treated factor VIII concentrate. *Lancet* 1985; **2**: 1–4.

5 Lim SG, Lee CA, Charman H, Tilsed G, Griffiths PD, Kernoff PB. Hepatitis C antibody assay in a longitudinal

study of haemophiliacs. *Br J Haematol* 1991; **78**: 398–402.

6 Makris M, Preston FE, Triger DR *et al*. Hepatitis C antibody and chronic liver disease in haemophilia. *Lancet* 1990; **335**: 1117–19.

7 Lawlor E, Johnson Z, Thornton L, Temperley I. Investigation of an outbreak of hepatitis A in Irish haemophilia A patients. *Vox Sang* 1994; **67** (Suppl. 1): 18–19.

8 Mannucci PM, Gdovin S, Gringeri A *et al*. Transmission of hepatitis A to patients with hemophilia by factor VIII concentrates treated with organic solvent and detergent to inactivate viruses. The Italian Collaborative Group. *Ann Intern Med* 1994; **120**: 1–7.

9 Evatt BL. Prions and haemophilia: assessment of risk. *Haemophilia* 1998; **4**: 628–33.

10 Nilsson IM, Berntorp E, Freiburghaus C. Treatment of patients with factor VIII and IX inhibitors. *Thromb Haemost* 1993; **70**: 56–9.

11 Martinowitz U, Schulman S, Gitel S, Horozowski H, Heim M, Varon D. Adjusted dose continuous infusion of factor VIII in patients with haemophilia A. *Br J Haematol* 1992; **82**: 729–34.

12 Varon D, Martinowitz U. Continuous infusion therapy in haemophilia. *Haemophilia* 1998; **4**: 431–5.

13 Lusher JM, Arkin S, Abildgaard CF, Schwartz RS. Recombinant factor VIII for the treatment of previously untreated patients with hemophilia A. Safety, efficacy, and development of inhibitors. Kogenate Previously Untreated Patient Study Group. *N Engl J Med* 1993; **328**: 453–9.

14 Addiego J, Kasper C, Abildgaard C *et al*. Frequency of inhibitor development in haemophiliacs treated with low-purity factor VIII. *Lancet* 1993; **342**: 462–4.

15 Hay CR, Colvin BT, Ludlam CA, Hill FG, Preston FE. Recommendations for the treatment of factor VIII inhibitors: from the UK Haemophilia Centre Directors' Organisation Inhibitor Working Party. *Blood Coagul Fibrinolysis* 1996; **7**: 134–8.

16 Gringeri A, Santagostino E, Mannucci PM. Failure of recombinant activated factor VII during surgery in a hemophiliac with high-titer factor VIII antibody. *Haemostasis* 1991; **21**: 1–4.

17 Mannucci PM. Desmopressin (DDAVP) in the treatment of bleeding disorders: the first 20 years. *Blood* 1997; **90**: 2515–21.

18 Shouval D. Vaccines for prevention of viral hepatitis. *Haemophilia* 1998; **4**: 587–94.

19 Wilde JT, Lee CA, Collins P, Giangrande PL, Winter M, Shiach CR. Increased bleeding associated with protease inhibitor therapy in HIV-positive patients with bleeding disorders. *Br J Haematol* 1999; **107**: 556–9.

20 Rickard KA. Guidelines for therapy and optimal dosing of coagulation factor for treatment of bleeding and surgery in haemophilia. *Haemophilia* 1995; **1** (Suppl.): 8–13.

21 Kobrinsky NL, Stegman DA. Management of haemophilia during surgery. In: Forbes CD, Adelort L, Madhok R, eds. *Haemophilia*. London: Chapman and Hall, 1997: 239–48.

2

Orthopaedic Surgery

CHAPTER 2

General Principles in Orthopaedic Surgery of Haemophilia

E C RODRIGUEZ-MERCHAN AND N J GODDARD

INTRODUCTION

The successful outcome of surgery in haemophilia depends upon a close working relationship between the orthopaedic surgeon and the haematologist. This chapter outlines the general principles involved in undertaking surgery in patients with haemophilia, the surgical technique, preoperative evaluation, the risk of infection after surgery in the HIV-positive patient and the risk of intraoperative transmission of blood-borne diseases.

PREOPERATIVE EVALUATION AND SURGICAL TECHNIQUE

Elective surgery for patients with haemophilia is now possible due to the increasing availability of factor concentrate. Prior to undertaking surgery it is important to establish the exact nature of the haemorrhagic disorder. It goes without saying that the bleeding disorder must be fully corrected before beginning surgery.

INDICATIONS FOR ORTHOPAEDIC SURGERY

The common indications for orthopaedic intervention surgery in patients with haemophilia have been outlined by Canale [1] and include the following:
• Chronic haemophilic synovitis (Fig. 2.1) that cannot be controlled by adequate factor replacement (synovectomies).
• Severe soft-tissue contractures that have been unresponsive to standard non-operative measures (tendon release, capsulotomy or osteotomy).
• Bony deformities that merit corrective osteotomy.
• A pseudotumour that may require surgical excision and perhaps grafting.
• Severe degenerative change in a joint with increasing disability and incapacitating pain (total joint replacement or arthroplasty).
Post and Telfer [2] emphasized that the surgery must be carried out carefully, with particular attention paid to haemostasis. It has been pro-

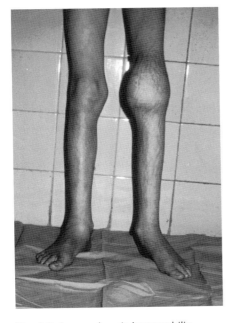

Fig. 2.1 Severe chronic haemophilic synovitis in a young person with haemophilia.

posed that as many procedures as possible should be carried out under the same anaesthetic in order to reduce the requirement for factor VIII replacement. The surgery itself should be carried out meticulously using a pneumatic tourniquet whenever possible. The wound should be closed carefully in layers, taking care to avoid dead space formation. Diathermy should be used sparingly. It is advisable to use deep wound drains for a minimum of 24–48 hours. Aspirin or similar nonsteroidal anti-inflammatory medications should be avoided postoperatively as they can interfere with platelet function. As far as possible, one should avoid intramuscular injections postoperatively for pain management.

Multiple joint involvement is frequent in adult patients with haemophilic arthropathy (Figs 2.2 and 2.3). It is not unusual to have two knees, or contralateral hip and knee, affected. Under these circumstances, it would be somewhat illogical to operate on one joint, leaving the other joint affected, thus impairing the ultimate functional outcome. Horoszowski *et al.* [3] advocated multiple joint surgery in a single operating session whenever possible. They reported on a series of 11 patients who underwent multiple joint operations in a single session (generally bilateral knee replacements) in patients with haemophilia. There are obvious advantages to this, the most important of which is the restoration of normal biomechanics of the affected limbs, but the reduction in the length of the rehabilitation period combined with the need for only one operative session requiring factor replacement and extensive analgesia are also important considerations.

Martinowitz *et al.* [4] have extensive experience in the use of fibrin sealant as a haemostatic agent when operating on patients with haemophilia. They reported on a series of 23 patients where they used a combination of fibrin sealant and continuous infusion of factor replacement. They found a significant reduction in blood loss in haemophilic patients, using this combination, compared with non-haemophilic patients in the absence of the fibrin sealant. In addition, and encouragingly, there was a significant reduction in the requirements for factor VIII replacement, leading to cost savings [4].

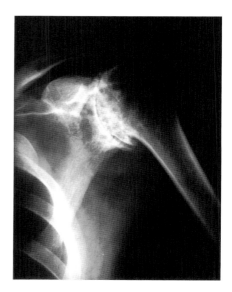

Fig. 2.2 Advanced haemophilic arthropathy of the shoulder. The joint is severely damaged.

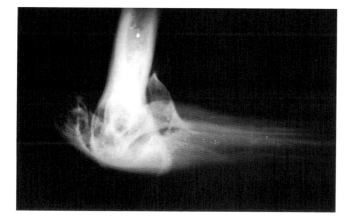

Fig. 2.3 Advanced haemophilic arthropathy of the elbow. The joint cartilage is totally destroyed and the bone ends are enlarged and deformed.

RISK OF INFECTION AFTER ORTHOPAEDIC SURGERY IN THE HIV-POSITIVE PATIENT

Unfortunately, a significant proportion of patients with haemophilia have become infected with the human immunodeficiency virus, and they are consequently at an increased risk of bacterial and opportunistic infection because of immunosuppression. In these patients the risk of postoperative infection following orthopaedic surgery is significantly increased [5]. Ragni *et al* [6] reported a series of 66 patients with a CD4 count of ≤ 200 cells/mm^3 undergoing 74 orthopaedic procedures. They found postoperative infection in 10 patients (a rate of 13%) up to 5 months. In five of these patients preoperative infection had preceded joint infection. The most frequently isolated organism was *Staphylococcus aureus* (60%) and the knee was the most commonly affected joint (90%). In patients with HIV and haemophilia, the infection rate for arthroplasty appears to be increased 10-fold compared with other procedures.

Phillips *et al.* [7] reported a series of patients investigated at the Royal Free Hospital Haemophilia Centre in London between 1982 and 1994. The aim of this study was to look at whether orthopaedic interventions accelerated the fall of CD4 lymphocyte counts in patients with haemophilia infected by the HIV virus, and whether patients who underwent surgery had different rates of progression of AIDS or death when compared to patients not undergoing surgery. The objective was to establish whether physicians treating such patients should be cautious about advising surgery in haemophilic patients infected with HIV on the basis that it might be detrimental to their ultimate prognosis. The results showed that there were no significant differences in the rate of development of AIDS or mortality between patients who underwent surgery and those who did not. They concluded that elective joint replacement surgery on HIV-positive patients with haemophilia did not affect the progression of AIDS, nor did it adversely affect the death rate. They did, however, find that the risk of postoperative infection was 13% in HIV-positive patients with CD4 counts of ≤ 200 cells/mm^3.

Luck [8] reported that an HIV-positive non-haemophilic patient with a prosthetic implant is also at risk of late haematogenous implant infection as the disease progresses. Thus, medical attention and prophylactic antibiotics prior to dental work or urethral instrumentation should be standard practice in order to reduce the possibility of late infection in this group. He also felt that because the risk of surgical complication increases with progression of the disease, patients for planned surgery should be fully assessed as to their immunological status. The CD4 count, history of opportunistic infection, state of nutrition and general health probably provide the best background information for an assessment of the risk of subsequent postoperative complications [8].

INTRAOPERATIVE TRANSMISSION OF BLOOD-BORNE DISEASE

The transmission of blood-borne pathogens such as HIV and hepatitis B and C represent a substantial risk to healthcare workers looking after patients with such infections. Surgeons are obviously at an increased risk of contracting both HIV and hepatitis from such patients. The risk of contracting hepatitis B following exposure to contaminated blood is far greater than the risk of contracting HIV. Despite this, it is important to emphasize the risk of HIV transmission for two reasons; firstly, vaccination is undoubtedly effective in reducing the risk of infection with hepatitis B, and secondly, hepatitis B is fatal in less than 10% of cases. There is, however, no effective vaccine against HIV, and if contracted it can ultimately lead to the development of AIDS and, possibly, death [9].

Of the haemophiliacs who received pooled, untreated factor VIII preparations, 70% are HIV-positive, as are up to 90% of severe haemophiliacs. Sadly, many of these patients have subsequently died. The high incidence of infection with HIV has resulted in a stressful and potentially fearful atmosphere among patients, relatives and medical staff. The risk of transmission of HIV to orthopaedic surgeons and operating theatre staff is significant. The American Academy of Orthopedic Surgeons' taskforce [10] recommended that every effort should be made to reduce the potential for transmission of AIDS/HIV whenever possible. They have recommended the following precautions to be taken in the operating room.

• Do not hurry an operation. Excess speed may result in injury. The most experienced surgeon should be responsible for the surgical procedure if the risk of injury to operating-room personnel is high.

• Wear surgical clothing that offers protection against contact with blood. Knee-high, waterproof, surgical shoe covers, waterproof gowns or undergarments and full head covering should be worn.

• Double gloves should be worn at all times.

• Surgical masks should be changed if they become moist or splattered.

• Protective eyewear (goggles or full-face shields) that covers exposed skin and mucous membranes should be used.

To avoid inadvertent injury to surgical personnel, the orthopaedic surgeon should observe the following:

• Use instrument ties and other 'no-touch' suturing and sharp instrument techniques when possible. Do not tie with a suture needle in your hand.

• Avoid passing sharp instruments and needles from hand to hand; instead, place them on an intermediate tray.

• Make a warning announcement when sharp instruments are about to be passed.

• Avoid having two surgeons suture the same wound.

• Take extra care when performing digital examination of fracture fragments or wounds containing wires or sharp instrumentation.

• Avoid contact with osteotomes, drill bits and saws.

• Use spacesuit-type clothing when splatter is inevitable, such as when irrigating large wounds or using power equipment.

• Routinely check gowns, masks and shoe covers of operating room personnel for contamination during the surgical procedure, and change as necessary.

If a member of the operating team is inadvertently pricked or cut, the wound should be washed immediately with iodine, soap and water. If the injured person has been immunized for hepatitis B (and has adequate titres), or is positive for hepatitis B surface antigen or antibody, no further treatment is necessary. Otherwise, two doses of hepatitis B immunoglobulin should be given, 5 ml immediately and 5 ml after 1 month.

The estimated risk of seroconversion per injury in orthopaedic surgery is approximately 0.4%. Although orthopaedic surgeons are at risk from contracting HIV and hepatitis from haemophiliacs, neither the practice of these surgeons, nor the care that the patients would normally expect to receive, should be adversely affected [9].

REFERENCES

1 Canale ST. Haemophilia. In: Canale ST, ed. *Campbell's Operative Orthopaedics*, 9th edn, Vol. 1, Chapter 24. St Louis: Mosby, 1998: 883–7.

2 Post M, Telfer MC. Surgery in hemophilic patients. *J Bone Joint Surg (Am)* 1975; **57A**: 1136–42.

3 Horoszowski H, Heim M, Schulman S, Varon D, Martinowitz U. Multiple joint procedures in a single operative session on hemophilic patients. *Clin Orthop* 1996; **328**: 60–4.

4 Martinowitz U, Schulman S, Horoszowski H, Heim M. Role of fibrin sealants in surgical procedures on patients with hemostatic disorders. *Clin Orthop* 1996; **328**: 65–75.

5 Rodriguez-Merchan EC. Management of orthopaedic complications of haemophilia. *J Bone Joint Surg (Br)* 1998; **80B**: 191–6.

6 Ragni MV, Crossett LS, Herndon JH. Postoperative infection following orthopaedic surgery in human immunodeficiency virus-infected hemophiliacs with CD4 counts < or = 200/mm³. *J Arthroplasty* 1995; **10**: 716–21.

7 Phillips AM. Sabin CA, Ribbans WJ, Lee CA. Orthopaedic surgery in hemophilic patients with human immunodeficiency virus. *Clin Orthop* 1997; **343**: 81–7.

8 Luck JV Jr. Orthopaedic surgery of the HIV-positive patient: complications and outcome. *Instruct Course Lect* 1994; **43**: 543–9.

9 Rodriguez-Merchan EC. Intraoperative transmission of blood-borne disease in haemophilia. *Haemophilia* 1998; **4**: 75–8.

10 American Academy of Orthopedic Surgeons' Task Force on AIDS and Orthopaedic Surgery Recommendations for the prevention of human immunodeficiency virus (HIV) transmission in the practice of orthopedic surgery. Chicago: The Academy, 1989.

CHAPTER 3

Blood-Induced Joint Damage: an Overview of Musculoskeletal Research In Haemophilia

G ROOSENDAAL, H M VAN DEN BERG, F P J G LAFEBER AND J W J BIJLSMA

INTRODUCTION

Haemophilia is an X-chromosome-linked disease characterized by an increased and lifelong tendency to haemorrhage due to a deficiency or functional defect of coagulation factor VIII or IX. The worldwide prevalence of haemophilia A is estimated to be 1 case in 10 000 males, whereas for haemophilia B the occurrence is 1 in 25 000 males. The clinical features of the joint problems associated with haemophilia A and B are similar. In severe haemophilia the factor VIII or IX coagulant activity is < 1 IU/dL. Patients with a coagulant activity between 2 IU/dL and 5 IU/dL are usually only moderately affected, while patients with levels above 5 IU/dL only have problems if they sustain major trauma. The higher the factor VIII or IX coagulant activity, the fewer the clinical problems.

In severe cases (45% of haemophilic patients), serious bleeding can occur spontaneously, especially in the larger joints. In severe haemophilia 85% of all bleeding events occur in joints, and 80% of these events affect the ankle, knee or elbow, with the hip and shoulder affected to a lesser extent. There is no satisfactory explanation as to why bleeds occur so frequently in joints compared with other sites, nor why there is a predisposition for the knee, ankle and elbow joints, but it has been suggested that mechanical factors are important in this respect. The direct symptoms or short-term effects of joint bleeding are pain, swelling, warmth and muscle spasm. With appropriate treatment the lesion settles in a few days as the blood is reabsorbed. The long-term effects of joint bleeding are more serious. Repeated episodes of intra-articular bleeding cause damage to the joint (haemophilic arthropathy), leading to deformity and crippling [1,2]. The delay between joint bleeding and the subsequent joint damage makes it difficult to establish the exact pathogenetic mechanism of haemophilic arthropathy.

Recurrent haemarthroses lead to specific changes in both synovium and cartilage, which finally result in total destruction of the joint. This process is called haemophilic arthropathy [3–8] and is the most common cause of morbidity in patients with haemophilia, greatly affecting their quality of life. Haemophilic arthropathy in general becomes evident at an early age (15–25), and because haemophilic patients nowadays have a normal life expectancy, the number of disease years per patient (years of joint disease) can be as high as 50. This is in contrast to other musculoskeletal diseases, such as osteoarthritis and rheumatoid arthritis, which usually start at an older age and as a consequence have less impact on people of working age and on social security costs.

However, when it comes to the *treatment* of the most common complication of haemophilia, haemophilic arthropathy, consensus is hard to find. Definitions of, for example, the severity of bleeding, the degree of joint damage or the type of synovitis are a source of debate. The treatment of (chronic) synovitis and joint damage varies enormously worldwide and is frequently based on tradition and local practice. The use of physiotherapy, immobilization, intra-articular corticosteroids, synoviorthesis with rifampicin or radiosynoviorthesis, open or arthroscopic synovectomy, laser synovectomy or general orthopaedic procedures all generate controversy and discussion. While some of the differences are related to the high costs of clotting factors needed for the treatment of haemophilic arthropathy, an important reason for these differences is a lack of knowledge about the mechanisms responsible for this condition.

The pathogenetic mechanisms of haemophilic arthropathy are not precisely known. It is generally accepted that there is a relationship between recurrent intra-articular bleeding and the long-term development of joint damage. However, little is known about the effects of blood on joint structures, for instance, the amount of blood or the number of bleeding episodes that initiate joint damage. Such questions are difficult to answer. Although investigators agree that a certain number of bleeding episodes eventually result in clinically evident synovial tissue changes and in cartilage damage, the question remains as to how many bleeding events are needed to start irreversible damage, whether it is clinically evident or not. More insight into this problem may lead to preventive measures for patients with haemophilia.

Synovial changes and the destruction of articular cartilage are the most prominent events in haemophilic arthropathy. Cartilage contributes to the extraordinary properties of joints and allows for the distribution of large compressive loads and stable movement of the joint with a very low level of friction. There are no reports indicating that the cartilage of patients with haemophilia (before joint destruction starts) is different from that of healthy people.

Several different types of joint disorder – degenerative (such as osteoarthritis), inflammation-mediated (such as rheumatoid arthritis) and blood-induced (such as haemophilic arthropathy) – result in cartilage damage and changes in synovial tissue. A number of mediators are involved in these changes, for example, enzymes, cytokines and oxygen metabolites. Current concepts, which are based on experimental *in vitro* studies and clinical experience, hold that the synovium becomes catabolically active because of exposure to blood components and as a result induces cartilage destruction. Synovial iron deposition, which is easily detectable by magnetic resonance imaging, is suggested to be indicative of the severity of haemophilic arthropathy. However, these concepts are based on a limited number of studies. In comparison to our knowledge about osteoarthritis and rheumatoid arthritis, little is known about the mechanisms of cartilage damage in haemophilic arthropathy. Possibly the pathophysiology is multifactorial in origin and includes degenerative cartilage-mediated and inflammatory synovium-mediated components.

INFLAMMATORY SYNOVIUM-MEDIATED ASPECTS OF HAEMOPHILIC ARTHROPATHY

It is recognized that the repeated extravasation of blood into the joint cavity is the factor responsible for synovial and cartilage changes [8,9]. Synovial changes are thought to precede cartilage changes. The progressive accumulation of iron from red blood cells removed from the joint cavity by synovial macrophages over time during successive intra-articular haemorrhages has been postulated to be the trigger for synovial inflammation. This synovial inflammation would ultimately lead to joint damage that becomes evident years after the first bleeding episode has occurred [10].

An important characteristic of synovial change is the deposition of iron (haemosiderin) in the synovium, both in the synovial lining and the supporting layer. Haemosiderin deposits in the lining appear as discrete granules, scattered throughout the cytoplasm of the cells. The haemosiderin deposits in the supporting layer appear as dense aggregates, both intracellular and extracellular. Because of an abundance of synovial iron deposits, the synovium appears macroscopically to be brownish (haemosiderotic). Experimental haemarthrosis induces synovial changes resembling those seen in human haemophilic patients. The haemosiderin deposits are thought to induce synovial hypertrophy (resulting in villi) and (in the subsynovial layer) neovascularization (resulting in increased vascularity). Another suggested effect of the haemosiderin deposits is an infiltration of the synovial membrane with lymphocytes, although follicles of lymphocytes (as can be seen in the synovial membrane of rheumatoid arthritis) have not been observed. In general, the morphological picture of the synovium differs with the age of patient and probably correlates with the number of intra-articular bleedings, being villous, proliferative and hyperaemic in younger patients, while in older patients a flat synovium with fibrosis can be seen. Compared to inflammatory arthropathies like rheumatoid arthritis there are only mild inflammatory changes.

Synovial iron deposits as a result of recurrent intra-articular haemorrhages are also found in other joint disorders such as pigmented villonodular synovitis, haemangiomas of the synovial membrane and haemosiderotic synovitis. These joint disorders all result in joint damage resembling haemophilic arthropathy, which suggests that synovial iron deposits indeed play an important role in the pathogenesis of blood-induced cartilage damage [11,12]. Accumulation of iron as a degradation product of haemoglobin may be a direct stimulus for the proliferation of synoviocytes and an attractant of inflammatory cells; the subsequent production of enzymes and cytokines could lead to the destruction of articular cartilage [13,14].

A recent study of patients with haemophilia who went for elective orthopaedic surgery of the knee found that in all patients the synovial tissue showed areas with an appearance of haemosiderin adjacent to areas of normal appearance [15]. This finding provided a model for an analysis of the effect of synovial iron deposits in synovial tissue. The macroscopic appearance corresponded closely to the histological iron deposits and, in addition, to the inflammatory and catabolic activity of the tissues. The results show that the iron deposits at localized sites in the synovium are associated with the production of pro-inflammatory cytokines and an ability to inhibit the formation of human cartilage matrix. This supports the hypothesis that iron plays a leading role in the induction of synovial changes and the consequent production of catabolic mediators harmful to articular cartilage. It is not clear whether haemosiderin is directly involved in the stimulation of cytokine production; it seems more likely that phagocytosis by synovial cells and blood macrophages released into the haemarthritic joint leads to the stimulation of cytokine production.

The inflammatory changes in haemosideritic synovial tissue, as determined histologically, are mild compared with those from tissue with inflammatory joint disease such as rheumatoid arthritis, but the production *in vitro* of catabolic mediators such as IL-1, IL-6 and TNFα is comparable to that found for synovial tissue from patients with rheumatoid arthritis [unpublished observations]. The potential for damage by haemosideritic synovial tissue underlines the importance of early diagnosis and treatment of chronic synovitis in haemophilic patients. Magnetic resonance imaging makes it possible to demonstrate hypertrophic synovial tissue with haemosiderin deposits in joints with chronic synovitis [16]. Apart from reducing the frequency of bleeding episodes, it can be suggested that synoviorthesis or early synovectomy may slow down joint deterioration in haemophilic arthropathy. The presence of significant synovial iron deposits may be an indication for synoviorthesis or synovectomy to reduce consequent joint damage.

DEGENERATIVE CARTILAGE-MEDIATED ASPECTS OF HAEMOPHILIC ARTHROPATHY

A considerable number of reports concerning blood-induced joint damage suggest that synovial changes have a leading role in the development of joint damage. In experimentally induced haemarthrosis, one of the earliest effects observed is proliferation and inflammation of the synovial tissue (synovitis). Synovial changes are thought to induce and therefore *precede* changes in cartilage. However, there are also observations which question whether this is the only and the initiating mechanism of joint damage in haemophilia [17]. They hold that intra-articular blood has a direct harmful effect on cartilage before, and independent of, synovial changes and suggest that joint damage may occur *before* synovial inflammation is evident; primarily there may be damage of articular cartilage with synovitis as a consequence.

The latter concept is substantiated by findings in a human *in vitro* model of haemarthrosis [18–20]. Biochemical and metabolic analyses showed that subtle but irreversible changes in chondrocyte metabolic activity occurred in human cartilage after a short exposure to blood *in vitro*. Clinically, these changes cannot be detected but they may play a role in the pathogenesis of blood-induced arthropathy. Human articular cartilage consists of a relatively small number of chondrocytes embedded in a relatively large amount of extracellular matrix that consists mainly of collagen and proteoglycan. There is a continuous turnover of these matrix components, with a delicate balance between synthesis and breakdown [21]. Several mediators, such as growth factors, enzymes, cytokines, oxygen metabolites and their natural inhibitors, are involved in maintaining this balance but are also involved in cartilage damage when there is an imbalance between synthesis and breakdown.

Results of these studies show that when human cartilage is subjected to a relatively short exposure of 4 days (the time for blood to evacuate naturally from a joint) to whole blood in concentrations up to 50% (blood concentration during haemarthrosis approaches 100%), long-lasting damaging effects are induced. There is marked inhibition of matrix formation (proteoglycan synthesis) and increased breakdown, that is, release of matrix components (proteoglycan release), resulting in a continuing loss of matrix (proteoglycan content). The initial biochemical changes seen in these studies were not accompanied by either histologically detectable or macroscopic changes. However, these studies reveal that cartilage changes induced by short-term exposure to whole blood result in continuing inhibition of proteoglycan synthesis, accompanied by a continuing decrease in proteoglycan content. In the long term, histological and macroscopic changes would probably follow.

To gain more insight into the mechanism of blood-induced cartilage damage it is crucial to know which blood components are responsible for cartilage changes. Human *in vitro* studies reveal marked inhibition of proteoglycan synthesis by mononuclear cells (MNC). This effect of MNC has been reported before, for instance, in studies of blood from patients with rheumatoid arthritis. The proposed mechanisms include, among others, effects of lysosomal enzymes and catabolic cytokines. However, none of these effects proved to be long lasting. In recent *in vitro* studies [22], whole blood showed long-lasting inhibition of proteoglycan synthesis and enhancement of glucosamynoglycan (GAG) release in contrast to isolated components. Only the combination of MNC and red blood cells (RBC) revealed effects comparable to whole blood. A possible explanation for the irreversible damage by this combination is the conversion of oxygen metabolites produced by the monocytes in the MNC population to the toxic hydroxyl radicals catalysed by iron supplied by RBC [22,23].

OTHER CONCEPTS

These results, indicating a direct harmful effect of blood on cartilage, do not exclude the important role of reported synovium-induced cartilage damage. In addition to 'synovium related' changes (certainly important in the long run), cartilage damage may be induced initially by blood. This cartilage damage may in turn induce inflammatory responses. Recent canine *in vivo* studies support these concepts [24]. This work was undertaken to test the hypothesis, based on results of *in vitro* studies, that a short exposure to blood during a single or a limited number of bleeding events results in changes which inevitably lead to joint destruction.

Experimental cartilage changes

Results of canine studies show that canine cartilage exposed *in vivo* to whole blood for a relatively short time (4 days) exhibits long-lasting biochemical and histochemical changes of the cartilage matrix and changes in chondrocyte metabolic activity as well as alterations in the synovium. These changes are predictive of irreversible joint damage in the long term. The changes with respect to loss and content of proteoglycans persisted for at least 16 days. The total proteoglycan content remained low despite the enhanced synthesis of proteoglycans on day 16. The shift from an inhibition to a stimulation of proteoglycan synthesis from day 4 to day 16, while the decreased proteoglycan content remained low, suggests that the increase in proteoglycan synthesis was an ineffective attempt to repair cartilage. A similar ineffective enhancement of proteoglycan synthesis has also been described for osteoarthritic cartilage.

Swelling of cartilage is an early sign that is an important marker of osteoarthritic cartilage and is believed to be caused by disruption of the collagen network. The cross-linked three-dimensional fibrillar network of collagen is responsible for the tensile strength of cartilage, and disruption of this network by proteolytic enzymes, excessive mechanical loading and oxygen metabolites will lead to pathological conditions. In this canine *in vivo* study a slightly, but statistically significant, higher percentage of degraded collagen was detected in the injected joint compared to the control joint on day 4, indicating that even a short exposure to intra-articular blood can damage the collagen network, with a possible detrimental effect in time. Oxygen metabolites formed during intra-articular bleeding might be involved in this process. This would suggest that the short exposure to blood itself, and not the synovitis that was evident on day 16, is involved in this collagen-destructive process.

These canine *in vivo* findings concerning the effects of blood on cartilage proteoglycan and collagen are consistent with the findings of Convery *et al.* [25]. During the continuous presence of blood in 14 mongrel dogs they found morphological changes of the articular cartilage after 16 weeks, but there was a significant decrease in GAG content as early as 4 weeks. The total collagen content was significantly altered after 12 weeks. Biophysical analysis of the cartilage surface after 8 weeks showed that the tissue was more deformable and less resistant to shear than the control cartilage. In addition, Parsons *et al.* found in an animal model that the continuous presence of blood in the joint for 10 days resulted in cartilage which was significantly more compliant than normal [26], which they attributed to the loss of proteoglycan. We believe that intra-articular blood-induced collagen damage may also have been involved and that such changes take place after a relatively short exposure.

Experimental synovial changes

In this canine *in vivo* study the changes in synovial tissue shortly after exposure to blood were restricted to mild synovial inflammation. The synovial tissue did not have cartilage-damaging potential. Because cartilage changes were already evident at an early stage, this observation does not support the general concept that changes in synovial tissue are a prerequisite for, and precede, the changes in cartilage. On the contrary, it corroborates *in vitro* findings that cartilage changes occur after a short exposure to blood, before the involvement of synovial inflammation. Two weeks after exposure to blood, the inflammation of synovial tissue was accompanied by destruction of cartilage. Apparently, it takes time for the synovium to acquire cartilage-damaging activity, which might depend on the phagocytosis of blood cells, or on the accumulation of haemosiderin and subsequent production of cytokines and matrix metalloproteinases. Thus, blood first has a direct effect on cartilage, presumably as a result of the iron-catalysed formation of destructive oxygen metabolites. Whether these changes are essential for the subsequent synovial changes remains to be elucidated. Blood itself may bring about these synovial alterations. These recent studies show that synovitis is involved, but that it is not the only mechanism in the joint damage caused by intra-articular bleeding. This pathogenetic concept does not contradict the current concept of blood-induced cartilage damage in which synovial changes are thought to play an important role. Several pathological processes are possibly involved, some of them occurring in parallel and others sequentially.

CONCLUSIONS

The pathogenetic mechanism of haemophilic arthropathy is multifactorial and includes degenerative cartilage-mediated and inflammatory synovium-mediated components. Intra-articular blood first has a direct effect on cartilage, presumably as a result of the iron-catalysed formation of destructive oxygen metabolites, and then it affects the synovium. Thus, both processes occur in parallel, and while they influence each other they probably do not depend on each other. This concept resembles degenerative joint damage as found in osteoarthritis. These processes finally result in fibrosis and destruction of the joint. It is unknown whether and, if so, when a point of no return is reached. More insight into the mechanisms of haemophilic arthropathy may have consequences for the prevention and treatment of this complication in patients with haemophilia. Research has yet to fully unravel the mechanism of haemophilic arthropathy and to define a possible point of no return.

SUMMARY

Haemophilia is an X-chromosome-linked disease characterized by an increased tendency to haemorrhage. Due to recurrent haemarthroses specific changes occur in synovium and cartilage. This process is called haemophilic arthropathy. The pathogenetic mechanisms involved are not precisely known. Current concepts, which are based on experimental *in vitro* studies and clinical experience, hold that the synovium becomes catabolically active because of the exposure to blood components and as a result induces cartilage destruction. A considerable number of reports concerning blood-induced joint damage suggest that synovial changes have a leading role in the development of the joint damage and therefore *precede* the changes in cartilage. However, there are also observations which question whether this is the only and the initiating mechanism of joint damage in haemophilia; intra-articular blood has a direct harmful effect on cartilage before synovial changes and this suggests that joint damage may occur before synovial inflammation is evident. Primarily, there may be damage of articular cartilage with synovitis as a consequence. These studies show that synovitis is involved, but that it is not the only mechanism in joint damage caused by intra-articular bleeding. These findings do not contradict the current concept of blood-induced cartilage damage in which synovial changes are thought to play an important role. Several pathological processes are possibly involved, some of them occurring in parallel and others sequentially. Possibly, intra-articular blood first has a direct effect on cartilage, and then it affects the synovium. Thus, both processes occur in parallel, and while they influence each other they probably do not depend on each other. This concept resembles degenerative joint damage as found in osteoarthritis.

REFERENCES

1 Creveld van S, Hoedemaker PJ, Kingma MJ, Wagenvoort CA. Degeneration of joints in haemophiliacs under treatment by modern methods. *J Bone Joint Surg (Br)* 1971; **53B**: 296–302.

2 Madhok R, Bennett D, Sturrock RD, Forbes CD. Mechanisms of joint damage in an experimental model of haemophilic arthritis. *Arthritis Rheum* 1988; **31**: 1148–55.

3 Stein H, Duthie RB. The pathogenesis of chronic haemophilic arthropathy. *J Bone Joint Surg (Br)* 1981; **63B**: 601–9.

4 Madhok R, York J, Sturrock RD. Haemophilic arthritis. *Ann Rheum Dis* 1991; **50**: 588–91.

5 Hoaglund FT. Experimental hemarthrosis: the response of canine knees to injections of autologous blood. *J Bone Joint Surg (Am)* 1967; **49A**: 285–98.

6 Zeman DH, Roberts ED, Shoji H, Miwa T. Experimental haemarthrosis in rhesus monkeys: morphometric, biochemical and metabolic analyses. *J Comp Pathol* 1991; **104**: 129–39.

7 Wolf CR, Mankin HJ. The effect of experimental hemarthrosis on articular cartilage of rabbit knee joints. *J Bone Joint Surg (Am)* 1965; **47A**: 1203–10.

8 Roy S, Ghadially FN. Pathology of experimental haemarthrosis. *Ann Rheum Dis* 1966; **25**: 402–15.

9 Mainardi CL, Levine PH, Werb Z, Harris ED. Proliferative synovitis in hemophilia: biochemical and morphologic observations. *Arthritis Rheum* 1978; **21**: 137–44.

10 Pelletier J-P, Martel-Pelletier J, Ghandur-Mnaymneh L, Howell DS, Frederick-Woessner J. Role of synovial membrane inflammation in cartilage matrix breakdown in the Pond-Nuki model of osteoarthritis. *Arthritis Rheum* 1985; **28**: 554–61.

11 Abrahams TG, Pavlov H, Bansal M, Bullough P. Concentric joints space narrowing of the hip associated with hemosiderotic synovitis (HS) including pigmented villonodular synovitis (PVNS). *Skeletal Radiol* 1988; **17**: 37–45.

12 France MP, Gupta SK. Non-haemophilic hemosiderotic synovitis of the shoulder: a case report. *Clin Orthop* 1991; **262**: 132–6.

13 Morris, CJ, Blake DR, Wainwright AC, Steven MM. Relationship between iron deposits and tissue damage in the synovium: an ultra structural study. *Ann Rheum Dis* 1986; **45**: 21–6.

14 Blake DR, Gallagher PJ, Potter AR, Bell MJ, Bacon PA. The effect of synovial iron on the progression of rheumatoid disease: a histologic assessment of patients with early rheumatoid synovitis. *Arthritis Rheum* 1984; **27**: 495–501.

15 Roosendaal G, Vianen ME, Wenting MJG, van Rinsum AC, van den Berg HM, Lafeber FPJG, Bijlsma JWJ. Iron deposits and catabolic properties of synovial tissue from patients with haemophilia. *J Bone Joint Surg (Br)* 1998; **80B**: 540–5.

16 Rodriguez-Merchan EC. Pathogenesis, early diagnosis, and prophylaxis for chronic hemophilic synovitis. *Clin Orthop* 1997; **343**: 6–11.

17 Roosendaal G, Van Rinsum AC, Vianen ME, van den Berg HM, Lafeber FPJG, Bijlsma JWJ. Haemophilic arthropathy resembles degenerative rather than inflammatory joint disease. *Histopathology* 1999; **34**: 144–53.

18 Roosendaal G, Vianen ME, van den Berg HM, Lafeber FP, Bijlsma JW. Cartilage damage as a result of hemarthrosis in a human in vitro model. *J Rheumatol* 1997; **24**: 1350–4.

19 Roosendaal G, Vianen ME, Marx JJM, van den Berg HM, Lafeber FPJG, Bijlsma JWJ. Blood induced joint damage: a human *in vitro* study. *Arthritis Rheum* 1999; **42**: 1025–32.

20 Lafeber FP, Vander Kraan PM, van Roy JL, Huber Bruning O, Bijlsma JW. Articular cartilage explant culture; an appropriate in vitro system to compare osteoarthritic and normal human cartilage. *Connect Tissue Res* 1993; **29**: 287–99.

21 Niibayashi H, Shimizu K, Suzuki K, Yamamoto S, Yasuda T, Yamamuro T. Proteoglycan degradation in hemarthrosis: intraarticular, autologous blood injection in rat knees. *Acta Orthop Scand* 1995; **66**: 73–9.

22 Bates EJ, Lowther DA, Handley CJ. Oxygen free-radicals mediate an inhibition of proteoglycan synthesis in cultured articular cartilage. *Ann Rheum Dis* 1984; **43**: 462–9.

23 Burkhardt H, Schwingel M, Menninger H, Macartney HW, Tschesche H. Oxygen radicals as effectors of cartilage destruction: direct degradative effect on matrix components and indirect action via activation of latent collagenase from polymorphonuclear leukocytes. *Arthritis Rheum* 1986; **29**: 379–87.

24 Roosendaal G, Tekoppele JM, Vianen ME, van den Berg HM, Lafeber FPJG, Bijlsma JWJ. Blood induced joint damage: a canine *in vivo* study. *Arthritis Rheum* 1999; **42**: 1033–9.

25 Convery FR, Woo SL, Akeson WH, Amiel D *et al*. Experimental hemarthrosis in the knee of the mature canine. *Arthritis Rheum* 1976; **19**: 59–67.

26 Parsons JR, Zingler BM, McKeon JJ. Mechanical and histological studies of acute joint hemorrhage. *Orthopedics* 1987; **10**: 1019–26.

CHAPTER 4

Biomechanical Research in Haemophilia

A SEUSER, T WALLNY, G SCHUMPE, H H BRACKMANN AND W J RIBBANS

INTRODUCTION

Bleeding episodes in patients with haemophilia occur mainly (80%) in the locomotor system. The progression of blood-induced arthropathy is much faster than that of normal osteoarthritis. With insufficient factor substitution the development of a 'target joint' is likely. The principal haemophilic joints are the knee, ankle and elbow. Much research has taken place in the field of morphologic pathology, surgery, conservative treatment and radiology with the development of scoring systems and new procedures [1–13]. The existing systems have never been evaluated or correlated to joint function. We know from biomechanical motion analysis of healthy persons and patients with osteoarthritis that the locomotor system is highly sensitive to external influences. Small changes in function can produce enormous joint loading that is not detectable by clinical or radiological examination.

A number of important biomechanical questions arise from the highly individual progression of haemarthropathy:

1 Is there a correlation between clinical or radiological scores and joint function?

2 Does motion analysis assist in making therapeutic decisions?

3 Can specific motion data be used to estimate the risk of bleeding into or loading of a joint?

4 Is there a specific, clinically undetectable, restriction of function that we can diagnose with motion analysis and help to optimize conservative treatment?

5 How sensitively does a haemarthropathic joint react to external manipulation (for example, training machines, silicone heel cushioning, intra-articular therapy)?

An analysis of the biomechanics of human movement is fundamental to understanding normal and pathological function. Although many parameters can be used to describe the biomechanics of human movement, there are several kinematic and kinetic parameters that are particularly relevant to the understanding of the pathomechanics of human movement. The kinematics of human movement (joint kinematics) is normally described in terms of relative angles between adjacent limb segments. In practice, human gait is most often described in terms of motion in the sagittal plane of adjacent limb segments (flexion–extension motion patterns) [14].

Joint kinetics is the study of the relationship between force and motion. The motion of the skeletal system is the result of a balance between external and internal forces. The external forces of the skeletal system include gravity, inertia and foot–ground reaction forces during walking. Internal forces are created by muscular contraction, passive soft-tissue stretching and bone contact in joint articulations. At any instant during walking or any activity of daily living, the external forces and moments must be balanced by internal forces and moments. Joint kinetic studies include: interpretation of joint moments, factors influencing joint moments, moment magnitudes during the activities of daily living, and direct measurements of joint loading during function [14–17].

ULTRASOUND TOPOMETRY

On-line motion analysis was performed with the Original Ultrasound Topometer (UST, Bonn, Germany). This analysis system is based on measurement of the elapsed time of ultrasound impulses from a transmitter to four receivers [18,19] fixed in a frame. Knowing the four elapsed times of each ultrasound impulse from transmitter to receiver, the computer calculates the exact location of the transmitter with an accuracy of < 1 mm. As many as 12 different ultrasound transmitters can be used simultaneously. The small ultrasound transmitters are fixed on anatomically relevant points. For joint analysis we use three transmitters above and three below the joint. We place the transmitters only on bony parts to decrease the influence of muscle movement. All recorded data can be processed with special software, providing analysis of the relative joint angles, angular velocity and angular acceleration to be shown in any of three dimensions. In addition, we can measure the roll and glide mechanism of the knee joint related to the joint angle.

THE KNEE

The functional key for understanding the kinematics of the knee is the role and glide mechanism [20,21]. The roll and glide mechanism is a product of all the joint structures including ligaments, cartilage, menisci, bones and, most importantly, the muscles. It represents the basics of the inner joint function in muscle-controlled joints such as the knee joint. We measure the specific changes of the roll and glide mechanism by measuring the tilt of the tibia during knee flexion, indicating rolling on the fixed femur. If the tibia keeps its position during the whole range of movement, it represents pure gliding. Normally, we find between 20° and 30° of tibial tilt distributed throughout the range of movement (Fig. 4.1a). The roll and glide ratio during knee motion is dependent on the different loading situations. We produce more rolling if we push a weight with our foot (closed chain) and more gliding by pushing it with the anterior part of the tibia (open chain). With increasing weight the rolling increases as well (Fig. 4.1b).

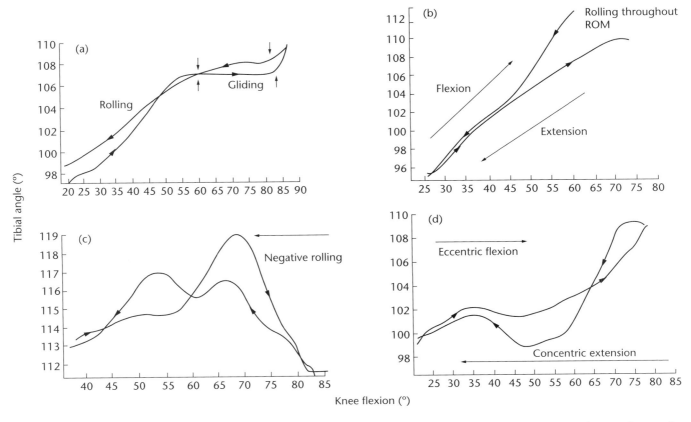

Fig. 4.1 Roll and glide curves. Tibial angle versus knee flexion. (a) Roll and glide curve in normal individual on leg press machine with unilateral loading of 10 kg. Note gliding motion especially during flexion between 60° and 85°. (b) The same individual with maximum loading. Note rolling motion throughout the range of movement. (c) Left knee of the same patient, graded Pettersson 0 but with disturbed kinetics: rolling between 50° and 70° of flexion, negative rolling between 70° and 85° of flexion. (d) A different patient graded as Pettersson 8 but with a good distribution of rolling throughout the range of movement.

We examined patients in different stages of haemarthropathy under specific loading conditions. They performed a unilateral exercise programme on a leg press machine [22] with increasing weight starting with 10 kg up to an individual maximum. An additional endurance test was performed with 60% of the maximum weight. The test ended when the patient felt exhausted. All haemophiliacs showed a diminished rolling and increased gliding motion. Repeated trials with the same weight showed a high degree of variation in the roll and glide curve, a sign of disturbed coordination. In the severely disturbed joints we detected 'negative rolling' similar to the wheels of a car that drives up a steep hill and then rolls backwards.

Increased gliding and 'negative rolling' (Fig. 4.1c) indicated a disturbed inner knee motion with the loss of polycentric motion and a sagittal loading of the joint. We were able to demonstrate that the biomechanical data from motion analysis did not correlate with clinical scores and radiographic findings. A 'Pettersson 8' knee joint does not necessarily have a disturbed inner knee function (Fig. 4.1d). Conversely, we saw 'healthy joints' (Pettersson score 0) with just one bleeding episode but highly disturbed inner joint motion. The roll and glide mechanism characterizes the inner knee motion and aids in detecting functional disturbances and in optimizing conservative treatment. We can identify the exact location of the disturbance at different times during the knee flexion cycle and use the information for effective treatment. Control analysis will show the changes and indicate the need for surgery if the monocentric character of the joint cannot be influenced by conservative treatment due to severe structural damage.

In another study, we used the roll and glide mechanism to investigate the influence of intra-articular hyaluronic acid on the knee joint. The controversial role of intra-articular hyaluronic acid on joints has been extensively reported [23–32]. Motion analysis was performed in addition to two knee scores and the Pettersson score. Whereas the clinical and radiological scores did not show significant changes, the roll and glide curves before and after therapy did. Although the monocentric character of the curves did not improve, we saw a significant reduction of 'negative rolling', a significant improvement in coordination and an increase in the range of movement. This apparent positive influence of the hyaluronic acid on the health of the synovium correlated with the subjective improvement felt by the patient.

In addition to the roll and glide curves, angular velocity and acceleration (Fig. 4.2) give us a deeper understanding of joint loading. From physics, we know that force equals mass times acceleration. If the mass is constant, acceleration is proportional to the acting forces! Sudden acceleration or force peaks can harm the joint because the muscles are not fast enough to react and protect! The normal distribution of joint velocity and acceleration under load in one extension–flexion cycle is symmetric (Fig. 4.2b). The maximum values for angular velocity and the maximum values of angular acceleration are similar in extension and flexion. Loss of this distribution is pathognomonic for poorly balanced joints. In the hyaluronic acid study we were able to demonstrate that the angular velocity and acceleration were restored symmetrically after therapy.

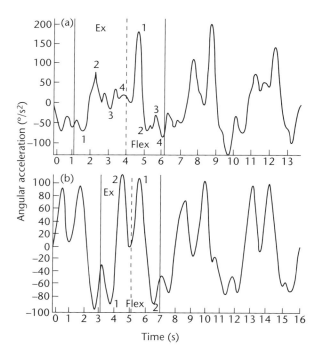

Fig. 4.2 Angular acceleration of a patient with severe haemarthropathy on the leg press machine. (a) Before treatment: note loss of rhythm and increased values for acceleration during flexion ($200°/s^2$) versus extension ($80°/s^2$) in the same cycle. (b): After treatment with hyaluronic acid the patient showed motion symmetry in all measured extension–flexion cycles. Ex = extension; Flex = flexion.

In patients with haemophilia there is a disturbed balance between load and stability under different loading conditions of the joints. During everyday activities, as well as during exercise, care must be taken to minimize negative stress on the joints. We were able to demonstrate that these patients should not use selective extension–flexion training machines that provide exercises in an *open chain*. Training in a *closed chain,* for example, on a leg press, is most suitable to achieve a maximum training benefit with a minimum of negative impact on the knee joint.

A comparison of results from walking on a treadmill at 3 and 5 km/h and jogging at 7 km/h, of isokinetic training in the open chain, and of leg press training in a closed chain, revealed that leg press training leads to the lowest acceleration values. This form of exercise produces only one-seventh of the acceleration during walking at a speed of 3 km/h. The highest values for angular acceleration were produced during isokinetic training in the open chain. Closed chain exercise shows all the biomechanical characteristics of normal gait and offers, importantly, a minimal angular acceleration. In cases of previously damaged haemophilic joints, maximum training has to be achieved with a minimum of physical stress to the joint.

There have been no investigations into the role of active rotation in the knee joint published in the haemophilia and/or biomechanical literature. We examined 10 healthy persons to get a better understanding of the normal rotational capacity of the knee joints, and compared the results with the knee joints of 10 patients with haemophilia in different stages of haemarthropathy graded using the Pettersson score. The patients were asked to perform a maximum external rotation with the knee bent at 90°. Next, they were asked to extend the knee joint slowly, keeping the maximum rotation during the whole extension arc. The same procedure was performed with maximum internal rotation. Both knees were examined.

The knee joint showed a specific rotation pattern. The average rotational capacity for external rotation of a normal knee in our 20 knees was 30±3°. It showed a sigmoid curve characterized by a maximum rotational capacity at 80±10° of flexion. We saw a rapid linear decrease towards extension with nearly no rotation in full extension. The average rotational capacity for the internal rotation of a normal knee was 31±4° in our trial. Again, it showed a sigmoid curve characteristic with a maximum rotational capacity at 90±9° of flexion. We saw an initial rapid loss of rotational capacity with a slower linear decrease towards extension and virtually no rotation in full extension. Even slight injuries have a long-term influence on joint kinematics. A knee joint with a rotational injury 3 weeks previously and no overt sign of symptoms showed remarkable changes in rotation. Rotation in both directions showed a loss of curve characteristics and diminished ability to rotate. Repeated trials showed large variations in the curve characteristics.

In haemophilic patients the knees are even more disturbed. For example, a patient with a Pettersson score of 7 in the left knee and an extension deficit of 10° had external rotation of 28° with only a slight loss of curve characteristic. The internal rotation was reduced by 10°. The right knee had a Pettersson score of 0 and an extension deficit of

5°. We observed 17° external and 18° internal rotation. The functional capacities of the knee did not mirror clinical or radiographic scores. External rotation of the knee seems to be more involved than internal rotation. The less involved knee joint requires the same intensive therapy as the affected knee to improve its biomechanical profile (see section on 'The elbow', p. 33).

THE ANKLE

Shock absorption becomes very important in damaged joints with destroyed cartilage and progressive muscular imbalance as in haemarthropathy. The ankle joint is not predictable in its reaction to external stresses. Biomechanical trials using gait analysis showed that silicone heel cushions do have not the predicted shock-absorbing effect on the ankle joint during gait [33–43].

We examined 20 ankles of 10 haemophilic patients in different stages of haemarthropathy of the ankle. Patients with acute bleeding, chronic synovitis, pain, flexion or extension contraction of the ankle joint or other acute illnesses were excluded. Clinical examination was used to measure the range of motion of the tibiotalar and the subtalar joint. Radiographs of the ankle were taken and the Pettersson score was used for interpretation. All the patients showed differences to normal ankle motion during stance due to their different stages of haemarthropathy.

The gait pattern changed dramatically with a silicone heel cushioning. When walking on the treadmill at a velocity of 2 km/h the angular velocity of the ankle was found to be increased when wearing heel cushioning, producing twice the acceleration at the ankle joint. The influence of heel cushioning diminished with restricted ankle motion. Ankles in late stages of haemarthropathy, severe radiographic changes and markedly restricted range of motion in the tibiotalar and subtalar joints were not influenced by wearing a heel cushion. Their gait pattern with and without the heel cushion was the same. Those end-stage joints had lost the capacity to react any more to external forces. Gait analysis of the corresponding knee joints, however, showed that compensation took place proximally and resulted in 'false movements', higher angular velocities and accelerations and therefore higher loading of these joints. The better the condition of the ankle, the bigger and more detrimental was the influence of heel cushioning on ankle joint and gait pattern.

Silicone is a very flexible material. When it is put under pressure it is compressed and stores potential energy. At the moment of pressure release, the stored energy will again produce kinetic energy. This kinetic energy is able to influence the motion of the ankle during gait. As the energy is not strong enough to lift the heel, the first impact is on the advancement of the tibia relative to the talus and on subtalar motion. The muscles are not fast enough to react adequately to the unusual situation. Therefore, they cannot act and stabilize the foot but have to react to the external force produced by the kinetic energy of the heel cushioning. This reaction is uncoordinated and produces higher joint angles, a higher angular velocity and a higher angular acceleration in the ankle joint. A higher acceleration is related to a higher loading of the joint. This additional movement and the excessive dorsiflexion take extra time to happen, producing a longer contact time of the heel. This influences the whole gait cycle.

A haemophilic joint which already shows subclinical changes due to former joint bleedings is not able to compensate the additional forces produced by the heel cushioning (even if there is no clinical evidence of motion restriction or muscle weakness). In an ankle joint with a low degree of haemarthropathy, there is a distinct difference in comparison with normal gait due to a subtle loss of soleus elasticity and tibialis anterior dysfunction. The muscles cannot react in time and, at its natural limits, movement of the joint is restricted by passive structures such as ligaments and the joint capsule. Without muscular control, the ankle joint is loaded with shear forces and the uncoordinated motion may cause impingement of the synovial tissue, which is a potentially major determinant for joint bleeding in haemophilia.

THE ELBOW

The radiohumeral joint is the site of 80% of the first symptoms in the elbow joint, and 40% of patients who develop restriction in elbow flexion show a diminished rotational capacity as well. These changes appear difficult to control even with intensive conservative treatment [44–49].

We examined rotation of the elbow joint. The results show that there is a particular distribution pattern for the whole range of rotation throughout the extension–flexion arc of the elbow. In the healthy control group, there is a nearly linear increase in supination capacity with increasing flexion, and a decrease of pronation. During elbow extension, pronation capacity is increasing and supination decreasing. The mean of maximum pronation was 102° in maximum extension and 78° in maximum flexion. A maximum of 117° of supination was reached at a flexion of 130° and a minimum of 72° in complete extension (Fig. 4.3a).

In the haemophilic elbow, we detected abnormalities in both magnitude and curve characteristic (Figs 4.3b and c). There was no correlation between clinical or radiological findings. Even elbows with 'Pettersson 0' joints showed changes in distribution of rotation and diminished rotational range of movement (Fig. 4.3b). We have to conclude that even slight disturbances in the elbow joint, causing clinically undetectable changes in muscle and ligaments, will result in a functional pathology. Early physiotherapy with special attention to rotation throughout the whole flexion is mandatory to prevent progressive and irreversible joint damage.

Even if there is no motion restriction in the extension–flexion arc, there may already be a severe loss of rotational ability. From a biomechanical point of view, the knee and elbow need maximum ability to rotate to keep the surfaces congruent throughout the whole range of motion. Loss of rotation disturbs the natural inner joint kinematics and produces shear forces which increase the loading of the joint and may lead to more bleeding episodes. Physiotherapy therefore needs to focus on rotational motion in every bending position of the knee (Fig. 4.1) and elbow joint.

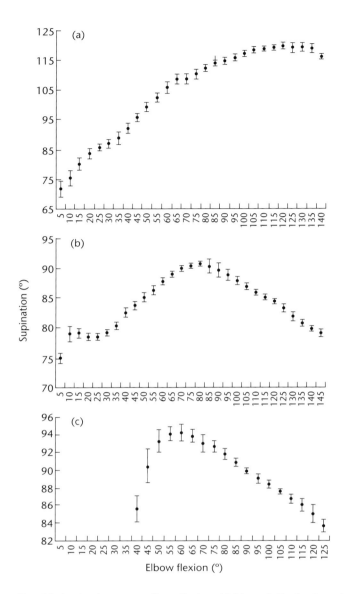

Fig. 4.3 Supination versus elbow flexion. (a) Normal distribution with nearly linear increase of supination during flexion. (b) Patient graded Pettersson 0: almost normal start till 80° of flexion, then loss of supination ability instead of a further increase. Range of movement for supination is also diminished. (c) Patient graded Pettersson 1 with extension restricted to 35°. Linear increase of supination till 65°, then decrease till the end of flexion. Error bar = mean ± SD.

CONCLUSION

Biomechanical research in haemophilia is still in its infancy. As haemophilic arthropathy presents a variety of symptoms, we need to examine more patients in order to understand more about the functional pathology of joints. The existing biomechanical motion data teach us that there are more complex aspects of joint kinetics than can be understood from superficial clinical or radiological observation. Biomechanical diagnosis and motion analysis are of growing importance, especially in chronic illnesses. To understand the locomotor system, we need a lot more information than the traditional diagnostic scoring systems can offer. As we deal with dynamic problems, motion analysis will be a useful tool for objectively planning and monitoring successful therapy.

REFERENCES

1 Arnold WD, Hilgartner MW. Hemophilic arthropathy. *J Bone Joint Surg (Am)* 1977; **59**: 287–305.

2 Atkins RM, Henderson NJ, Duthie RB. Joint contractures in the hemophilias. *Clin Orthop* 1987; **219**: 97–106.

3 Erlemann R, Pollmann H, Adolph J, Peters PE. Die hämophile Arthropathie unter besonderer Berücksichtigung des Ellenbogengelenkes. *Radiologie* 1990; **30**: 116–23.

4 Hamel J, Pohlmann H, Schramm W. Verteilung und Ausmaß der hämophilen Arthropathie bei Erwachsenen mit schwerem Faktor VIII-Mangel. *Z Orthop* 1988; **126**: 574–8.

5 Johnson RP, Babitt DP. Five stages of joint disintegration compared with range of motion in hemophilia. *Clin Orthop* 1987; **201**: 36–106.

6 Pettersson H, Ahlberg A, Nilsson IM. A radiographic classification of hemophilic osteoarthropathy. *Clin Orthop* 1980; **149**: 153–9.

7 Rodriguez-Merchan EC. Effects of hemophilia on articulations of children and adults. *Clin Orthop* 1996; **328**: 7–13.

8 Seuser A, Effenberger W, Oldenburg J, Brackmann HH. Zwölfjahresergebnisse der klinischen und radiologischen Ellenbogenscores bei Kindern mit schwerer Hämophilie. In: Scharrer I, Schramm W, eds. *26. Hämophilie-Symposium Hamburg*. Berlin: Springer, 1995.

9 Seuser A, Klein H, Wallny T, Schumpe G, Brackmann H-H, Kalnins W. Grundlagen des medizinischen Bewegungstrainings für Hämophile. In: *27. Hämophilie-Symposium Hamburg*. Berlin: Springer, 1996: 266–7.

10 Seuser A, Oldenburg J, Brackmann HH. Pathogenese, Diagnose und orthopädische Therapie der hämophilen Gelenkarthropathie. In: *Hämostaseologie: Molekulare und zelluläre Mechanismen, Pathophysiologie und Klinik*. Berlin: Springer, 1999: 198–9.

11 Syrbe G, Linde P. Ein-Jahresanalyse von Blutungsergebnissen von 223 Hämophilen in der DDR. *Folia Haematol Int Mag Klin Morphol Blutforsch* 1990; **117**: 519–25.

12 Kalnins W, Klein H. Konzept der krankengymnastischen Behandlung der hämophilen Arthropathie. In: Scharrer I, Schramm W, eds. *26. Hämophilie-Symposium Hamburg*. Berlin: Springer, 1995.

13 Seuser A, Brackmann HH, Oldenburg J, Effenberger W. Orthopaedic outcome of the knee and ankle joints of children and adolescents with severe hemophilia A: a 12 year follow up. Presented at the *3rd Musculoskeletal Congress of the World Federation of Hemophilia*, Herzliya, Israel, 1995 (abstract).

14 Andriachi TP, Sum J, Yoder D. Biomechanics and gait. In: Kadders JR, ed. *Orthopaedic Knowledge Update 5*. Rosemont, IL: American Academy of Orthopaedic Surgeons, 1996: 29–40.

15 Cochran GVB. *A Primer of Orthopaedic Biomechanics*. New York: Churchill Livingstone, 1982: 268–93.

16 Kadaba MP, Ramakaishnan HK, Wootten Me, Gainey J, Gorton G, Cochran GVB. Repeatability of kinematic, kinetic and electromyographic data in normal adult gait. *J Orthop Res* 1989; **7**: 849–60.

17 Perry J. *Gait Analysis, Normal and Pathological Function*. Thorofare, Slack, USA, 1992: 51–87.

18 Schumpe G. *Differenzierung der funktionellen Kniebewegung von hämophilen Patienten mittels Ultraschall-Topometrie*. Dissertation, Bonn Rheinische Friedrich-Wilhelms-Universität, Bonn, 1982.

19 Seuser A, Schumpe G, Gäbel H. Quantifizierung von rehabilitativen Therapiemaßnahmen und Qualitätssicherung durch die Verlaufskontrolle mittels Ultraschalltopometrie. *Wien Med Wschr* 1994; **110**: 15–18.

20 Radin EL, Orr RB, Kelman JL, Paul IL, Rose RM. Effects of prolonged walking on concrete on the knees of sheep. *J Biomech* 1982; **15**: 487–92.

21 Schumpe G. *Biomechanische Aspekte am Kniegelenk*. PhD thesis, Bonn Rheinische Friedrich-Wilhelms-Universität, Bonn, 1984.

22 Seuser A, Schumpe G, Eickhoff HH, Brackmann H-H, Oldenburg J. Analyse der Kniekinematik bei Patienten mit Hämarthopathie beim Leg Press Training. In: *24. Hämophilie-Symposium Hamburg*. Berlin: Springer, 1993: 150–4.

23 Carrabba M. The intra-articular treatment of osteoarthritis of the knee: a comparative study between hyaluronic acid and orgotein. *Europ J Rheumatol Inflammation* 1992; **12**: 47–57.

24 Dahlberg, L. Intraarticular injections of hyaluron in patients with cartilage abnormalities and knee pain: a one-year double-blind, placebo-controlled study. *Arthritis Rheum* 1994; **27**: 521–8.

25 Dougados M. High molecular weight sodium hyaluronate in osteoarthritis of the knee: a 1 year placebo-controlled trial. *Osteoarthritis Cartilage* 1993, **1**: 97–103.

26 Graf J. Intra-articular treatment with hyaluronic acid of the knee joint: a controlled clinical trial vs. mucopolysaccharide polysulfuric acid ester. *Clin Exp Rheumatol* 1992; **11**: 367–72.

27 Jones AC. A comparative study of intra-articular hyaluronic acid and intraarticular triamcinolone hexaceto-

nide in the treatment of osteoarthritis of the knee. *Osteoarthritis Cartilage* 1993; **1**: 71–4.

28 Lohmander LS. Intra-articular hyaluron injections in the treatment of osteoarthritis of the knee: a randomised, double-blind, placebo controlled multicentre trial. Hyaluronan Multicentre Trial Group. *Ann Rheum Dis* 1996; **55**: 424–41.

29 Pozo MA. Reduction of sensory responses to passive movements of inflamed knee joints by hylan, a hyaluronan derivative. *Exp Brain* 1997; **116**: 3–9.

30 Puttick MP. Acute local reactions after intraarticular hylan for osteoarthritis of the knee. *J Rheumatol* 1995; **22**: 1311–4.

31 Schneider U. Wirkungsweise von Hyaluronsäure bei Gonarthrose beider Kniegelenke im Rechts-/Links-Vergleich. Untersuchung mit Dynamometrie, Sauerstoff-partialdruck, Temperatur und Lequesne-Score. *Z Orthop* 1997; **135**: 341–7.

32 Weh L. Arthrose modifizieren mit Hyaluronsäure. *Extracta Orthopaedica* (Sonderdruck 6), 1994; **17**: 22–3.

33 Cerny K, Perry J, Walker JM. Effect of an unrestricted knee–ankle–foot orthosis on the stance phase of gait in healthy persons. *Int Orthop* 1990; **13**: 1121–7.

34 Clark TE, Frederick EC, Cooper LB. Biomechanical measurement of running shoe cushioning properties. In: Nigg BM, Kerr BA, eds. *Biomechanical Aspects of Sport Shoes and Playing Surfaces.* Canada: University of Calgary, 1983: 25–33.

35 Kaelin X, Denoth J, Stacoff A, Stuessi E. Cushioning during running – material test contra subject tests. In: Perren, S, Schneider E, eds. *Biomechanics: Current Interdisciplinary Research.* Dordrech: Martinus Nijhoff, 1985: 651–6.

36 Kapandji IA. Funktionelle Anatomie der Gelenke: Obere Extremität. Stuttgart: Enke, 1985.

37 Katoh Y, Chao EYS, Laughman RK, Schneider E, Morrey BF. Biomechanical analysis of foot function during gait and clinical applications. *Clin Orthop* 1983; **177**: 23–33.

38 Perry J. Anatomy and biomechanics of the hindfoot. *Clin Orthop* 1983; **177**: 9–16.

39 Seuser A, Schumpe G, von Deimling U. Bewegungsanalyse zur Erkennung von Ermüdungserscheinungen und deren Auswirkungen auf die innere Kinematik des Kniegelenkes. In: Liesen HEA, ed. *Regulations- und Repairmechanismen.* 33. Deutscher Sportärztekongreß Paderborn. Köln: Deutscher Ärzte-Verlag, 1993: 429–31.

40 Seuser A, Wallny T, Klein H, Ribbans WJ, Schumpe G, Brackmann HH. Gait analysis of the hemophilic ankle with silicone heel cushion. *Clin Orthop* 1997; **343**: 74–80.

41 Sutherland D, Cooper L, Danial D. The role of the plantar flexors in normal walking. *J Bone Joint Surg (Am)* 1980; **62A**: 354–63.

42 Voloshin A, Wosk J. An *in vivo* study of low back pains and shock absorption in the human locomotor system. *J Biomech* 1982; **15**: 21–7.

43 Wright DG, Desai SM, Henderson WH. Action of the subtalar and ankle joint complex during the stance phase of walking. *J Bone Joint Surg (Am)* 1964; **46A**: 361–82.

44 Gamble JG, Vallier H, Rossi M, Glader B. Loss of elbow and wrist motion in hemophilia. *Clin Orthop* 1996; **328**: 94–101.

45 Morrey BF, An KN, Stormont TJ. Force transmission through the radial head. *J Bone Joint Surg (Am)* 1988; **70A**: 250–6.

46 Sojbjerg JO. The stiff elbow. *Acta Orthop Scand* 1996; **67**: 626–31.

47 Spanagel M, Seuser A, Schumpe G, Effenberger W, Brackmann HH. Pro- und Supination des hämophilen Ellenbogens: Eine biomechanische Studie. In: Scharrer I, Schramm W, eds. *26. Hämophilie-Symposium Hamburg.* Berlin: Springer, 1995: 293–7.

48 Stroyan M, Wilk KE. The functional anatomy of the elbow complex. *J Orthop Sport Phys Ther* 1993; **17**: 279–88.

49 Werner FW, An KN. Biomechanics of the elbow and forearm. *Hand Clin* Nr. 4; Wiesbaden München: Selecta, 1994; **10**: 357–73.

CHAPTER 5
Haemophilic Haemarthroses

E C RODRIGUEZ-MERCHAN AND N J GODDARD

INTRODUCTION

Haemarthrosis is undoubtedly the most common and potentially most disabling manifestation of haemophilia, and it is the complications of such bleeding episodes that will bring the patient to the attention of the orthopaedic surgeon. A haemarthrosis is frequently preceded by the patient's perception of an aura or tingling sensation in the joint. Such haemarthroses may occur spontaneously or as a result of trauma (Fig. 5.1). The bleeding into the joint will cause the patient to place the joint in a position of maximum volume, i.e. least pressure. This is generally in slight flexion. Any movement beyond this is painful and restricted. A basic examination generally reveals the presence of a haemarthrosis, particularly if the joint is subcutaneous, as in the knee. However, ultrasound or magnetic resonance imaging may be helpful in determining the presence of deep-seated haemarthroses or muscle bleeds, for example, in the psoas tendon or around the hip.

The majority of patients with haemophilia around the world are treated by standard blood replacement therapy or on-demand therapy. The amount of factor consumed per annum per patient per kilogram varies between 500 and 2000 units, and treatment should be aimed at reducing spontaneous haemarthroses. Thus, long-term prophylaxis is the measure most likely to produce the best orthopaedic outcome. The goals of treatment in patients with haemophilia are essentially to reduce the tendency for repeated haemarthroses, to preserve a functional range of motion and to reduce the tendency for muscular atrophy [1]. The increasing introduction of continuous prophylactic clotting factor replacement has been reported to slow the natural history of the development of haemophilic arthropathy. Experience from Sweden has shown that continuous prophylaxis beginning in childhood has prevented the development of haemophilic arthropathy if the concentration of the patient's deficient factor is prevented from falling below 1% of normal [2]. This can be achieved with the administration of 25 to 40 units per kg three times weekly in patients with classic haemophilia A, and 25 to 40 units per kg twice weekly in patients with haemophilia B.

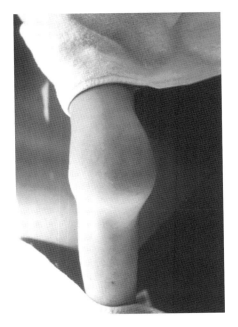

Fig. 5.1 Severe haemarthrosis on the right knee in a young person with haemophilia.

THE EFFECTS OF HAEMARTHROSIS ON SYNOVIUM AND ON JOINT CARTILAGE

Safran *et al*. [3] performed an experimental study in order to investigate the effect of a single injection of unpreserved blood on joint stiffness and synovium and cartilage histology in the ankle joints of rabbits at 10 and 28 days following injection. Their results demonstrated that the presence of blood in an otherwise normal joint did not lead to ultimate compromise in the integrity of the cartilage or the joint function. Therapeutic aspiration of an acute post-traumatic haemarthrosis does not appear to be necessary for the prevention of long-term problems.

Roosendaal *et al*. [4] later investigated the direct effect of blood and blood components on human cartilage *in vitro*. They showed that whole blood anticoagulated with heparin, coagulated blood, mononuclear cells, red cells and plasma in this order of potency increased proteoglycan synthesis in a dose-dependent manner. The effect of the combination of mononuclear cells and red cells in concentration equivalent to those in whole blood was significantly greater than the effects of the isolated components alone and did not differ from that of whole blood. They found that cartilage exposed to this combination for more than 4 days exhibited irreversible inhibition of proteoglycan synthesis. The effect was similar to that of whole blood and the opposite to that of the individual components or other combinations.

If a single joint becomes the site of a recurrent haemarthrosis, this is generally referred to as a target joint. When the joint fails to recover fully between bleeding episodes there is hypertrophy of the synovium, and the joint becomes permanently warm and swollen. Arnold and Hilgartner [5] found that hydrolytic enzymes increase in both haemophilic synovium and the joint fluid. Acid phosphatase and catepsin D may also play a role in maintaining chronic inflammation in the synovium.

The release enzymes responsible for the breakdown of protein have a destructive effect not only on the free blood but also, as might be expected, on the synovium, the cartilage and the bone itself. The role of iron deposition in the pathophysiology of haemophilic arthropathy has not been fully established. Stein and Duthie [6] described well-defined cytoplasmic deposits of iron (siderosomes) in the synovial cells, the subsynovial tissues and in chrondrocytes of the superficial layers of the articular cartilage. The haemosiderin staining of the synovium and the cartilage bears testimony to the destructive elements of the proteolytic enzymes.

Roosendaal *et al*. [7] obtained synovial specimens from patients with haemophilia and found that the haemosiderotic deposit in the tissue was often adjacent to macroscopically normal tissue in the same joint. Samples from both affected and unaffected synovial tissue were analysed histologically and biochemically in order to determine the catabolic activity. This showed that in patients with haemophilic arthropathy local synovial iron deposits were associated with increased catabolic activity. As early as 4 days after the onset of a single haemarthrosis, the synovium often shows focal areas of the villus formation. Recurrent haemarthroses stimulate the synovium, which in turn hypertrophies within the joint. This hypertrophic synovial tissue comes to occupy space and is likely to be further injured and cause new bleeding. This process initiates, and is responsible for, the chronic synovitis found within the joints of patients affected with haemophilia. Radiological evaluation of affected joints shows a pronounced increase in the density of the joint space and the recesses caused by accumulation of fluid or, alternatively, the hypertrophic synovium.

Ultrasound is a safe and reliable diagnostic technique for distinguishing synovial hypertrophy from a simple effusion or haemarthrosis. Magnetic resonance imaging may also be used as an alternative diagnostic aid in the case of synovial proliferation or joint effusion in patients with haemophilia (Fig. 5.2). The hypertrophic synovium is characterized by villus formation, marked increase in vascularity and chronic inflammatory cells (Fig. 5.3).

The cells in the synovium can absorb a limited amount of iron once the quantity is exceeded. However, the cells may disintegrate and release lysosomes which not only destroy the adjacent articular cartilage but result in further inflammation of the synovium. Blood from break-

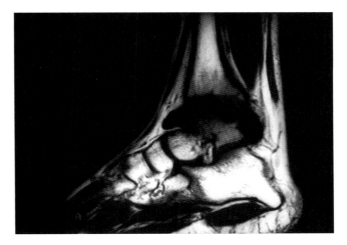

Fig. 5.2 Magnetic resonance imaging of an ankle showing an intense degree of haemophilic synovitis.

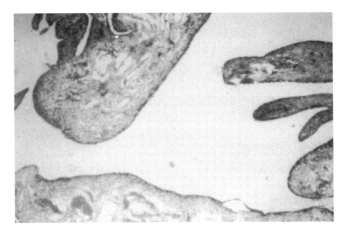

Fig. 5.3 Knee synovium from a person with haemophilia. Note a late stage of hypertrophic synovitis.

down products also has an adverse effect on the chondrocytes. The abnormal synovium will act in a similar manner to that of arterio-venous fistula, producing an increase in blood supply in the area of the growth plates. This inflammatory reaction causes accelerated ossification and growth of the epiphyses leading to osseous problems and epiphyseal overgrowth in young patients (Fig. 5.4).

Such bone hypertrophy can in turn lead to leg length discrepancies, angular deformity and alteration in structures, especially of the developing skeleton. The symptoms of chronic haemophilic arthropathy classically develop in patients with haemophilia during the second and third decades. In patients in whom growth has been completed and the epyphyses fused, the major effect is seen on the articular cartilage. As damage of articular cartilage progressively worsens, there is a progressive deterioration in the joint surface, with movement becoming increasingly limited and painful. Radiographs show a narrowing of the joint space and reduction and irregularity of the previously congruent joint surfaces [8].

TREATMENT OF HAEMARTHROSIS

The optimal treatment of an acute haemarthrosis involves a combination of factor replacement, joint aspiration (when appropriate), analgesia, rest and supervised rehabilitation. As outlined in the initial chapters, the care involves a team approach led by the haematologist, but including input from orthopaedic surgeons and physiotherapists. Simple bleeding episodes can be managed at home using self-administered factor replacement.

In order to control an acute haemarthrosis, the optimal factor level should be 30–50 IU/dL. To achieve such a level in a patient with severe haemophilia, 15–25 IU/kg of factor VIII and 30–50 IU/kg of factor IX may be required. A single treatment may not be sufficient for a major bleeding episode [9].

Nonsteroidal anti-inflammatory medications are relatively contraindicated in patients with haemophilia. Thus, analgesic agents (paracetamol, codeine) should be used to provide adequate analgesia. In addition, the joint should be rested. A sling may be appropriate for an upper limb injury, and care should be taken to avoid aggravating the condition, for instance by lifting or carrying heavy items. Lower limb injuries may require immobilization in a splint and a period of restricted weight bearing and use of crutches.

The role of joint aspiration remains somewhat controversial with certain centres practising this on a routine basis and others avoiding it when at all possible. Our preference is to aspirate the joint at an early opportunity in order to minimize the potential for late cartilage damage and synovial hypertrophy (Fig. 5.5). It is a relatively straightforward matter to aspirate a subcutaneous joint such as the knee, ankle or elbow. Aspiration of the hip, however, should only be undertaken under some form of imaging, either image intensifier or ultrasound. We recommend aspiration of a tense, painful joint which shows no improvement following adequate replacement of factor.

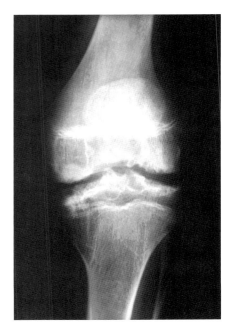

Fig. 5.4 Anteroposterior radiograph of the knee of a 14-year-old boy showing severe haemophilic arthropathy.

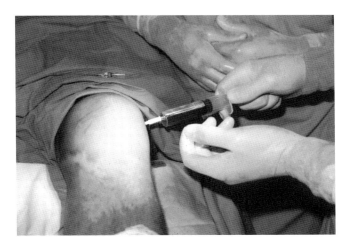

Fig. 5.5 Joint aspiration (arthrocentesis) of a haemophilic knee.

A haemarthrosis in the hip is generally apparent from the clinical picture of a patient holding his or her hip somewhat flexed and externally rotated [10]. Ultrasound distinguishes between a haemarthrosis, an intraperitoneal haemorrhage, a subperiosteal bleed, a bleed into the soft tissues around the hip, or a psoas haematoma. Heim *et al.* [10] reported two cases in which an acute haemarthrosis into the hip resulted in a flexion contracture associated with severe intractable pain unresponsive to narcotic agents. Simple aspiration of the joint produced dramatic pain relief and restored early mobility.

Although children with haemophilia tend to be accustomed to repeated injections, repeated joint aspirations can induce a sensation of fear lasting for long periods. Greene [11] advocated the use of topical anaesthetic patches prior to aspirating the joint. Immediately before aspiration, further local anaesthetic should be infiltrated deep down to the capsule. A large-bore needle should be used, and following aspiration of the haemarthrosis a compression bandage should be applied for 24–48 hours before beginning supervisory rehabilitation with a physiotherapist.

In patients who are HIV-positive one must also bear in mind the possibility of a septic arthritis. A painful, swollen joint mimicking a simple haemarthrosis may be the effect of a septic arthritis. A particularly high index of suspicion is warranted if adequate factor replacement fails to relieve the symptoms, and especially if there are signs of systemic infection. Under these circumstances joint aspiration, and culture of the aspirate, is mandatory. Appropriate antibiotic therapy may cure a septic arthritis, but it may be necessary to irrigate the joint arthroscopically at a later stage [12]. Major haemarthroses should be treated aggressively in order to prevent late onset haemophilic arthropathy.

REFERENCES

1 Rodriguez-Merchan EC. Pathogenesis, early diagnosis, and prophylaxis for chronic hemophilic synovitis. *Clin Orthop* 1997; **343**: 6–11.

2 Nilsson IM, Berntorp E, Löfqvist T, Pettersson H. Twenty-five years' experience of prophylactic treatment in severe hemophilia A and B. *J Intern Med* 1992; **232**: 25–32.

3 Safran MR, Johnston-Jones K, Kabo JM, Meals RA. The effect of experimental hemarthrosis on joint stiffness

and synovial histology in a rabbit model. *Clin Orthop* 1994; **303**: 280–8.

4 Roosendaal G, Vianen ME, Van den Berg HM *et al.* Cartilage damage as a result of hemarthrosis in a human *in vitro* model. *J Rheumatol* 1997; **24**: 1350–4.

5 Arnold WD, Hilgartner MW. Hemophilic arthropathy. *J Bone Joint Surg (Am)* 1977; **59A**: 287–305.

6 Stein H, Duthie RB. The pathogenesis of chronic haemophilic arthropathy. *J Bone Joint Surg (Br)* 1981; **63B**: 601–9.

7 Roosendaal G, Vianen ME, Wenting MJG *et al.* Iron deposits and catabolic properties of synovial tissue from patients with haemophilia. *J Bone Joint Surg (Br)* 1998; **80B**: 540–5.

8 Rodriguez-Merchan EC. Effects of hemophilia on articulations of children and adults. *Clin Orthop* 1996; **328**: 7–13.

9 Ribbans WJ, Giangrande P, Beeton K. Conservative treatment of hemarthrosis for prevention of hemophilic synovitis. *Clin Orthop* 1996; **343**: 12–18.

10 Heim M, Varon D, Strauss S, Martinowitz U. The management of a person with haemophilia who has a fixed flexed hip and intractable pain. *Haemophilia* 1998; **4**: 842–4.

11 Greene WB. The role of orthopaedists in the prevention of haemophilic arthropathy. *Haemophilia* 1996; **2** (Suppl. 1): 1.

12 Rodriguez-Merchan EC, Magallon M, Manso F, Martin-Villar J. Septic arthritis in HIV positive haemophiliacs: four cases and a literature review. *Int Orthop* 1992; **16**: 302–6.

CHAPTER 6

Chronic Haemophilic Synovitis

E C RODRIGUEZ-MERCHAN AND N J GODDARD

INTRODUCTION

Recurrent haemarthroses will inevitably lead to significant hypertrophic synovitis in patients with haemophilia. If the synovitis is not controlled, there will be progressive cartilage degradation, ultimately resulting in haemophilic arthropathy with significant functional impairment. The degree of haemophilic synovitis is directly related to an increase in bleeding frequency in the affected joint. It is possible to diagnose synovitis at an early age by means of frequent reviews of patients in their haemophilia centres.

Sometimes standard conservative measures, such as factor replacement and physiotherapy, do not break the vicious cycle of haemarthrosis–synovitis–haemarthrosis (Figs 6.1 and 6.2). Under these circumstances it has been postulated that synovectomy, either chemical, radioactive or surgical (open or arthroscopic), can in turn reduce the bleeding tendency and so delay the onset of haemophilic arthropathy.

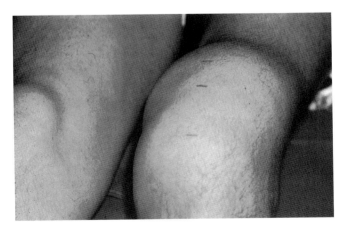

Fig. 6.1 Clinical view of the knees of a young boy with haemophilia. Note the severe degree of haemophilic synovitis in his left knee.

NON-OPERATIVE SYNOVECTOMY (SYNOVIORTHESIS)

The term synoviorthesis (medical synovectomy) is commonly used to describe the intra-articular injection of a substance that will restore inflamed and/or hypertrophic synovium to normal. A number of preparations have been proposed, all with some success, including corticosteroids, osmic acid, rifampicin and radioactive isotopes.

Chemical synoviorthesis with rifampicin

Caruso, in the 1980s, was one of the first workers to use rifampicin as a chemical agent for the treatment of the synovitis associated with rheumatoid arthritis [personal communication, Pietrogrande, 1987]. Rifampicin was chosen for its proteolytic and fibrinolytic properties. Despite encouraging early results there was, however, a high failure rate.

Caviglia *et al.* [1] further evaluated the efficacy of rifampicin in an animal model and in the clinical situation. The animal study demonstrated that an induced haemarthrosis of 8 weeks' duration is sufficient to produce a state of synovitis, with the synovium showing the characteristic pattern of inflammatory infiltrate. There was no such effect on the control joint which had been injected with physiological saline. After 10 weeks the synovium showed signs of regeneration, and by 16 weeks the joints injected with saline solution showed the same pattern microscopically as the rabbits treated with rifampicin.

In the clinical study [1], the affected joint was aspirated and the volume replaced with up to 2 g of rifampicin mixed with 1 cm^3 lidocaine (2%). This protocol was repeated weekly for ten cycles or until the synovitis had receded. Their results were encouraging with 40 patients having excellent results (21 ankles, 6 knees and 13 elbows), and eight patients with good results (two ankles, two knees and four elbows). They concluded that synoviorthesis with rifampicin appeared to be an effective method for the treatment of haemophilic synovitis, especially in small joints (elbows and ankles) and in younger children. They recommended a maximum number of ten injections for the knees and up to five for elbows and ankles before the procedure should be abandoned.

Radioactive synoviorthesis

Ahlberg [2] was the first to report his experience with synoviorthesis in haemophiliacs, aimed at destroying the diseased synovium by using a radioisotope. He reported an improvement of synovitis and cessation of haemorrhage in 95% of the joints injected. Radiation from radioactive isotopes causes fibrosis in the subsynovial connective tissue of the joint capsule and of the synovial villi. It also affects the complex vascular system of the synovial membrane, resulting in the closure of some vessels. There does not appear to be any detrimental effect on the articular cartilage.

There is a theoretical risk of inducing malignant disease and chromosomal changes in blood cells, but to date there have been no reports of locally induced cancer in any patient treated with radioactive synoviorthesis. It has been reported that the risk of gene mutation is negli-

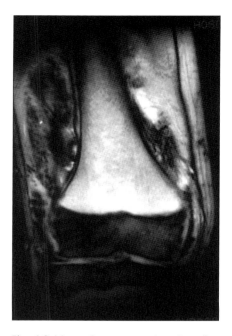

Fig. 6.2 Magnetic resonance imaging of a haemophilic knee. Note the enormous degree of haemophilic synovitis.

gible [3]. The ideal radioisotope for synoviorthesis should be easy to obtain, nontoxic and chemically pure. The isotope should be a beta-emitter since beta rays have a relatively shallow depth of penetration. It should have a short half-life to minimize whole-body irradiation, should leakage occur. Ideally, it should be administered in a homogeneous colloid suspension with a particle size of 100 nm.

During the period 1974–76, we treated 100 affected joints in 64 haemophilic patients with a single dose of gold-198 [4]. A dose of 5 mCi was used in patients under 15 years of age and 10 mCi in patients over 15 years of age. The results were mixed with 8 good, 23 fair and 7 poor results at an average follow-up of 14 years in 38 male haemophiliacs. Patients with symptoms of less than 1 year's duration had a greater percentage of good results than those with symptoms for longer than 1 year.

We felt that gold-198 was an effective agent for radiation synovectomy, particularly in the early stages of the disease where there were minimal radiographic changes. It appeared to reduce the incidence of haemarthrosis and to slow the rate of evolution of radiographic changes. Our results showed that joint function was prolonged, but that there was ultimately gradual deterioration of the joint with the passage of time.

Between 1977 and 1992, Rivard et al. [5] performed 92 synoviortheses on 48 patients using colloidal phosphorus-32 chromic phosphate. Their regime consisted of using 1 mCi for knees and 0.5 mCi for other joints. The frequency and degree of bleeding was reduced in the majority of patients with a follow-up of 1–15 years. However, they found that despite the reduced bleeding tendency there was a progressive deterioration of the radiographic appearance of the affected joints.

The complications reported included extra-articular leakage of the isotope but, with no incidence of induced radioactive burns, this was slight. Chromosome breakages were noted but interestingly these occurred almost exclusively in patients who were seropositive for HIV and in whom the CD4-lymphocyte count was decreased. In three patients there was a subacute inflammatory reaction which developed within hours of the synoviorthesis, persisting for up to 6 months.

Between 1992 and 1994, a prospective study was performed in two centres comparing chemical synovectomy using repeated weekly injections of rifampicin and radioactive synovectomy using yttrium-90 [6]. The study involved 35 haemophilic patients suffering from chronic haemophilic synovitis with 38 affected joints. It was found that rifampicin injections were painful and that several repeated injections at weekly intervals proved to be necessary in order to be effective. Yttrium proved to be very effective, but it is expensive and not readily available. Weighing up the advantages and disadvantages, the authors concluded that rifampicin was the agent of choice for the elbows and ankles, but that yttrium-90 was preferable for the knees.

Löfqvist et al. [7] have shown that radioactive synoviorthesis is invaluable in the management of chronic haemophilic synovitis in those patients with factor inhibitors who might otherwise be difficult to treat. Although their results were inferior to those for patients with haemophilia and no inhibitors, they felt that radioactive synovectomy should be considered not only because of its ease, but also the induced decrease in joint bleeding frequency that it brings about.

OPERATIVE SYNOVECTOMY

Open synovectomy was advocated in 1969 as a method of managing haemophilic synovitis of the knee [8]. Subsequent experience has consistently shown a reduction in the frequency of haemarthrosis after synovectomy of the elbow, of the knee and of the ankle.

Elbow synovectomy

Following reports of elbow synovectomy by Gilbert and Glass [9], we opted for a combination of synovectomy and resection of the radial head in 15 young patients with haemophilia. The indications for surgery were: severe pain and bleeding in the elbow despite appropriate, episodic replacement therapy, and hypertrophy of the radial head and a significant loss of forearm rotation. The age at operation was 21–27 years. We concluded that synovectomy combined with radial head excision is an effective and long-lasting method to achieve improvement of function with minimal risk [10]. It does not appear to jeopardize the possibility of subsequent surgery and can delay the need for more radical operations such as ulno-humeral Haas fascial arthroplasty or prosthetic elbow arthroplasty.

LeBalch *et al.* [11] published encouraging results of simple synovectomy without radial head resection in a large series of predominantly younger patients (only 10 patients were older than 14 years). This more limited procedure is probably more suited to the younger patient without significant deformity of the radial head.

Knee synovectomy

We have reported on our experience of knee synovectomy in 27 patients with chronic haemophilic synovitis [12]. An open technique was used in 18 cases, the remaining nine were performed arthroscopically. The average age at the time of operation was 13 years in both groups. The open group was followed up for an average of 15 years and the closed for 5 years (Figs 6.3 and 6.4).

Synovectomy by either route significantly reduced bleeding episodes, but associated cofactors were shown to be the age of the patient at the time of operation, the severity of the haemophilia, the radiographic stage and the completeness of synovectomy.

As arthroscopic techniques developed in the 1970s it was clear to us that there was less postoperative morbidity, particularly stiffness, with arthroscopic surgery, especially of the knee. It has been reported that arthroscopic synovectomy is effective in reducing recurrent haemarthrosis and maintaining range of motion [13,14]. Additional procedures (meniscal resections, cartilage shaving, removal of loose bodies or complete débridement) can easily be performed at the same time, so enhancing the ultimate result. Postoperative continuous passive motion

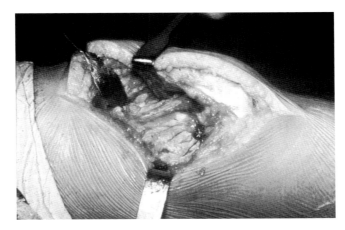

Fig. 6.3 Intraoperative view of an open surgical synovectomy of the knee.

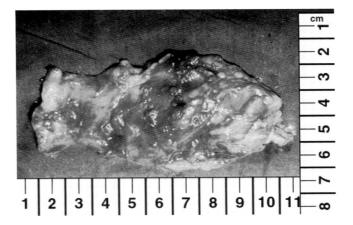

Fig. 6.4 Macroscopic view of the synovium excised during an open surgical synovectomy of the knee.

is beneficial and speeds recovery, but certain problems may be anticipated with younger children.

Arthroscopic synovectomy has proved to be effective in removing inflamed synovium and decreasing the incidence of recurrent haemarthroses, but in common with other methods of treatment joint deterioration continues but probably at a lesser pace.

Ankle synovectomy

The majority of synovectomies performed have been for knee or elbow disease, since these are the most commonly affected joints. The ankle remains a problem, however, and Greene [15] analysed the results of synovectomy of the ankle in five patients who had haemophilia with an average age at the time of operation of 9 years and average duration of follow-up of 5 years. The operation was performed via an anteromedial, an anterolateral and a posterior incision. In comparison with the complications encountered after synovectomy of the knee or the elbow, the rehabilitation process after synovectomy of the ankle was relatively straightforward. It was concluded that synovectomy of the ankle was a useful procedure in patients with haemophilia who have hypertrophic synovitis and recurrent haemarthrosis.

PHYSIOTHERAPY AND ORTHOTICS

Buzzard [16] emphasized the important role of the physiotherapist in the prevention and treatment of the sequelae of recurrent haemarthroses. No one particular method of treatment has been shown to eradicate haemorrhages; however, there are protocols that can help. Electrotherapy, splints, ice, pulsed short-wave diathermy, ultrasound, transcutaneous nerve stimulation, hydrotherapy and exercise are extremely important, especially in developing countries where blood products are scarce.

Heim *et al.* [17] have stressed the importance that orthotics may play in both a protective and preventive role, especially with regard to the knee. There are a plethora of commercial knee orthoses available.

In cases of ankle arthopathy or instability, an orthosis or shoe adaptation may be useful in alleviating pain or during rehabilitation. Shock absorbing viscoheels in shoes seem to reduce the bleeding frequency and pain [18] in the ankle. However, this must be tempered by the experience of Seuser *et al.* [19] who reported that silicone heel cushioning or other shock absorbing devices were not useful for prevention and treatment of chronic haemophilic synovitis, and may cause additional deterioration of the ankle.

SUMMARY

In the authors' experience, synovectomy (by any method) significantly reduces the tendency to bleeding episodes, but does not halt the radiographic deterioration of joints [20]. Thus, synoviorthesis should be the first choice for patients with persistent synovitis of the joints. If two to three consecutive synoviortheses at 3–6-month intervals fail to halt synovitis, a surgical synovectomy should be considered as an alternative for the treatment of chronic haemophilic synovitis.

REFERENCES

1 Caviglia HA, Fernandez-Palazzi F, Maffei E *et al*. Chemical synoviorthesis for hemophilic synovitis. *Clin Orthop* 1996; **343**: 30–6.

2 Ahlberg A. Radioactive gold in the treatment of chronic synovial effusion in hemophilia. In: Ala F, Denson KWE, eds. *7th Congress of the World Federation of Hemophilia*. Amsterdam: Excerpta Medica, 1971: 212–15.

3 Erken EHW. Radiocolloids in the management of hemophilic arthropathy in children and adolescents. *Clin Orthop* 1991; **264**: 129–35.

4 Rodriguez-Merchan EC, Magallon M, Martin-Villar J *et al*. Long-term follow-up of haemophilic arthropathy treated by Au-198 radiation synovectomy. *Int Orthop* 1993; **17**: 120–4.

5 Rivard GE, Girard M, Belanger R *et al*. Synoviorthesis with colloidal P chromic phosphate for the treatment of hemophilic arthropathy. *J Bone Joint Surg (Am)* 1994; **76A**: 482–8.

6 Rodriguez-Merchan EC, Caviglia HA, Magallon M, Perez-Bianco R. Chemical synovectomy vs. radioactive synovectomy for the treatment of chronic haemophilic synovitis: a prospective short-term study. *Haemophilia* 1997; **3**: 118–22.

7 Löfqvist T, Petersson C, Nilsson IM. Radioactive synoviorthesis in patients with hemophilia with factor inhibitor. *Clin Orthop* 1997; **343**: 37–41.

8 Storti E, Traldi A, Tossatti E, Davoli PG. Synovectomy: a new approach to haemophilic arthropathy. *Acta Haematol* 1969; **41**: 193–205.

9 Gilbert MS, Glass K. Hemophilic arthropathy of the

elbow. *Mt Sinai J Med* 1977; **44**: 389–96.

10 Rodriguez-Merchan EC, Galindo E, Magallon M *et al.* Resection of the radial head and partial open synovectomy of the elbow in the young adult with haemophilia: long-term results. *Haemophilia* 1995; **1**: 262–6.

11 LeBalch A, Ebelin T, Laurian Y *et al.* Synovectomy of the elbow in young hemophilic patients. *J Bone Joint Surg (Am)* 1987; **69A**: 264–9.

12 Rodriguez-Merchan EC, Galindo E, Ladreda JMM, Pardo JA. Surgical synovectomy in haemophilic arthropathy of the knee. *Int Orthop* 1994; **18**: 38–41.

13 Wiedel JD. Arthroscopic synovectomy of the knee in hemophilia: 10- to 15-year followup. *Clin Orthop* 1996; **328**: 46–53.

14 Eickhoff HH, Koch W, Raderschadt G, Brackmann HH. Arthroscopy for chronic hemophilic synovitis of the knee. *Clin Orthop* 1997; **343**: 58–62.

15 Greene WB. Synovectomy of the ankle for hemophilic arthropathy. *J Bone Joint Surg (Am)* 1994; **76A**: 812–19.

16 Buzzard BM. Physiotherapy for the prevention and treatment of chronic hemophilic synovitis. *Clin Orthop* 1997; **343**: 42–6.

17 Heim M, Martinowitz U, Horoszowski H. Orthotic management of the knee in patients with hemophilia. *Clin Orthop* 1997; **343**: 54–7.

18 Heijnen L, Roosendaal G, Heim M. Orthotics and rehabilitation for chronic hemophilic synovitis of the ankle: an overview. *Clin Orthop* 1997; **343**: 68–73.

19 Seuser A, Wallny T, Klein H *et al.* Gait analysis of the hemophilic ankle with silicone heel cushion. *Clin Orthop* 1997; **343**: 74–80.

20 Rodriguez-Merchan EC, Magallon M, Galindo E, Lopez-Cabarcos C. Hemophilic synovitis of the knee and elbow. *Clin Orthop* 1997; **343**: 47–53.

CHAPTER 7

On the Safety of Synoviorthesis in Haemophilia

F FERNANDEZ-PALAZZI AND H A CAVIGLIA

INTRODUCTION

It is well known that haemarthrosis is the most frequent bleeding episode in haemophilia, occurring in the musculoskeletal system. It arises from the lax subsynovial venous plexus where a lack of thromboplastic activity has been demonstrated [1]. It follows that we can prevent haemarthrosis acting on the synovial membrane by resecting or by fibrosing it. Resection (synovectomy) was first performed by Storti *et al.* [2] who thus pioneered preventive orthopaedic surgery in haemophilia. Synovectomy can also be carried out arthroscopically or by laser surgery. Fibrosis of the synovial membrane (synoviorthesis) can be achieved with a sclerosing material, either a chemical such as osmic acid or rifampicin, or a radioactive colloid such as gold-198, rhenium-196 or yttrium-90. When a surgical synovectomy is performed, it requires hospitalization and only one or two joints can be operated on at a time; a high level of antihaemophilic factor (AHF) coverage is required, up to 100% on the day of surgery, 50% for the first week and 30% for 4 weeks. The surgical approach for this procedure is through either a medial parapatellar incision or a double medial and lateral incision, with an overall success rate of 75–80%. A reduction in the range of movement results in most cases, caused by osteoarthritic changes and capsular scarring.

Many authors have reported satisfactory results of surgical synovectomy in haemophilia from centres in North and South America [2–6]. Outcomes of arthroscopic synovectomy have been reported from centres in the United States and from several teams in Europe [3,4]. Arthroscopic synovectomy is less surgically aggressive, but postoperative bleeding still occurs and requires a high level of AHF coverage. Finally, synovectomy by laser beam has been reported from Israel [7].

SYNOVIORTHESIS

Synoviorthesis by means of a chemical agent such as osmic acid was first used in rheumatoid arthritis, and had the drawback of being very painful and destroying the articular cartilage. Rifampicin was also used in rheumatoid arthritis by Caruso [personal communication, Pietrogrande, 1987] with unsatisfactory results because in rheumatoid arthritis, unlike haemophilia, the synovial membrane is involved in the disease. Rifampicin is an antibiotic that has an antiprotease action and an inhibitory action on fibrinolysis, thus it brings about fibrosis of the synovium. We introduced the use of rifampicin as a method of synoviorthesis. We utilized a dose of 500 mg in 10 mL of local anaesthetic for the knee, 500 mg in 5 mL of anaesthetic for shoulders, and 250 mg in 1 mL of anaesthetic for elbows and ankles, to be injected intra-articularly once a week for 5–7 weeks according to results, followed by a compression bandage and immediate mobilization. In order to indicate a synoviorthesis we developed a grading system (Table 7.1).

Synoviorthesis with rifampicin

Our experience consists in treating 38 patients with 39 joints injected [8] (Table 7.2). Objective evaluation was performed according to the following scale:

- *Excellent:* 'Dry joint'; recuperation of function; no haemarthrosis; no synovitis.
- *Good:* Clinical improvement; synovitis; diminution of haemarthrosis; recovery of function.
- *Fair:* Synovitis; diminution of haemarthrosis; no recovery of function.
- *Poor:* Synovitis; recurrence of haemarthrosis.

The patient was asked to score the result from his or her ('subjective') point of view, between 1 and 10, and scores were graded as poor (1–3), fair (4–6), good (7–8) and excellent (9–10). The results obtained are combined in Table 7.2.

In conclusion, synovectomy with rifampicin is a good method for use in selected cases of grade II severity. It has the drawback of requiring multiple injections and being painful; nevertheless, pain diminishes after the third injection. The treatment is contraindicated in acute cases, chronic 'full' joint and enlarged joints with chronic synovitis.

Radioactive synoviorthesis

The current preferred method for synoviorthesis is to use a radioactive colloid. Since Ahlberg and Petterssen reported their first cases [9] with

Table 7.1 Grading system developed by the present authors to indicate suitability of synoviorthesis.

Stage	Indications
I Transitory synovitis	With no post-bleeding sequelae. Synoviorthesis is indicated as preventive if there are more than two episodes of haemarthrosis in 6 months.
II Permanent synovitis	With persistent thickening of the synovial membrane and diminution of range of motion. Synoviorthesis is mandatory.
III Chronic arthropathy	As for grade II plus muscular atrophy and axial deformities of the limb. Synoviorthesis is helpful.
IV Fibrous or osseous ankylosis	Synoviorthesis is contraindicated.

Table 7.2 Results of synoviorthesis with rifampicin, scored by patients (subjective) and clinical evaluation (objective) [8].

	Total	Knee	Elbow	Ankle
Status of joints before synoviorthesis				
Grade I	21	13	4	4
Grade II	16	7	5	4
Grade III	2	2	–	–
Total (grades I–III)	39	22	9	8
Subjective opinion after synoviorthesis				
Excellent	21	11	6	4
Good	15	8	3	4
Fair	2	2	–	–
Poor	1	1	–	–
Objective evaluation				
Excellent	20	11	6	3
Good	17	9	3	5
Fair	1	1	–	–
Poor	1	1	–	–

radioactive gold-198, other radioisotopes with little gamma radiation (such as rhenium-186) or no gamma radiation (yttrium-90) have been used first in Argentina and Venezuela, Spain and other European countries, South Africa, and lately in the United States.

The procedure is performed by an intra-articular injection of a radioactive colloid that will fibrose the synovial membrane, thus constricting the subsynovial venous plexus and preventing haemarthrosis. It is carried out on an ambulatory basis and as many as 16 cases can be treated in one sitting. It requires very low AHF coverage to raise factor levels to 30% above coagulation level for 72 hours. In our unit, we first obtain images of the inflamed joint with technetium Tc 99m for reference purposes, raise AHF to 15% and then perform an intra-articular injection of local anaesthetic followed by injection of the radioactive colloid and immobilization with plaster of Paris for 4 days. If we use a colloid with gamma rays (gold-198), a gammagram and scintigraphy are needed to confirm that the material is confined to the injected joint. Before removing the needle from the joint, it is irrigated with anaesthetic to avoid skin burns. We perform regular follow-ups every 6 months, with a Tc 99m scan to measure the reduction of inflammation in the joint; evaluation of recurrence, AHF requirements and length of treatment. Finally, a chromosome study confirms the presence or absence of chromosomal damage [10].

The dosage employed for synoviorthesis was 5 mCi in 10–15 mL of physiological saline for knee joints, 4 mCi in 5 mL physiological saline for shoulders, 2–3 mCi in 3 mL physiological saline for elbows and 2 mCi in 3 mL physiological saline for ankles. Radioactive synoviorthesis was performed on 79 patients; two joints were injected in the same patient on three occasions and the same joint was injected twice on four occasions, making a total of 86 joints (Table 7.3).

Table 7.3 The present authors' experience with radioactive synoviorthesis.

Series	Date	Isotope	No. of joints	Knee	Elbow	Ankle	Shoulder
I	September 1976	Gold-198	10	5	3	2	–
II	May 1977	Gold-198	10	7	3	–	–
III	February 1980	Gold-198	10	8	1	1	–
IV	December 1980	Gold-198	10	5	5	–	–
V	November 1982	Rhenium-186	10	6	2	1	1
VI	September 1993	Rhenium-186	10	5	1	2	2
VII	October 1996	Yttrium-90	10	7	–	1	2
VIII	December 1997	Yttrium-90	16	8	3	5	–
Total			86	53	21	11	1
Grade I			31	20	3	8	–
Grade II			34	23	8	3	–
Grade III			16	10	5	–	1

Results

The treatment was successful in most cases, with 30 reporting no haem-arthrosis, 14 being markedly improved and only five failures (knees) that went on to be treated by a surgical synovectomy. The requirement for AHF fell by 67–94.5%. When a haemarthrosis did recur, it subsided with local measures such as ice or compression. The length of time required for treatment of haemarthrosis following synoviorthesis was 1–4 days compared with a previous mean of 8 days and a maximum of 25 days of treatment.

CHROMOSOME STUDIES

In order to assess the safety of radioactive synoviorthesis, a series of chromosome studies were performed using banding and fluorescence techniques in non-irradiated haemophilic individuals and at 1–2 years and 5–6 years after treatment. The first study, in 1978 at 1–2 years follow-up, examined 354 metaphases (mp) after synoviorthesis with gold-198, where breakage lesions appeared in 61 mp (17.2%) and fragmented chromosomes in 13 mp. Of these, only six were premalignant lesions (1.7%) (two dicentrics, two markers, one triradius and one segregated chromosome). The second study, in 1982 at 5–6 years follow-up of the same irradiated patients, examined 649 metaphases. At this stage, breakages were found in 21 cases (3.2%), segregated in one and fragmented in one, with no premalignant lesions. Those present in the earlier study had completely disappeared (Table 7.4A). We also performed a third study in non-irradiated haemophiliacs on 282 mp, obtaining one breakage and two acrocentric segregations with no premalignant lesions.

Therefore, we can conclude that all chromosomal changes attributable to the radioactive material injected have disappeared within a few years of the treatment and are thus transitory. These findings are similar to those noted after other types of drug therapy such as nonsteroidal anti-inflammatory drugs, aspirin, and so on, and some infectious diseases (for example, presence of virus).

Table 7.4 Chromosomal studies assessing effects of radioactive synoviorthesis [10].

A. Effects of gold-198	Study I 1978 1–2 yrs post-therapy		Study II 1982 5–6 yrs post-therapy		Study III Non-irradiated subjects	
	No.	%	No.	%	No.	%
Metaphases studied	354		649		282	
Non-specific structural changes	61	17.23	21	3.24	2	0.71
Fragmented chromosomes*	6	1.69	0	0	0	0

B. Effects of rhenium-186	Group A Pre-treatment		Group B 5–7 months post-therapy	
	No.	%	No.	%
No. of patients	11		7	
Metaphases studied	272		159	
Total abnormal cells	13	4.77	19	11.94
Aneuploidy	13	4.77	17	10.69
Fragmented chromosomes†	0	0	2	1.25

*Premalignant lesions; †no premalignant abnormalities.

Chromosome studies performed before and after radioactive synoviorthesis with rhenium-186 showed no premalignant chromosomal abnormalities such as markers, segregations, triradiates, dicentrics and others. This is in contrast to the previous studies with gold-198. The participants were in two groups: group A comprised 11 haemophiliacs before radioactive injection and group B comprised 7 of the 11, examined 5–7 months after treatment (Table 7.4B).

DISCUSSION

Radioactive synovectomy (synoviorthesis) has turned out to be one of the most successful preventive measures against haemarthrosis. Since the first report of radioactive synovectomy in haemophilia of Ahlberg and Petterssen in 1979, many centres have adopted this procedure as the one of choice for fibrosing the synovial membrane to prevent further haemarthrosis. Since 1976, we have performed 86 radioactive synoviortheses in 79 patients aged between 6 and 40 years with a mean age of 10 years (45 patients were under 12 years of age). The knees were injected in 53 cases, elbows in 21 cases, ankles in 11 and shoulders in 1 case. The procedure was performed in 8 sittings of 10 patients each, except the last one with 16. The synoviorthesis is carried out by means of an intra-articular injection of the radioactive material, preceded by a local anaesthetic. The clinical result of this procedure is an excellent outcome with no further bleeding for 80% of patients. In cases of failure, a new injection can be given in the same joint after a 6-month interval, or an injection for the same purpose in another joint.

One of the criticisms against this method is the possible chromosomal damage induced by the radioactive material. In our centre, two studies have been carried out in order to see whether these possible changes are permanent, and both have demonstrated that chromosomal changes are reversible. The radioactive material used in these synoviortheses was gold-198. In 1978, 354 metaphases were studied, with the finding of 61 ruptures (17.2%, non-premalignant) and six structural changes (1.69%) considered premalignant (Table 7.4A). In this connection, any number below 2% is considered not to be dangerous. A further study was performed in 1982, in the same group of patients, yielding a result of 21 ruptures (3.34%) and no structural changes. This demonstrated that the possible premalignant changes disappeared with time.

A third study was performed on a series of 11 patients who received radioactive synoviorthesis with rhenium-186 in November 1991 (Table 7.4B). We performed for comparison a chromosomal study just before and 6 months after treatment, and the results confirmed that the changes which could be attributed to the radiation appear equally in non-irradiated patients, and those related to the radiation disappear with time, never reaching the danger level of 2%. In the group treated with rhenium-186 we studied an additional 130 metaphases, finding identical results and no structural changes.

Although only time can give a definite answer, it seems that radioactive synovectomy is safe and brings great benefit to patients with haemophilia. The procedure is easy, not aggressive, requires low antihaemophilic factor cover, can be done on an ambulatory basis, enables many patients to be treated in one sitting, has an 80% success rate, and so far no long-standing structural chromosomal damage has been demonstrated that is attributable to the radioactive material.

SUMMARY

Synoviorthesis, either chemical with rifampicin or radioactive with colloids such as gold-198, rhenium-186 or yttrium-90, is an effective procedure for the prevention of recurrent haemarthrosis, acting on the synovial membrane by means of a fibrosis that constricts the subsynovial venous plexus and thus prevents future bleeding. The authors have achieved overall 85 excellent clinical results, totally comparable with results reported for surgical synovectomy. The chromosomal studies performed on these irradiated patients, regardless of the radiocolloid isotope used, demonstrated no premalignant chromosomal abnormalities from the treatment. Its low cost, ease of procedure, possibility of a number of patients being treated in one session on an ambulatory basis and effective clinical results recommend this procedure as the one of choice for treating recurrent haemarthrosis in haemophilia.

REFERENCES

1 Astrup T, Sjolin L. Thromboplastic and fibrinolytic activity of human synovial membrane and fibrous capsular tissue. *Proc Soc Exp Biol Med* 1958; **97**: 852.

2 Storti E, Traldi E, Davoli RG. Synovectomy: a new approach to hemophilic arthropathy. *Acta Haematologica* 1969; **41**: 193.

3 Fernandez-Palazzi F. Synovectomy in haemophilia. When and How? Presented at the *21st Congress of the World Federation of Haemophilia*, Mexico, 1994; 29.

4 Wiedel JD. Arthroscopy synovectomy in hemophilic arthropathy of the knee. *Scand J Haematol* (Suppl.) 1984; **40**: 263.

5 Silvelo L, Bussi L, Baudo F, De Cataldo F. Results of synovectomy of the knee in haemophilia. *Haematology* 1974; **1**: 81.

6 Pietrogrande V, Torri G. Sinovectomia quirúrgica. In:

Fernández-Palazzi F, ed. *Sinovectomia en Artropatía Hemofilica.* Caracas: Di grafica Gomez, 1986: 61.

7 Horoszowski H, Heim M, Seligsohn M, Martinowitz U, Farina I. Use of the laser scalpel in orthopaedic surgery on hemophilic patients. In: Seligsohn M, ed. *Haemophilia.* Sussex: Castle House, 1981.

8 Fernandez-Palazzi F. Treatment of acute and chronic synovitis by non-surgical means. *Haemophilia* 1998; **4**: 518.

9 Ahlberg A, Pettersson, H. Synoviorthesis with radioactive gold in hemophiliacs. *Acta Orthop Scand* 1979; **50**: 513.

10 Fernandez-Palazzi F, de Bosch N, de Vargas A. Radioactive synovectomy in hemophilic haemarthrosis: follow-up of 50 cases. *Scand J Haematol* 1984; **33**: 291.

CHAPTER 8

Intra-articular Corticosteroid Therapy for Haemophilic Synovitis of the Knee

E C RODRIGUEZ-MERCHAN, A VILLAR, M QUINTANA SR AND J GAGO

INTRODUCTION

In the treatment of rheumatic synovitis, intra-articular injection of methylprednisolone has been shown to be effective for periods lasting weeks or months [1–4]. Such injections have also been used in haemophilic synovitis, although this procedure has commonly been seen as an empirical treatment with only short-term effects [5–6]. In contrast, the value of ultrasonography (echography) in diagnosing haemophilic synovitis of the knee joint has been clearly demonstrated [7]. The purpose of this prospective study was to investigate the efficacy of intra-articular methylprednisolone for the treatment of chronic haemophilic synovitis of the knee 5 years after completion of treatment.

METHODOLOGY

Ten patients aged 18–30 years (mean age 25 years) with severe haemophilia A were enrolled in the study. The criterion for selection was haemophilic synovitis on clinical examination, confirmed by ultrasonography. The degree of haemophilic synovitis was measured by ultrasonography on a five-point scale from 0 to 4, where 0 indicated the absence of synovitis and grade 4 indicated severe synovitis. All patients had synovitis of grade 3 or 4 prior to commencing treatment. In each patient there was a clear correlation between clinical signs and ultrasound findings. Before the procedure a radiographic assessment was carried out according to the Pettersson and Gilbert scale [8].

Factor VIII levels were raised to 50% of normal before injection and maintained at this level for 7 days. Treatment consisted of penetrating the joint, aspiration of the synovial fluid and injection of methylprednisolone (80 mg). Each step was carried out under aseptic conditions using the same needle. After the procedure, a compression bandage was applied for 48 hours, after which patients were permitted to move the joint as much as they wished. Assessment by ultrasound was carried out at 1, 3, 6 and 12 months following treatment and thereafter on a yearly basis.

RESULTS

At 24–48 hours post-injection, nine patients reported a subjective improvement in the perception of pain. This improvement persisted at 12 weeks of follow-up, although only seven patients continued to report the improvement 1 year after treatment. At 5 years of follow-up, all patients reported pain levels to be the same as, or worse than, before the procedure. Results were graded on a five-point scale from 0 (excellent) where no synovitis was present at any time during the study to 4 (poor) where the degree of synovitis did not decrease. According to this scale, at 1 year of follow-up there were four excellent results, three good results, two fair results and one poor result. At 5 years of follow-up all the results were poor. There was a clear correlation between clinical results and ultrasound findings. However, there was no correlation between the radiographic assessment before the procedure and the results. The main findings of this study are summarized in Table 8.1.

DISCUSSION

Some authors have used intra-articular injections of corticosteroids for the treatment of haemophilic synovitis, although their long-term effects have not been investigated [5,6]. After an initial study by Shupak *et al.* [5] in 1988, which showed satisfactory short-term results, our intention was to perform a pilot prospective study to investigate the role of intra-articular injections of corticosteroids, initially in the short-term and later with long-term follow-up.

The primary objective of the study was to investigate a less aggressive procedure for the treatment of haemophilic synovitis, given that the alternative methods were synoviorthesis (intra-articular injections of radioactive materials) and surgical synovectomy (open or arthroscopic). Our results have shown that the index procedure has a role to play in the treatment of chronic haemophilic synovitis, with satisfactory short-term effects lasting approximately 1 year, after which time efficacy decreases (Fig. 8.1a–d).

Table 8.1 Results in 10 patients with severe haemophilia A treated with intra-articular injection of 80 mg methylprednisolone [6].

Case	Side affected	Age (years)	Degree of synovitis before treatment (score: 0–4)	Radiographic score before treatment (score: 0–13)	Results at 1 year follow-up	Results at 5 years follow-up
1	Right	26	3	5	Excellent	Poor
2	Right	25	3	6	Good	Poor
3	Left	26	4	5	Excellent	Poor
4	Left	18	3	7	Fair	Poor
5	Right	25	3	6	Good	Poor
6	Left	24	4	8	Poor	Poor
7	Right	30	3	5	Excellent	Poor
8	Right	26	3	6	Good	Poor
9	Right	24	4	7	Fair	Poor
10	Right	26	3	5	Excellent	Poor

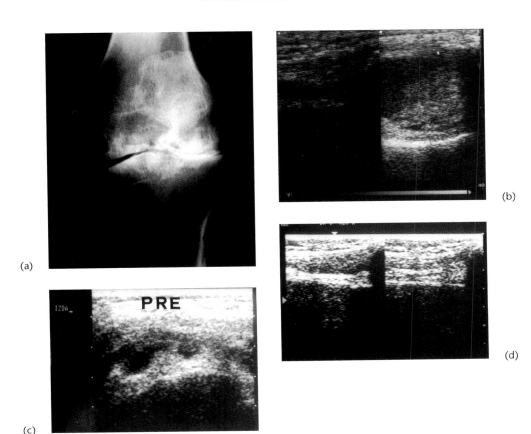

(a)

(b)

(c)

(d)

Fig. 8.1 Imaging studies of a 26-year-old male haemophilic patient (case 3): (a) anteroposterior radiograph of the left knee showing advanced degree of haemophilic arthropathy; (b) echogram showing grade 4 haemophilic synovitis; (c) echogram of the same knee showing large synovial nodules (arrow); (d) echogram at 1 year follow-up after treatment with intra-articular injection of 80 mg methylprednisolone, showing near total disappearance of synovitis (degree 0 to 1).

SUMMARY

This prospective study evaluated the effectiveness of intra-articular methylprednisolone (80 mg) in 10 knees of 10 haemophilic patients with chronic synovitis. The patients were radiographically and ultra-sonographically evaluated before starting any kind of treatment, and thereafter evaluation continued periodically until completion of the 5-year follow-up period. One year after injection the improvement in pain levels was still satisfactory, but pain levels increased again shortly thereafter. Five years after completion of treatment, all results were poor. Our current belief is that injection of intra-articular methylprednisolone should be used in highly immunosuppressed patients with severe haemophilic arthropathy, as a simple procedure that can alleviate articular pain for a defined period of time.

Acknowledgements
The authors wish to thank Arancha de Orbe MD of the Radiographic Department of La Paz University Hospital, Madrid, for performing the echographic studies.

REFERENCES

1 Gray RG, Tenenbaum J, Gotleib NC. Local corticosteroid injection treatment in rheumatic disorders. *Semin Arthritis Rheum* 1981; **10**: 4–8.

2 Hollander JL, Jessar RA, Brown EM Jr. Intrasynovial corticosteroid therapy: a decade of use. *Bull Rheum Dis* 1961; **11**: 239–43.

3 Hollander JL. Arthrocentesis technique and intrasynovial therapy. In: McCarty DJ, ed. *Arthritis and Allied Conditions*. Philadelphia: Lea & Febiger, 1985: 541–9.

4 Stolzer BC, Barr JH Jr, Margolis HM *et al.* Intra-articular injections of adrenocorticosteroids in patients with arthritis. *Penn Med J* 1962; **65**: 911–6.

5 Shupak R, Teitel J, Garvey MB *et al.* Intra-articular methylprednisolone therapy in hemophilic arthropathy. *Am J Hematol* 1988; **27**: 26–30.

6 Rodriguez-Merchan EC, Villar A, Orbe A, Magallon M. Therapy with intra-articular methylprednisolone in the hemophilic chronic synovitis of the knee. *Rev Clin Esp* 1994; **194**: 40–2.

7 Rodriguez-Merchan EC, Gago J, Orbe A. Ultrasound in the diagnosis of the early stages of haemophilic arthropathy of the knee. *Acta Orthop Belg* 1992; **58**: 122–6.

8 Pettersson H, Gilbert MS. *Diagnostic Imaging in Hemophilia*. Berlin: Springer-Verlag, 1985.

CHAPTER 9

Intra-articular Hyaluronic Acid for Haemophilic Arthropathy of the Knee

T WALLNY, H H BRACKMANN, H SEMPER, L PERLICK, W EFFENBERGER, L HESS AND A SEUSER

INTRODUCTION

In osteoarthritis, pain relief is the major goal of traditional pharmacological treatment. Besides nonsteroidal anti-inflammatory drugs or intra-articular steroids, two other classes of slow-acting drugs have been defined: symptomatic slow-acting drugs for treatment of osteoarthritis (SYSADOA) and disease-modifying osteoarthritis drugs (DMOADs) [1]. Since the end of the 1930s [2], intra-articular injections have been used for the treatment of arthropathies. Different drugs have been tried with varying degrees of success, including corticosteroids, osmic acid, procaine, aprotinin, orgotein and, lastly, hyaluronic acid, for which a prolonged effect is claimed.

Hyaluronic acid and sodium hyaluronate are both also known as hyaluron or hyaluronan. Hyaluronic acid is a natural substance of high molecular weight belonging to the group of saccharide bipolymers which are the building blocks of cartilage and synovial fluid. The molecule, which was isolated in 1934 by Meyer and Palmer, is found physiologically in the human body in the umbilical cord, synovium, vitreous and skin. It has been used in medicine since 1960 and is now categorized as a SYSADOA [3].

The active constituent in the preparation which we used (Hyalart®, Bayer, Leverkusen, Germany) is prepared from cockscombs. The highly viscous liquid has to be given intra-articularly. Hyaluronic acid has been licensed and used successfully since 1989 in the treatment of osteoarthritis of the knee. The positive effects are presumably brought about by an improvement of the functional characteristics of the joint fluid and the hyaluronic acid layer on the surface of the articular cartilage. The natural production of hyaluronic acid, which is reduced in patients with arthritis [4], can, when supplemented, normalize the concentration and the molecular weight in the synovial fluid [5]. *In vivo* studies of this drug administered intra-articularly found that patients' symptoms of pain, swelling and restriction of movement are improved [6,7].

In summary, the following effects can be assumed:
- increased viscosity

- protection against enzymatic damage because of buffering of enzymes
- binding of radicals and effect on cytokine levels
- increase in endogenous hyaluronic acid production
- analgesia
- increase in the shock absorption function of the synovium [5–13].

Because of these characteristics, hyaluronic acid intervenes in several of the complex pathogenic mechanisms involved in the development of haemophilic arthropathy and also influences the symptom complexes which occur. Despite the possibilities offered by modern orthopaedic surgery, the treatment of haemophilic arthropathy is not always satisfactory, as not all patients can be referred for operative procedures when conservative therapy has failed. There is therefore a need to examine less invasive treatments for this group of patients. Fernandez-Palazzi *et al.* [14] were the first to use hyaluronic acid in patients with haemophilia (treating two shoulders, one knee and one ankle), but there are no reports on larger groups of patients. The present study reports our experience with 20 haemophilic knees treated with this medication.

METHODOLOGY

In a prospective study, after clinical examination, plain radiographs, magnetic resonance imaging and ultrasound topometric motion analysis, one ampoule of 20 mg hyaluronic acid (Hyalart) was injected under sterile conditions into the knee joint once a week for 5 weeks. Seventeen patients with severe haemophilia A and three with severe haemophilia B were included, all of whom (average age 41 years, range 29–60 years) had pain caused by the arthropathy. Seven of them were HIV-positive and 14 had chronic hepatitis C.

The score of the Advisory Committee of the World Federation of Haemophilia (WFH) and the Aichroth score for special evaluation of the knee were used. Apart from the plain radiological examination, all investigations were repeated 3 months after the first injection to monitor the therapy's success. In addition, patients was asked before treatment and 3 months after treatment to grade the knee pain using a visual analogue scale. No physiotherapy took place during this period. After an average period of 2 years the patients were re-evaluated using the WFH-score, the Aichroth-score and the visual analogue scale.

All patients were receiving long-term treatment of at least 1000–2000 units of factor VIII three times a week and, on the day of hyaluronic acid injection, a further 3000 units were given to prevent joint bleeding. The average WFH score for the affected knee was 8.3 points, and the average Pettersson score was 7 points. The average Aichroth score was 38 points prior to the treatment (theoretical maximum is 55 points). The study was authorized by the Ethics Committee of Bonn University.

RESULTS

Clinical results

After 3 months the average WFH score had improved from 8.3 to 7.6, the Aichroth score increased from 38 to 40 and the visual analogue scale for subjective experience of pain fell from 5.4 to 3.8 points. Subjectively, 14 of the 20 patients benefited, with an improvement in symptoms of up to 50%, while 5 patients stated within 3 months that they experienced no difference due to the treatment. The improved patients benefited particularly during joint-loading activities such as climbing stairs, walking for more than half an hour, and when starting to walk. In one patient there was a subjective worsening of symptoms. However, it should be borne in mind that improved load-bearing capacity of the knee can be limited by the simultaneous presence of arthropathy in the ankles. No correlation could be found between the success of therapy and poor clinical or radiological score.

Evaluation was repeated at 2-year follow-up in autumn 1999. One of the 14 patients who had experienced relief of symptoms required arthroscopic knee joint débridement 15 months after treatment. A second patient who improved for a period of 16 months is complaining of a subjective worsening now. The other 12 patients who improved have continued to benefit for up to 28 months (average 24 months). One patient with a chronic synovitis who did not improve with hyaluronic acid underwent radioactive synovitis with yttrium-90; the condition of the remaining five patients has remained unchanged. After 24 months follow-up, average scores were (excluding the two patients treated with arthroscopy and radioactive synovectomy): WFH score 7.5 points, Aichroth score 39 points and visual analogue scale 4.0 points (Fig. 9.1).

Magnetic resonance imaging

MRI scans were carried out 3 months after the first hyaluronic acid injection and showed no significant differences compared with the pretreatment scans.

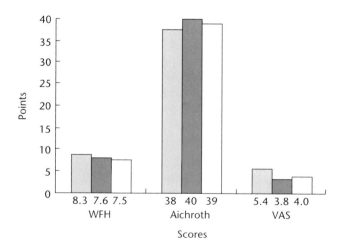

Fig. 9.1 Clinical results comparing effects of treatment with intra-articular injection of hyaluronic acid once a week for 5 weeks: light grey, before treatment; dark grey, 3 months after start of treatment; white, at 2-year follow-up. WFH, World Federation of Haemophilia; VAS, visual analogue scale.

DISCUSSION

Treatment with hyaluronic acid can be recommended in patients with haemophilia when conservative therapy has failed, especially when operative procedures are not possible, or the patient does not want them. The results shown here must be regarded as a clinical report. However, it was surprising that, with cartilage largely destroyed, nevertheless a positive effect on joint function could be achieved. The authors are conscious that they cannot explain the observed effects in this study. Although the objective and subjective parameters suggest an effect, it is difficult to show what mechanisms are responsible for the success of therapy, particularly in the medium and long term. After 2 years the continuous 'positive effect' cannot be attributed directly to hyaluronic acid. One possibility might be the temporary improvement in the 'joint milieu' which represents the basis for a less painful loading of the joint. A double-blind randomized study would give more information, but would not have been feasible with this study design. It is also doubtful whether injection of saline as a placebo into the knee joint of a patient who is HIV-positive would be ethically justifiable.

Several randomized, double-blind placebo-controlled trials confirm that intra-articular hyaluronic acid is effective in the treatment of osteoarthritis of the knee [4,7–9,11–13]. The treatment appears to be well tolerated, with only a few cases of transient cutaneous rashes or urticaria, which were not observed in our study. On the other hand, efficacy needs to be assessed critically; there are no long-term studies of the course of therapy, and no beneficial effects have been found when compared with placebo (in non-haemophilic patients) [15]. Leardini *et al.* [16] compared the effect of three injections of either hyaluronic acid or methylprednisolone acetate (40 mg) with a 1-year follow-up, and found no difference in efficacy. The high costs (of hyaluronic acid) and risks could not be justified when the success of therapy can be found only briefly, especially in haemophilia. We therefore do not anticipate any usefulness for prophylactic injections in the case of asymptomatic arthropathy.

SUMMARY

Hyaluronic acid has been used successfully in the treatment of osteoarthritis since 1989. There has been no experience in haemophiliacs in larger study groups, and we treated 20 patients with haemophilic arthropathy of the knee, by intra-articular injection of hyaluronic acid. The results showed subjective improvement in 14 patients, however, positive aspects were limited by arthropathy in adjacent joints. We recommend hyaluronic acid for haemophilic arthropathy of the knee when regular conservative therapy has failed and operative treatment is not feasible.

REFERENCES

1 Lequesne M, Brandt K, Bellamy N *et al.* Guidelines for testing slow acting drugs in osteoarthritis. *J Rheumatol* 1994; **21** (Suppl.): 65–71.

2 Desmarais, MHL. Value of intra-articular injections in

osteoarthritis. *Ann Rheum Dis* 1952; **11**: 277–81.

3 Maheu E. Hyaluronan in knee osteoarthritis: a review of the clinical trials with hyalgan. *Eur J Rheumatol Inflamm* 1995; **15**: 17–24.

4 Carrabba M, Paresce E, Angelini AM. The intraarticular treatment of the osteoarthritis of the knee: a comparative study between hyaluronic acid and orgotein. *Eur J Rheumatol Inflamm* 1992; **12**: 43–57.

5 Toyoshima H, Mamiki O, Morisaki N. Therapeutic efffects of intraarticular injection of high molecular weight hyaluronic acid on osteoarthritis of the knee. *Int Clin Pharm Ther Tox* 1982; **20**: 501–7.

6 Dahl LB, Dahl IMS, Engstrom-Lauret A. Concentration and molecular weight of sodium hyaluronate in fluid from patients with rheumatoid arthritis and other arthropathies. *Ann Rheum Dis* 1985; **44**: 817–22.

7 Dougados M. High molecular weight sodium hyaluronate in osteoarthritis of the knee: 1 year placebo controlled trial. *Osteoarthr Cart* 1993; **1**: 97–103.

8 Jones AC. A comparative study of intra-articular hyaluronic acid and intra-articular triamcinolone hexacetonide in the treatment of osteoarthritis of the knee. *Osteoarthr Cart* 1993; **1**: 71.

9 Graf J. Intra-articular treatment with hyaluronic acid of the knee joint: a controlled clinical trial versus mucopolysaccharide polysulfuric acid ester. *Clin Exp Rheumatol* 1992; **11**: 367–72.

10 Schneider U. The efficiacy of hyaluronic acid with osteoarthritis of both knees in right/left comparison. *Z Orthop* 1997; **135**: 341–7.

11 Lohmander LS. Intra-articular hyaluronan injections in the treatment of osteoarthritis of the knee: a randomised, double blind, placebo controlled multicentre trial. Hyaluronan Multicentre Trial Group. *Ann Rheum Dis* 1996; **55**: 424–31.

12 Pozo MA. Reduction of sensory responses to passive movements of inflamed knee joints by hylan, a hyaluronan derivative. *Exp Brain Res* 1997; **116**: 3–9.

13 Dahlberg L. Intraarticular injections of hyaluronan in patients with cartilage abnormalities and knee pain: a one-year double-blind, placebo-controlled study. *Arthritis Rheum* 1994; **37**: 521–8.

14 Fernandez-Palazzi F, Rivas Hernandez S, De Saez A, de Bosch NB. Treatment of the hemophilic chronic arthropathy by intraarticular injections of cortisone or hyaluronan. In: Melanotte PL, Africano A, eds. *International Symposium on Orthopaedic Problems in Haemophilia*. Castelfranco Veneto: M Maynery, 1994: 113–19.

15 Henderson EB, Smith EC, Pegley F, Blake DR. Intra-articular injections of 750 KD hyaluronan in the treatment of osteoarthitis: a randomized single centre double-blind placebo-controlled trial of 91 patients demonstrating lack of efficacy. *Ann Rheum Dis* 1994; **53**: 529–34.

16 Leardini G, Franceschini M, Mattara L, Bruno R, Perbellini A. Intra-articular sodium hyaluronate (Hyalgan) in gonarthrosis. *Clin Tri J* 1987; **24**: 341–50.

CHAPTER 10

Joint Débridement, Alignment Osteotomy and Arthrodesis

E C RODRIGUEZ-MERCHAN AND N J GODDARD

INTRODUCTION

Faced with a patient with severely disabling end-stage haemophilic arthropathy we should strive to restore long-term pain-free function with minimal associated risk. It may be possible in some circumstances to prolong function in a severely arthritic joint, which may benefit from judicious intra-articular steroid injections, with adequate haemostatic cover. Fortunately, as the disease progresses many end-stage joints gradually evolve to a form of auto-ankylosis, with an associated reduction of pain and bleeding episodes without any surgical intervention. Surgery should only be contemplated when lesser measures fail either to provide adequate pain relief or to preserve joint function, with resulting disability.

The usual surgical options available include joint débridement, osteotomy, arthrodesis and total joint replacement. Whenever possible, consideration should be given to performing multiple operations under the same anaesthetic, if this is deemed to be feasible, practical, safe and appropriate [1]. There are obvious advantages to this approach, the most important of which is the restoration of normal biomechanics for the functional limb, together with adequate control of pain and bleeding. In addition, the complication rate is shown to be less than expected, and the rehabilitation period relatively short.

JOINT DÉBRIDEMENT

Joint débridement may be indicated in younger patients where there is relative preservation of the joint architecture and congruity, when joint replacement is not considered to be a viable alternative. Some joints are obviously more amenable to surgical débridement and it is frequently performed in combination with synovectomy.

The knee

While it is accepted that total knee arthroplasty has become a safe and satisfying treatment for painful haemophilic arthropathy of the knee, it may not always be appropriate in the younger patient. Given the risks of accelerated wear and early loosening secondary to a more active lifestyle, and the ultimate need for revision surgery, it may be that one should consider more conservative surgical options. Soreff [2] reported three cases of joint débridement in haemophilic patients with late-stage arthropathy with no complications, who experienced satisfactory short-term pain relief.

Open-knee débridement requires a wide joint exposure, shaving of damaged cartilage, trimming of hypertrophic osteophytes, excision of the torn menisci (or torn portions) and removal of any loose bodies. In Madrid, we have performed joint débridement for advanced haemophilic arthropathy of the knee in 11 patients [3]. We routinely used a mid-line incision and a straightforward medial parapatellar approach, everting the patella. All scar tissue, meniscal remnants and osteophytes were removed, and the articular surfaces smoothed. A lateral retinacular release was performed while the patella was subluxated, followed by proximal or distal realignment.

The patients were mobilized (fully weight-bearing) as their pain allowed on the third post-operative day. At a mean follow-up period of 5.4 years (range 2–11 years), the clinical results were excellent in four cases, good in five and fair in two. These results lead us to conclude that under the right circumstances joint débridement should be considered as an alternative to knee replacement.

While this procedure cannot be considered as the final solution, it can provide adequate pain relief and restore functional activity until the patient reaches an age when a total knee arthroplasty is more acceptable. It therefore warrants consideration as a conservative treatment for haemophilic arthropathy of the knee for the young and middle-aged individual who is not ready or willing to accept the limitations of a total knee arthroplasty.

Some haemophilic patients develop large symptomatic juxta-articular cysts as a result of intraosseous haemorrhages, especially in the proximal tibia. These may threaten the integrity of the articular cartilage and require open curettage and grafting [4] (Fig. 10.1).

The ankle

Some patients develop a large anterior tibial osteophyte which is generally amenable to surgical excision, provided that the joint surfaces remain reasonably congruous. For those patients with anterior ankle pain, aggravated by dorsiflexion, excision of the anterior osteophytes (cheilectomy) may improve movement and comfort. This can be performed either open or arthroscopically, and may be combined with joint débridement and drilling of any osteochondral defects. As with the knee, though, the disease is progressive and the osteophyte may regrow [5], or there may be late collapse of the joint, requiring ankle fusion.

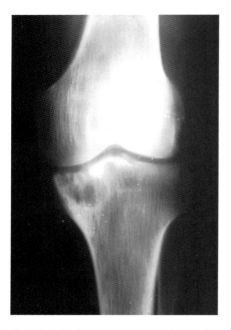
(a)

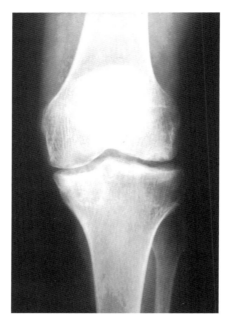
(b)

Fig. 10.1 (a) Preoperative view of a subchondral cyst in the proximal tibia of a 29-year-old man; (b) excellent result following open curettage and grafting.

REALIGNMENT OSTEOTOMY

Proximal tibial valgus osteotomy of the knee

Smith *et al.* [6] reported a series of six osteotomies of the knee for end-stage arthropathy in five patients. There were no complications (for example, infection, loss of mobility), pain relief was satisfactory and there was a reduction in the rate of haemarthroses. However, Luck's experience was markedly different, with major complications occurring in five of seven cases following high tibial osteotomy [7]. The reasons for this discrepancy are not immediately apparent, but it is probable that they may be related to technique, patient selection, and the fact that six of Luck's seven procedures were performed in the early days of elective reconstructive surgery on patients with haemophilia (1969–71).

Between 1975 and 1985, 14 haemophilic patients at the centre in Madrid underwent proximal tibial valgus osteotomy for severe genu varum [8]. The indications and criteria for inclusion were medial compartment pain, severe subjective pain, adequate peripheral vascularity in the limb, knee flexion of at least 90° and flexion contracture of <15°. The average age at operation was 32 years.

At operation, the proximal tibiofibular syndesmosis was excised and the deformity corrected by a lateral closing wedge tibial osteotomy. The position was held with two compression staples and a long leg plaster cast was applied (Fig. 10.2). Patients were then mobilized initially non-weight-bearing for two weeks. The cast was changed to a quadrilateral tendon-bearing (QTB) cast, so permitting weight-bearing for the subsequent six weeks.

Patients were followed up for at least 5 years and in our experience valgus osteotomy has yielded a favourable long-term result without se-

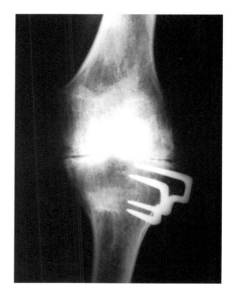

Fig. 10.2 Anteroposterior radiograph following proximal tibial valgus osteotomy; two staples were inserted and fixed to the proximal tibia, closing the osteotomy.

vere functional impairment or secondary aggravation of knee joint symptoms. When high tibial osteotomy fails to bring about a reduction from the preoperative pain level, a total knee replacement must be considered as the next choice for the treatment of haemophilic arthropathy of the knee.

Supramalleolar tibial osteotomy of the ankle

Pearce *et al.* [9] reported the results of supramalleolar varus osteotomy on seven ankles (in six patients) for haemophilic arthropathy and secondary valgus deformity. A 4 cm longitudinal incision was made immediately proximal to the medial malleolus. The distal tibial metaphysis was exposed subperiosteally, and a medially based wedge of cortex was excised using a reciprocating saw. The 10–15° cortical defect was then closed by angulating the bone and the position was held by a single staple. No fibular section was needed. In their series of seven ankles, symptoms were relieved and joint function was preserved after a simple osteotomy with minimal morbidity and no complications.

ARTHRODESIS

A successful arthrodesis will result in a pain-free joint, and so can lead to some restoration of function. As a working rule, though, the more distal the arthrodesis, the more likely one is to achieve successful outcome. Thus, for patients with severe ankle pain who have failed to respond to conservative treatment, an ankle arthrodesis may be indicated (Fig. 10.3), is well tolerated and will generally result in an increase in function. Many techniques have been described, including the use of internal fixation or external fixation, sliding grafts and cast immobilization techniques [5].

On the other hand, arthrodesis of the knee is less well tolerated, since it makes sitting, rising from a chair and the other activities of daily living somewhat awkward if not impossible. Knee arthrodesis has been recommended following infected total knee arthroplasty because of the low risk of reinfection, reliable pain relief and resultant knee stability. However, the indications for primary knee arthrodesis are rare nowadays, and it tends to be reserved for those patients with a failed total knee arthroplasty, including single-joint disease, young age, extensor mechanism disruption, a poor soft-tissue envelope, systemic immuno-compromise, and the presence of micro-organisms that require highly toxic antibiotic therapy or that are resistant to conventional antibiotics. Relative contraindications include bilateral knee disease, severe ipsilateral ankle or hip disease, severe segmental bone loss and contralateral extremity amputation [10].

SUMMARY

When advanced haemophilic arthropathy is present with severe disability, the aim should be to restore function, while at the same time minimizing the risk to the patient. Thus, surgery should be safe, timely

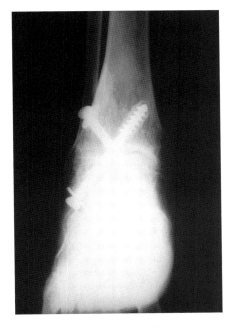

Fig. 10.3 Anteroposterior radiograph following ankle arthrodesis; two cannulated screws were inserted and fixed to the distal tibia.

and appropriate, with a predictable outcome and, whenever possible, carried out in combination with other procedures.

Joint débridement is an effective method to achieve this goal, especially around the elbow or ankle, and can be considered as an alternative to knee replacement in the younger age groups. Proximal tibial valgus osteotomy is a reliable treatment method for painful genu varum of the mobile haemophilic knee. Supramalleolar tibial varus osteotomy is an attractive alternative to the more commonly used surgical option of arthrodesis.

Finally, joint replacement, especially total knee replacement, can usually be relied upon to restore both mobility and function in a diseased joint. The potential benefits of joint replacement must, however, always be weighed up against the long-term sequelae, in particular, loosening and consequent revision surgery.

REFERENCES

1 Horoszowski H, Heim M, Schulman S *et al.* Multiple joint procedures in a single operative session on hemophilic patients. *Clin Orthop* 1996; **328**: 60–4.

2 Soreff J. Joint debridement in the treatment of advanced hemophilic arthropathy. *Clin Orthop* 1984; **191**: 179–82.

3 Rodriguez-Merchan EC, Magallon M, Galindo E. Joint debridement for haemophilic arthropathy of the knee. *Int Orthop* 1994; **18**: 135–8.

4 Rodriguez-Merchan EC. Management of the orthopaedic complications of haemophilia. *J Bone Joint Surg (Br)* 1998; **80B**: 191–6.

5 Ribbans WJ, Phillips M, Stock D, Stibe E. Haemophilic ankle problems: orthopaedic solutions. *Haemophilia* 1995; **1**: 91–6.

6 Smith MA, Urquhart DR, Savidge GF. The surgical management of varus deformity in haemophilic arthropathy of the knee. *J Bone Joint Surg (Br)* 1981; **63B**: 261–5.

7 Luck JV. Surgical management of advanced hemophilic arthropathy. *Prog Clin Biol Res* 1990; **324**: 241–56.

8 Rodriguez-Merchan EC, Galindo E. Proximal tibial valgus osteotomy for hemophilic arthropathy of the knee. *Orthop Rev* 1992; **21**: 204–8.

9 Pearce MS, Smith MA, Savidge GF. Supramalleolar tibial osteotomy for haemophilic arthropathy of the ankle. *J Bone Joint Surg (Br)* 1994; **76B**: 947–50.

10 Hanssen AD. Management of the infected total knee arthroplasty. In: Engh GA, Rorabeck CH, eds. *Revision Total Knee Arthroplasty*. Baltimore: Williams & Wilkins, 1997: 371–93.

CHAPTER 11

Total Hip Arthroplasty

E C RODRIGUEZ-MERCHAN, M ORTEGA-ANDREU AND G ALONSO-CARRO

INTRODUCTION

End-stage haemophilic arthropathy is further complicated by arthrofibrosis and loss of motion as the hypertrophic synovium is replaced by dense fibrous scar tissue. Arthropathy of the hip is moderate in frequency but is less common than ankle, knee or elbow arthropathy. It has two modes of onset. In childhood, rapidly progressive severe arthropathy may result from a single haemarthrosis because of increased intracapsular pressure leading to osteonecrosis of the capital femoral epiphysis [1] (Fig. 11.1). More often, hip arthropathy is the result of chronic synovitis similar to that which occurs in other joints. Between the second and fourth decades many haemophilic patients develop severe articular destruction. At this stage, possible treatments include arthrodesis and arthroplasty. For the hip, total hip arthroplasty remains the best solution [2].

Teitelbaum [3] reviewed pelvic radiographs of 34 patients complaining of pain in the hip (64 hips) from a population of 175 patients seen at one haemophilia centre. Sixteen (80%) of 20 hips that had an open

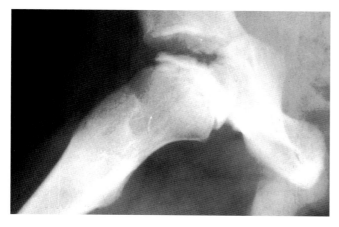
(a)

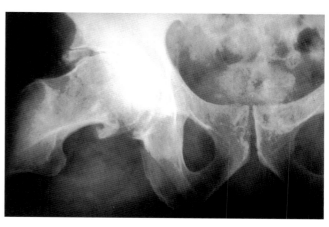
(b)

Fig. 11.1 Radiographs of the right hip of a boy with severe haemophilia. (a) At 12 years of age an intense collapse of the epiphysis in the anterior and superior quadrant with sparing of the posterior aspect of the femoral head can be noted; (b) radiograph taken at 31 years of age showing a severe degree of haemophilic arthropathy.

proximal femoral epiphysis had a valgus deformity, but none had osteo-arthritic changes. Fifteen (31%) of 48 skeletally mature hips had degenerative changes, including protusio acetabuli in eight hips. Thus, end-stage haemophilic arthropathy necessitating arthroplasty is infrequent in the hip.

There are few reports of the results of total hip arthroplasty in patients with haemophilia. The indication for a total hip arthroplasty in young patients who have haemophilic arthropathy of the hip should be severe disabling pain occurring both during activity and at rest that is unresponsive to non-operative treatment.

REPORTED SERIES AND RESULTS

The first important series was published by Luck and Kasper of the Orthopaedic Hospital, Los Angeles, USA in 1989 [4], announcing that the first prosthetic arthroplasty of the hip in a haemophiliac in the United States was a cup arthroplasty performed by J. Vernon Luck in 1968. Luck and Kasper reported that between 1968 and 1982, three more cup arthroplasties and ten primary, cemented hip arthroplasties were performed at the Orthopaedic Hospital by six different surgeons. Prostheses varied with the surgeon and include Müller (five cases), Ausfranc-Turner (two cases), Charnley (one case), Harris (one case) and Wagner resurfacing (one case). Since 1982, two cementless primary hip arthroplasties had been performed.

Eight patients had required revision, and one required an excision arthroplasty. The revisions included three cup arthroplasties because of pain and bleeding, three cemented total hips for aseptic loosening, two cemented total hips for infection, and one Wagner resurfacing for a fracture of the femoral head sustained in a fall 5 years postoperatively. One patient had a Girdlestone resection arthroplasty for a *Pseudomonas aeruginosa* infection. Thus, five of nine conventional, cemented total hip arthroplasties had failed over the last 16 years. Including the three cup arthroplasties, eight revisions had been performed. Seven of these patients were symptom-free. One patient developed *Serratia marcescens* infection 1 year after revision. In another of the revision cases, there was radiographic evidence of component loosening. This cup arthroplasty was revised to a cemented Charnley low-friction prosthesis in 1972. The femoral component loosened at 3 years and subsided, but it had stabilized and remained asymptomatic over the last 12 years.

The long-term experience of Luck and Kasper with various types of hip prostheses can be rated as only fair, with a revision rate of about 60% over 20 years. However, the clinical status of all patients was quite satisfactory in that all were free from hip pain and were capable of unlimited, unassisted, community ambulation. They were substantially better than they had been prior to their initial hip surgery. End-stage hip disease in haemophilic patients poses an unsolved problem. Primary cemented prostheses have a 33% aseptic failure rate 5–14 years after operation, which is higher than would be expected in a comparable group of patients with another form of polyarthritis. One reason for the loosening of cemented hip prostheses in haemophilic patients may be the increased stresses of a stiff-legged gait.

In 1992, Nelson *et al.* [5] reported the experience of the Nuffield Orthopaedic Centre, Oxford, UK. From 1969 until 1985, 39 total hip arthroplasties were performed in 38 patients for haemophilic arthropathy. The median age of the patients at operation was 48 years. In 21 patients, 22 hip replacements were reviewed clinically and radiographically, with a median follow-up of 7.6 years. Five of the 22 hips had been revised and three were likely to require revision in the near future. The incidence of revision was compared to other studies of total hip arthroplasty in young patients and the influence of HIV infection was examined. Total hip arthroplasty was believed to be an appropriate operation for disabling haemophilic arthropathy.

As haemophilic arthropathy infrequently affects the hip joint, Kelley *et al.* [6] in 1995 reported a multicentre retrospective study to determine the results of hip arthroplasty in haemophilic patients. Thirty-four hip arthroplasties were performed in 27 male patients at four major haemophilia centres between October 1972 and September 1990 in the United States.

The mean age of patients at the time of operation was 38 years (range 15–73 years). Four patients were seropositive for HIV at the time of the operation, and 16 patients were seropositive at the latest follow-up examination. Nine patients (33%) died before the latest review, seven of whom had been seropositive for HIV. The mean duration of follow-up was 8 years, with a minimum of 2 years for all patients who were still alive at the latest review.

Surgery was carried out as follows: 26 total hip arthroplasties performed with cement, six total hip arthroplasties performed without cement, one total hip arthroplasty in which the femoral component was inserted with cement and the acetabular component was inserted without it (so-called hybrid arthroplasty), and one bipolar arthroplasty performed with cement. There were no early infections after these 34 primary arthroplasties. Three late infections occurred around prostheses inserted with cement, all of which led to a resection arthroplasty. Six (21%) of the 28 cemented femoral components and six (23%) of the 26 cemented acetabular components were revised because of aseptic loosening.

Of the 24 cemented femoral components for which radiographs were available and which were still in place at the time of latest review or at the time of death, ten were definitely loose, two were probably loose, five were possibly loose and seven had no evidence of loosening. Of the 23 cemented acetabular components for which radiographs were available and which were still in place at the time of review, ten were definitely loose, seven were probably loose, three were possibly loose, and three were not loose. None of the cementless prostheses were loose. There was a high rate of loosening of the cemented hip prosthesis in this series. There was also a high rate of mortality overall, and a high rate of late deep infection in the patients who were seropositive for HIV. Kelley *et al.* advised caution when a total hip arthroplasty is considered for a patient with haemophilia. Despite the aforementioned complications, Kelley *et al.* stated that total hip arthroplasty has a continuing role in the treatment of haemophilic arthropathy in patients who have severe pain and disability.

During 1973–88, at the University Hospital, Malmö, Sweden, 13 total hip replacements were performed in 11 haemophilic patients with a mean age of 46 years. According to Löfqvist *et al.* [7], the indication for surgery was disabling pain due to advanced haemophilic arthropathy. The surgical technique was the same as for other patients: cemented Charnley prostheses were inserted, using the transtrochanteric approach. The mean duration of follow-up was 7 years. Five hips became loose within 6 years, and a further one after 13 years. Four hips were revised, two of them due to infection in patients who were also seropositive for HIV. At the latest follow-up, ten patients were alive, six had no hip pain, and seven could walk a distance of at least 1000 metres. Although these results were inferior to those obtained in arthrosis, total hip replacement should be considered in patients with haemophilia. Löfqvist *et al.* concluded that this group of patients can expect a fairly high frequency of aseptic loosening after total hip replacement. HIV-positive patients also seem to have an increased infection rate. However, according to their findings, they concluded that total hip replacement is of value in some haemophilic individuals.

In 1998 Heeg *et al.* [8] evaluated the long-term results of three total hip arthroplasties. One hip was revised after 9 years for aseptic loosening.

During 1976–99, six total hip arthroplasties were performed in six haemophilic patients at La Paz University Hospital, Madrid, Spain (Fig. 11.2). The indication for total hip arthroplasty in people with haemophilia was severe disabling pain, both during activity and at rest, that was unresponsive to non-operative treatment. The mean age of the patients was 42 years (range 35–47). Four Harris-Galante hybrid prostheses (acetabular component without cement and a precoated femoral component with cement), one uncemented isoelastic prosthesis

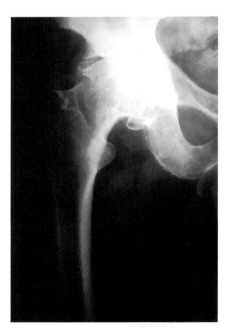 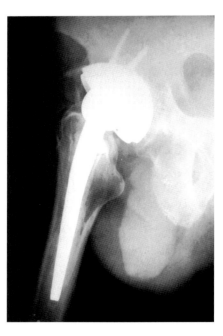

(a)   (b)

Fig. 11.2 Radiographs of a 35-year-old man with severe haemophilic arthropathy (a) before and (b) 7 years after a hybrid total hip arthroplasty.

and one cemented Charnley arthroplasty (for an ankylosed hip; see next section in this chapter) were used in these procedures. At the time of the index hip arthroplasty, no patient was known to be seropositive for HIV. The mean duration of follow-up for all the patients was 7 years (range 1–15 years). One patient (the one with the isoelastic prosthesis) died before the time of this review, and five were alive. So far, both clinical and radiographic results are satisfactory.

Studies from several haemophilia centres suggest that between 33% and 92% of patients with haemophilia A, and between 14% and 52% of persons with haemophilia B, carry the HIV antibody [9]. In two studies of hip arthroplasty for haemophilic arthropathy with more than 20 patients and more than 5 years' follow-up, approximately 50% of the patients were known to be seropositive for HIV, contributing to an overall mortality rate at median 7-year follow-up of 20% to 33% [5,6]. Patients with CD4 levels of greater than 500 cells/mm^3, a positive reaction with anergy testing to intradermal skin antigens, platelet count greater than 60 000, total leukocyte count greater than 1000, serum albumin greater than 25 g/L, and no history of opportunistic infections of neoplasm have a postoperative complication risk similar to the general population.

In addition to thorough preoperative medical preparation of the patient, considerable surgical preparation is also required. Depending on the age at which significant bleeding began, the proximal anatomy of the femur can be distorted and, in the most severe cases, there can be an extremely small femoral medullary canal, valgus and excessive anteversion of the head and neck, and protrusio acetabuli [10].

TOTAL HIP ARTHROPLASTY IN THE ANKYLOSED HIP

Converting a hip that has had an arthrodesis or is ankylosed to a total hip replacement commonly results in relief of pain in the lower back and knee, improved mobility of the hip, and correction of leg length discrepancy. The complications and failures are significantly more numerous than after conventional arthroplasty. The operation is technically difficult, and careful preoperative planning and experience are important factors in achieving a successful result. We have implanted a cemented Charnley total hip prosthesis in a 48-year-old man with mild haemophilia (factor VIII level of 4 IU/dL) in his right spontaneously ankylosed hip [11].

At the time of surgery he was anti-HCV (hepatitis C virus) positive, anti-HIV negative, and no circulating inhibitors were encountered. The indication for surgery was long-lasting intractable low back and ipsilateral knee pain. At 14-month follow-up, relief of pain had been achieved as well as correction of limb-length discrepancy, with a good result according to the Mayo Clinic hip score (Fig. 11.3). Doses of 50 IU per kg body weight of recombinant factor VIII (Recombinate; Baxter, Glendale, California, USA) were used during the 2-week stay in the hospital. The dosage was adjusted according to the recovery of factor VIII, with an overall factor consumption of 68 000 IU. As far as we know, this is the first case reported in the literature of a person with haemophilia in whom a spontaneous hip ankylosis has been satisfactorily converted

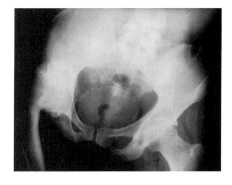

(a)

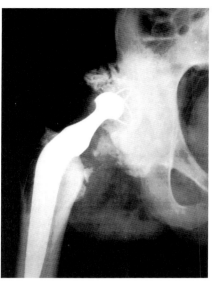

(b)

Fig. 11.3 (a) Preoperative anteroposterior view of the pelvis of a 48-year-old man with haemophilia. Note the severe degree of pelvic obliquity as well as spontaneous ankylosis of the right hip; (b) view at 14 months after a cemented Charnley total hip prosthesis.

with a total hip arthroplasty with a short-term follow-up. However, a much longer follow-up is still needed to ascertain the efficacy of this surgical procedure in haemophilia.

CONCLUSION

Caution is advised when total hip arthroplasty is considered for a person with haemophilia. The results are inferior to those obtained in osteoarthritis, and the incidence of complications is higher for those who are seropositive for HIV. Despite the complications, this operation has a continuing role in the treatment of haemophilic arthropathy in patients who have severe pain and disability. Total hip arthroplasty in people with haemophilia should only be performed in major centres with experience in managing these patients.

REFERENCES

1 Rodriguez-Merchan EC, Ortega F, Galindo E, Magallon M, Lopez-Cabarcos C. Legg-Calvé-Perthes disease in hemophilia. *Contemp Orthop* 1992; **25**: 472–9.

2 Rodriguez-Merchan EC. Editorial. Management of the orthopaedic complications of haemophilia. *J Bone Joint Surg (Br)* 1998; **80B**: 191–6.

3 Teitelbaum S. Radiologic evaluation of the hemophilic hip. *Mt Sinai J Med* 1977; **44**: 400–1.

4 Luck JV Jr, Kasper CK. Surgical management of advanced hemophilic arthropathy. An overview of 20 years' experience. *Clin Orthop* 1989; **242**: 60–82.

5 Nelson IW, Sivamurugan S, Latham PD, Matthews J, Bulstrode CJ. Total hip arthroplasty for hemophilic arthropathy. *Clin Orthop* 1992; **276**: 210–3.

6 Kelley SS, Lachiewicz PF, Gilbert MS, Bolander ME, Jankiewicz JJ. Hip arthroplasty in hemophilic arthropathy. *J Bone Joint Surg (Am)* 1995; **77A**: 828–34.

7 Löfqvist T, Sanzén L, Petersson C, Nilsson IM. Total hip replacement in patients with hemophilia. *Acta Orthop Scand* 1996; **67**: 321–4.

8 Heeg M, Meyer K, Smid WM, Van Horn JR, Van der Meer J. Total knee and hip arthroplasty in haemophilic patients. *Haemophilia* 1998; **4**: 747–51.

9 Sethr-Green JK, Evatt BL, Lawrence DN. Acquired immuno deficiency syndrome associated with hemophilia in the United States. *Instr Course Lect* 1989; **38**: 357–65.

10 Lachiewicz PF, Kelley SS. Systemic diseases resulting in hip pathology. In: Callaghan JJ, Rosenberg AG, Rubash

HE, eds. *The Adult Hip*. Philadelphia: Lippincott-Raven, 1998: 437–50.

11 Rodriguez-Merchan EC, Blanco M, Sanjurjo MJ, Magal-lon M. Joint replacement for a spontaneously ankylosed hip in a haemophilic patient. *Haemophilia* 1999; **5**: 69–72.

CHAPTER 12

Total Knee Arthroplasty

E C RODRIGUEZ-MERCHAN AND J D WIEDEL

INTRODUCTION

Patients with haemophilia commonly have a severe degree of knee joint destruction by the time they become adults, having suffered repeated articular bleeding episodes since the very early years of life. On many occasions such patients must face the orthopaedic surgeon because of the pain and severe functional disability related to advanced haemophilic arthropathy affecting the knee joints. With the success of total knee arthroplasties in patients with osteoarthritis and the availability of factor concentrates allowing major surgical procedures to be performed safely in haemophilia, total knee arthroplasty has become the treatment of choice in patients with chronic haemophilic arthropathy of the knee. The primary indication for total knee arthroplasty is severe, disabling pain that is unresponsive to medical treatment. Deformity and poor functional range of motion, particularly a severe flexion contracture of the knee, are contributing indications and may in themselves, without severe pain, justify the operation. In general, upper age limits are determined by patients' overall physiological status; while the lower age limits may be restricted because of the unrealistic demands of many patients.

REVIEW OF THE LITERATURE

In 1985 Lachiewicz et al. [1] published the results of 24 total knee arthroplasties in 14 patients with the following complications: two late infections, one subcutaneous haematoma, one case of haemolytic anaemia and one patient who developed an inhibitor. The average age was 35 years and the follow-up was 2–9 years. Results were excellent in fifteen knees, good in six, fair in one and poor in two (patients suffering from deep infection).

In 1988 Karthaus and Novakova [2] reported eleven total knee arthroplasties in eight patients with a follow-up of 2–8 years. Ten patients suffered postoperative complications: epistaxis, haemarthroses, anaphylactic reaction, urinary tract infection with haematuria, recurrent phlebitis at the site of venous puncture, and fever of a few days' duration. No surgical wound infection was found. Results were excellent or good in nine knees, fair in one and poor in one. Every patient reported subjective improvement in the degree of pain.

In 1989, Wiedel *et al.* [3] published a series of 97 total knee arthroplasties in 76 patients, showing a progressive increase of acute infections. They also noted that HIV-positive patients were prone to develop infections. In 1993, Gregg-Smith *et al.* [4] published a report on septic arthritis in haemophilia. They concluded that there was a high risk of secondary infection in HIV-positive patients and, therefore, recommended total knee arthroplasty be reserved for a very carefully selected group of patients.

In 1994, Birch *et al.* [5] published a letter in which they referred to 15 total knee arthroplasties with only one infection in an HIV-positive patient (occurring 5 years after the surgical procedure, following a haemarthrosis associated with a dental extraction). Eight patients were HIV-positive but only one was infected postoperatively. Thus, these authors favoured the use of total knee arthroplasty, emphasizing that such a procedure did not increase the risk of postoperative infection. However, they also stated that in patients with a low CD4 count the progression of HIV infection was likely to occur. In 1996, Löfqvist *et al.* [6] published an account of six cases of total knee arthroplasty with only one infection (in an HIV-positive patient) who eventually required a knee arthrodesis. Phillips *et al.* [7] in 1997 also reported 14 total knee arthroplasties with satisfactory results.

Recently, Thomason *et al.* [8] published results of 23 total knee arthroplasties in 15 patients. The mean follow-up period was 7.5 years, with a minimum of 4 years for the eight patients who were alive at the time of their review. Seven patients had died before the report was written, and all were seropositive for HIV. Using the Hospital for Special Surgery knee scoring system, the results were excellent in one knee, good in three, fair in two, and poor in 17. There were two early and two late deep infections, all occurring in patients who were seropositive for HIV. One knee had been revised for aseptic loosening.

In a study by Ragni *et al.* [9] carried out at 115 centres in 37 states of the USA, the rate of postoperative infection in HIV-positive haemophilic patients with a CD4 count of <200 cells/mm^3 was higher than in the non-haemophilic population. In a series of 27 total knee arthroplasties eight patients (30%) became infected. Such figures are considerably higher than the rate of infection in the non-haemophilic population (1–2%). Ragni *et al.* concluded that the indication for a total joint arthroplasty should be based on a careful analysis of the balance between risks and benefits. The present authors agree with them, and our view is that a knee joint arthroplasty is a surgical procedure with an excessive risk of postoperative infection, especially in HIV-positive haemophilic patients with a CD4 count of <200 cells/mm^3. It should not be forgotten that about 80% of the haemophilic population in developed countries is HIV-positive because they unfortunately received contaminated factor concentrates in the early 1980s.

Thus, taking into account the existing controversy over the risk of postoperative infection in the HIV-positive haemophilic patient, and the high rate of unsatisfactory results that have been reported, our view is that total knee arthroplasty is a surgical procedure that should be considered only for selected cases. We agree with Thomason *et al.* that, while total knee arthroplasty may be a useful treatment for the relief of pain attributable to end-stage haemophilic arthropathy, there is a high rate of complication, especially in patients who are seropositive for HIV. Considerations of life expectancy, age and immunological status are of paramount importance in the decision to undertake a total knee arthroplasty in haemophilia.

The alternative to total knee arthroplasty is joint débridement. In 1994, we reported 11 open knee débridements in 11 patients suffering from advanced haemophilic arthropathy of the knee [10]. Follow-up was for an average of 5.4 years (range 2–11 years), and the mean age of patients was 28.7 years (range 25–42 years). The results were also evaluated by the Hospital for Special Surgery disability score sheet. The clinical results were excellent in four, good in five and fair in two. Débridement should, therefore, be considered in the young person with haemophilia in order to avoid, or delay, total knee arthroplasty. Joint débridement represents an alternative to knee replacement which may give the patient years of life without pain. When débridement fails to relieve pain, replacement must be considered, but in a recent unpublished review of our results, débridement has been shown to be satisfactory for a mean period of 9 years (range 7–15 years). No patient who underwent débridement subsequently required a total knee arthroplasty.

AUTHORS' EXPERIENCE

Methodology

A retrospective review was carried out of 37 total knee arthroplasties, which were performed on 26 men between March 1975 and November 1995. Twenty-three men had classic type A haemophilia and three had type B haemophilia. Inhibitor screening and haematological workup were performed preoperatively. Screening for haemolysis involved checking daily haematocrits until measured factor levels and infusion of factor were stable.

All patients and their radiographs were evaluated by the authors. The Hospital for Special Surgery knee rating scale was used as follows: 85–100 excellent, 70–84 good, 60–69 fair, and less than 60 was poor. All patients were managed by a regional haemophilia centre, and when appropriate, by an infectious disease service.

Prior to 1986, haematological management consisted of titrating factor levels to 100% by bolus 1 hour prior to surgery. The levels were maintained at 30–60% factor level postoperatively, usually by bolus methods, for 7–21 days, with a gradual taper of factor level based on demands at physiotherapy. After 1986, patients were titrated to 120% factor level by bolus 1 hour prior to surgery and 80–100% levels by continuous infusion postoperatively for 3–7 days. The continuous infusions were then changed to bolus infusions designed to maintain factor levels at no less than 40–60%.

Patients with human immunodeficiency disease were evaluated to ensure their medical status was stable. A CD4 count of at least 200 cells/mm^3

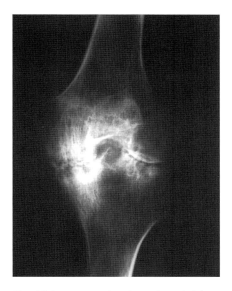

Fig. 12.1 Preoperative view of a painful knee with severe haemophilic arthropathy. A total knee arthroplasty was indicated.

was considered appropriate for surgical treatment. The primary indication for total knee arthroplasty was disabling pain unresponsive to non-operative therapy such as rest, physiotherapy, nonsteroidal anti-inflammatory drugs and analgesics. Radiographically, there was irregularity of the subchondral surface, narrowing of cartilage space, erosions and incongruity of joint margins. Of 26 patients, 16 had a prior surgical history of arthroscopic or open synovectomy.

Prostheses were utilized according to manufacturer specifications and included: 14 PCA knees (Howmedica, Rutherford, New Jersey), nine Intermedics knees (Intermedics Orthopedics, Austin, Texas), four UCI knees (University of California at Irvine, Irvine, California), two Miller-Galante II knees (Zimmer, Warsaw, Indiana) (Figs 12.1–12.3), two RAM knees (Dow-Corning-Wright, Arlington, Tennessee), two 3M knees (3M Company, St. Paul, Minnesota), one Townley knee (DePuy, Warsaw, Indiana) and one Kinematic knee (Howmedica, Rutherford, New Jersey). Starting in 1987, cementless fixation was considered as an alternative, based upon the stability of the press fit and the quality as well as quantity of bone surface area in contact with the prosthesis.

Postoperative closed suction drainage was routinely used. A compressive dressing was left in place for 2–3 days postoperatively. From 1980, a continuous passive motion machine was utilized immediately postoperatively. Blood transfusion was required in nine patients, averaging 4.6 units. All patients received prophylactic antibiotics with cephazolin, or vancomycin if a severe penicillin allergy was noted.

RESULTS

Overall, the results were classed as 84% good to excellent (22 of 26 patients), 8% fair (two patients) and 8% poor (two patients) using the Hospital for Special Surgery knee rating system. The mean pain score improved dramatically from 11 preoperatively to 28 postoperatively (a score of 30 indicating no pain). Functionally, patients improved from a mean of 12 preoperatively to 17 postoperatively (a score of 22 representing the maximum points for function). The Hospital for Special Surgery assessment improved from a mean of 43 points preoperatively

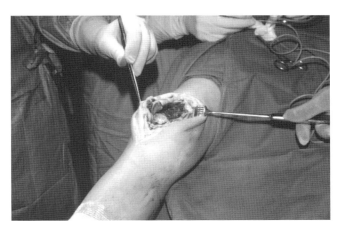

Fig. 12.2 Intraoperative view showing a black-stained synovium and severe articular destruction.

to 83 postoperatively. Additionally, the range of motion of the knee was a mean 57° preoperatively and improved to 75° postoperatively.

The actual range of motion, which was a mean 18° of extension to 75° of flexion preoperatively, improved to a mean 5° of extension to 80° of flexion postoperatively. Flexion contractures improved from 5–50° preoperatively to 5–30° postoperatively. The score for Hospital for Special Surgery flexion deformity improved from a mean of 3 preoperatively to 7 postoperatively (with 10 being no deformity).

Seventeen patients were HIV-positive. Nine have died from complications of acquired immunodeficiency disease. Their mean survival time was 113.8 months (9.6 years) after surgery, with a range of 3–16 years. Patients who tested positive for HIV tolerated their surgery well, as demonstrated by no significant decline in the HIV health scale.

HIV health scale used by the authors

I Asymptomatic
II Mild fungal or bacterial infection
III Recurrent or severe fungal or bacterial infection
IV Significant or life-threatening opportunistic infections such as cytomegalovirus, *Pneumocystis carinii* pneumonia, or toxoplasmosis.

Mean CD4 counts were measured at 368 cells/mm³ preoperatively and 343 cells/mm³ postoperatively.

Although the frequency of recurrent haemarthroses is usually much less in adults with advanced destructive changes, 62% of patients (16 of 26) gave a preoperative history of recurrent haemarthrosis ranging from one or two per year to two or three per month. During hospital admission, the total quantity of factor given ranged from 23 500 units to 111 292 units per patient.

After discharge from hospital, only three patients indicated that they experienced infrequent, recurrent (one to two per year) haemarthroses, which responded well to factor administration. However, two patients required a partial synovectomy to control frequent, recurrent bleeding episodes which persisted after total knee arthroplasty.

Complications were classified as early or late postoperative complications. Overall, there were 28 complications in 35 joint replacements, including haemarthrosis, arthrofibrosis, superficial wound infection, joint sepsis, wound dehiscence, peroneal nerve palsy and loosening of the prosthesis.

Early complications included severe haemarthrosis in five patients (two out of seventeen prior to 1986 and three of eighteen after 1986); four were treated uneventfully with arthroscopic washout and one with open lavage. Two partial peroneal nerve palsies, which were recognized in the immediate postoperative period, resolved. Failure to gain mobility, which required treatment with manipulation under anaesthesia, occurred in 12 patients (13 of 17 knees) prior to 1986, and in four patients (four of eighteen knees) after 1986. This may reflect the change to more aggressive factor replacement. When manipulation under anaesthesia was performed, this generally took place within 1–2 weeks of the total knee arthroplasty. The decision to manipulate was based on

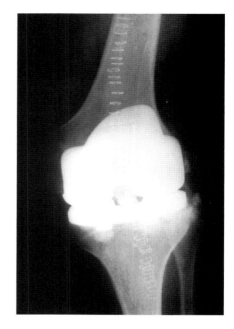

Fig. 12.3 Postoperative view after the implantation of a Miller-Galante II hybrid total knee prosthesis (with uncemented femoral component and pegged cemented tibial component).

no further gain in flexion beyond 60–70° during this 2-week postoperative period. One wound dehiscence occurred during manipulation under anaesthesia.

Infection is the late complication of most concern. A superficial wound infection occurred in one patient and resolved with irrigation, débridement and antibiotics. Of more concern were bilateral deep articular infections, which developed in two patients who tested positive for HIV and had CD4 counts of <200 cells/mm^3 at the time of occurrence. The onset of infection was delayed and occurred 2 years after each respective total knee arthroplasty. In each case, there was a documented source of distant infection (dental abscess, sinusitis or contaminated needle use). The first patient, who received a right cemented component in 1983 and a left uncemented component in 1986, developed a documented pneumococcus infection in both knees in 1988. Initially, the bilateral knee infection responded to arthroscopic irrigation and parenteral antibiotics. However, in 1990, *Staphylococcus aureus* was cultured from the right knee of the same patient, and a two-stage salvage procedure was performed with a good outcome. In the second patient, bilateral total knee arthroplasty was performed in 1982, with the right side uncemented and the left side cemented. Subsequently, in 1984 and 1988, *Staphylococcus aureus* was cultured from both knees. Eventually, this patient went on to attempted knee fusion ending in nonunions, but very functional resection arthroplasties.

Two knees were revised for loosening, one with progressive bone–implant interface radiolucency and the other with varus subsidence of the tibial component to approximately 20°. The index arthroplasties, both uncemented implants, lasted for 11 and 12 years, respectively.

CONCLUSION

In the era of total joint replacements in orthopaedics, it is obvious that a total knee replacement should be indicated in haemophilic patients suffering from severe knee pain and disability. However, the expected high risk of infectious and non-infectious postoperative complications is worrying. The authors do not imply that a total knee arthroplasty is never indicated in a haemophilic patient today, but the orthopaedic surgeon should consider the risks and benefits very carefully. The patient's age, his life expectancy and immunological status should be considered before suggesting a total knee replacement. If a total knee arthroplasty is contraindicated, knee-joint débridement is a possible alternative. In the absence of contraindications to prosthetic replacement, total knee replacement is the procedure of choice to correct deformity, relieve pain and improve the function of the knee.

It is in the best interests of the patient to be managed in a haemophilia centre where a comprehensive team approach can be provided. The medical status, physical disability, age and projected activity levels are the major factors in determining treatment for the patient with unilateral or bilateral haemophilic arthropathy of the knee. In more severely involved knees of patients with haemophilia, flexion contracture is a common deformity. In addition, valgus, external rotation deformity and posterior subluxation of the tibia may exist. The surgeon must have the expertise and experience to correct these deformities sufficiently when performing a total knee arthroplasty. A properly performed soft-tissue release which achieves a balance between the medial and lateral ligamentous structures and the posterior capsule can provide stability to the knee with a semi-constrained prosthesis. In cases with severe deformity requiring resection of the posterior cruciate ligament, a posterior cruciate substituting prosthesis may be necessary.

SUMMARY

Total knee arthroplasty provides considerable benefits in the majority of haemophilic patients, with marked pain relief and improvement in function and flexion contractures [3,11,12]. The procedure can, however, be associated with a high number of complications. The alternatives to total knee arthroplasty are knee débridement or arthrodesis, which may increase demand on other joints and which patients generally dislike.

REFERENCES

1 Lachiewicz PF, Inglis AE, Insall JN, Sculco TP, Hilgartner MW, Bussel JB. Total knee arthroplasty in hemophilia. *J Bone Joint Surg (Am)* 1985; **67A**: 1361–6.

2 Karthaus RP, Novakova IRO. Total knee replacement in haemophilia. *J Bone Joint Surg (Br)* 1988; **70B**: 382–5.

3 Wiedel JD, Luck JV, Gilbert MS. Total knee arthroplasty in the patient with hemophilia: evaluation and long-term results. In: Gilbert MS, Greene WB, eds. *Musculoskeletal Problems in Hemophilia*. National Hemophilia Foundation, 1989: 152–7.

4 Gregg-Smith SJ, Pattison RM, Dodd CAF, Giangrande PLF, Duthie RB. Septic arthritis in haemophilia. *J Bone Joint Surg (Br)* 1993; **75B**: 368–70.

5 Birch NC, Ribbans WJ, Goldman E *et al.* Letter. Knee replacement in haemophilia. *J Bone Joint Surg (Br)* 1994; **76B**: 165–6.

6 Löfqvist T, Nilsson IM, Petersson C. Orthopaedic surgery in haemophilia: 20 years' experience in Sweden. *Clin Orthop* 1996; **332**: 232–41.

7 Phillips AM, Sabin CA, Ribbans WJ, Lee CA. Orthopaedic surgery in hemophilic patients with human immunodeficiency virus. *Clin Orthop* 1997; **343**: 81–7.

8 Thomason HC III, Wilson FC, Lachiewicz PF, Kelley SS. Knee arthroplasty in hemophilic arthropathy. *Clin Orthop* 1999; **360**: 169–73.

9 Ragni MV, Crossett LS, Herndon JH. Postoperative infection following orthopaedic surgery in human immunudeficiency virus-infected hemophiliacs with CD4 counts <200/mm^3. *J Arthroplasty* 1995; **10**: 716–21.

10 Rodriguez-Merchan EC, Magallon M, Galindo E. Joint debridement for haemophilic arthropathy of the knee. *Int Orthop* 1994; **18**: 135–8.

11 Cohen I, Heim M, Martinowitz V, Chechick A. Orthopaedic outcome of total knee replacement in haemophilia A. *Haemophilia* 2000; **6**: 104–9.

12 Rodriguez-Merchan EC, Wiedel JD. Total knee arthroplasty in the HIV-positive haemophilia patient. *Haemophilia Forum*, 20 March 2000.

CHAPTER 13

Muscular Bleeding, Soft-tissue Haematomas and Pseudotumours

E C RODRIGUEZ-MERCHAN AND N J GODDARD

INTRODUCTION

More than 10% of bleeding complications in haemophilia occur within the muscles. Prompt treatment of an intramuscular bleed with clotting factors reduces the potential soft tissue complications and conservative orthopaedic management usually resolves the episode without any long-term sequelae. However, repeated and unresolved intramuscular haematomas may lead to the serious but fortunately rare complication of a pseudotumour.

INTRAMUSCULAR BLEEDING AND SOFT-TISSUE HAEMATOMAS

Intramuscular bleeds are generally associated with direct trauma and the diagnosis is usually quite obvious due to the presence of pain, swelling, local warmth and frequently an overlying bruise. The vast majority of these muscle bleeds resolve spontaneously with no detrimental functional sequelae, but one must always carefully assess the patient to ensure that there is no danger of neurovascular compromise [1].

The extent and nature of the haematoma can be readily assessed by ultrasound, which is a reliable and inexpensive diagnostic aid. It is useful in demonstrating not only the size and distribution but can also determine whether the contents are in liquid or in solid form. Magnetic resonance imaging and computed tomography (CT) scans, while obviously more precise, are expensive.

Treatment is generally conservative and relies upon restoration of normal clotting by administration of factor replacement. The limb is rested in a position of function and elevated if appropriate. Adequate analgesia is provided. Following the initial acute phase, physiotherapy should begin early in the rehabilitation in an attempt to restore full function, bearing in mind that secondary bleeds may subsequently occur.

The muscles of the forearm and of the lower leg in particular are enclosed in tight fascial compartments, and even a relatively small bleed can cause a disproportionate rise in intracompartmental pressure and risk the onset of compartment syndrome, which if left untreated can progress to the classical Volkmann's ischaemic contracture [2]. It is important to differentiate between compartment syndrome and arterial occlusion, and if there is any doubt it is a relatively straightforward undertaking to measure the intracompartmental pressures. Under certain circumstances a trend of rising pressure is significant, rather than an absolute maximum. Confirmed compartment syndrome is a surgical emergency and requires prompt decompression. A single incision, if too small, may risk an incomplete decompression, and long incisions should be made whenever appropriate in order to achieve adequate decompression of all affected compartments [3]. It is safer dealing with late scarring as a result of a compartment decompression rather that the sequelae of an inadequate decompression.

The complications of compartment syndrome are well known and include reduced function of the nerves that traverse the compartment and late onset of ischaemic muscle contractures. Nerve decompression and later excision of fibrosed and contracted scar tissue may be effective in the management of late complications.

Bleeding into deeply situated muscles may be somewhat difficult to diagnose. Probably the most frequently affected muscle is the iliopsoas which classically presents with a painful flexion deformity of the hip, with any attempt to extend the hip joint resulting in an increase in the level of pain and a compensatory lumbar lordosis. It may also be associated with abdominal pain mimicking acute appendicitis, and signs of compression of the femoral nerve with reduction in sensation over the anterior aspect of the thigh.

A bleed into iliopsoas has a similar clinical picture to an intra-articular bleed into the hip joint. It is important to distinguish between the two as the treatment differs considerably. Fortunately, ultrasound nicely differentiates the presence of a haemarthrosis in the hip joint, so distinguishing this from an iliopsoas bleed (Fig. 13.1). An intra-articular bleed generally responds promptly to correction of any factor deficiency and possibly aspiration. An iliopsoas bleed does not usually respond promptly to infusion of factor concentrate and a flexion contracture of the hip may persist for several weeks. Secondary haemorrhages into the same area are common and prophylactic treatment is advisable under these circumstances. The leg should be rested and full weight-bearing should be avoided, with care taken not to adversely stress the hip.

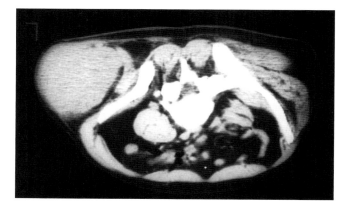

Fig. 13.1 CT scan showing an iliopsoas haematoma; note the enlargement of the right iliopsoas muscle.

In the presence of HIV infection or AIDS, any common bacteria may result in sepsis, and abscess formation should be suspected especially in patients who are immunocompromised and where the symptoms fail to respond to correction of normal clotting. Spontaneous infection of tissues has been reported in two HIV-positive patients with haemophilia [4] (Fig. 13.2).

Treatment of an abscess follows conventional lines with incision and drainage, prompt administration of appropriate intravenous antibiotics, especially when the CD4 count is low, and early rehabilitation.

PSEUDOTUMOURS

In 1965, Fernandez de Valderrama and Matthews [5] first described a haemophilic pseudotumour as a progressive cystic swelling involving muscle. This they felt was the result of recurrent haemorrhage and was generally accompanied by radiographic evidence of bone involvement. They emphasized that the condition should be differentiated from simple bone cysts which occur in the fascial envelope of the muscle without evidence of radiographic change.

The presence of a slowly enlarging mass in the limb or especially the pelvis, in a patient with haemophilia, should raise the suspicion of the possibility of a pseudotumour, although there have been rare reports of malignant tumours simulating a pseudotumour. Koepke and Browner [6] described a chondrosarcoma of the scapula and recently, in the centre in Madrid, we have had a liposarcoma presenting as a pseudotumour during an operation to remove a suspected haemophilic lesion.

The pattern of formation of a pseudotumour differs according to its anatomical site [7,8]. The majority of pseudotumours are seen in adults and occur in the long bones, where repeated and unresolved haematomas lead to subsequent encapsulation and calcification, with progressive enlargement of the mass and subsequent erosion of the adjacent bone. The muscles most frequently affected are iliacus, vastus lateralis and soleus. These have a large area of origin in common, they act across joints with a large range of motion, and insert into bones so as to en-

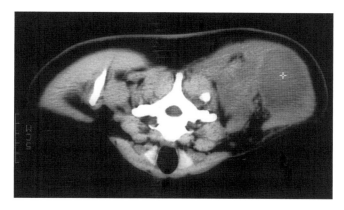

Fig. 13.2 CT scan of the left shoulder of an HIV-positive patient with haemophilia, showing a spontaneously infected soft-tissue haematoma (an abscess with multiple loculation).

hance their lever effect. Indirect trauma to these muscles is the most likely cause of bleeding into them.

Gilbert [8] has described two different clinical features for proximal and distal pseudotumours. Proximal pseudotumours occur more frequently in the proximal axial skeleton, especially around the femur and the pelvis. They probably commence in the soft tissues and then secondarily erode the bones from the outside. They have a slow evolution. They occur more frequently in adults and do not respond to conservative treatment. They generally present as a painless, firm, expanding mass which may appear to be multilocular, non-tender and adherent to the deeper structures. Such pseudotumours frequently remain painless and asymptomatic, until the patient presents later with a pathological fracture.

The radiological features are typical with a large soft-tissue mass and areas of adjacent bone destruction (Fig. 13.3). Calcification within the mass is a frequent finding. Pseudotumours of the ilium may cause significant bony erosion with little new periosteal bone formation.

Distal pseudotumours predominantly affect younger, skeletally immature patients. They are seen more commonly in children and adolescents and are generally the result of direct trauma. In this group of patients it is not unusual to see such tumours distal to the wrist and the ankle. Unlike the proximal lesions, these distal pseudotumours develop rapidly and appear to be secondary to an intraosseous haemorrhage. They are seen especially in the small cancellous bones such as the calcaneus, talus and metatarsals of the feet, but seldom in the carpus. Occasionally, this appearance and resolution of these pseudotumours has been reported following radiotherapy [9].

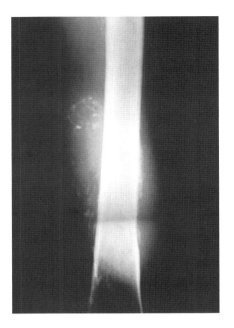

Fig. 13.3 Radiograph of a pseudotumour in the middle third of the thigh with soft-tissue calcification.

Pathology

A pseudotumour is basically an encapsulated haematoma. It has a thick, fibrous capsule surrounding the haematoma which may be in varying states of organization (Figs 13.4 and 13.5). Calcification and later ossifi-

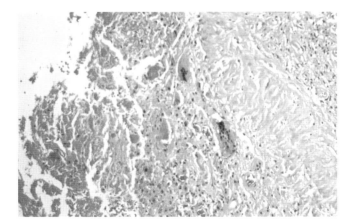

Fig. 13.4 Photomicrograph of a pseudotumour after removal. Internal zone containing degenerating haematic material and both fibrous and histiocytic proliferation; two multinucleate foreign body cells can be seen more medially.

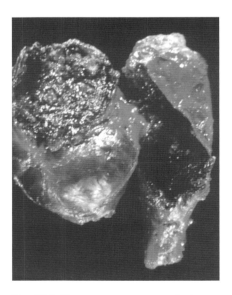

Fig. 13.5 The gross appearance of a large pseudotumour after removal.

cation may be seen within its wall. Smaller cysts may have a thinner but less adherent capsule containing more fluid blood.

The nature of the classic pseudotumour was accurately described by Duthie *et al.* [10] on analysing an amputation specimen. Sequential longitudinal sections showed that the haemorrhage was mainly extra-osseous and loosely enclosed in fibrous tissue. There was evidence of extensive subperiosteal bleeding and reactive new bone formation which expands both externally and internally, leading to extensive destruction of the involved bone. Histological examination showed the presence of subperiosteal woven bone. There were accumulations in the inflammatory cells, many of which were histiocytes containing copious amounts of siderin.

Treatment

These lesions are not common and, at the centre in Madrid, we have treated only 17 pseudotumours in a group of 450 patients [11]. In the early days before the advent of replacement therapy, the majority of proximal tumours were treated conservatively by a combination of immobilization and factor VIII replacement. This regime, however, generally failed to prevent progression of the lesion, and although regression was occasionally seen there were no true cures and recurrence and/or progression is the rule.

Distal pseudotumours in children, however, respond well to long-term replacement therapy and cast immobilization, and frequently resolve. With the increasing availability of factor replacement, surgical removal of proximal lesions is now a realistic proposition. Large proximal pseudotumours in adults should be removed surgically as soon as is practical following their diagnosis unless there are overwhelming contraindications. Initial assessment must include plain radiography, ultrasound and CT scanning in order to determine the extent of the lesion. Selective arteriography is used to demonstrate the vascularity of pseudotumours in the limb in an attempt to plan the surgical approach, and also to permit preoperative arterial embolization so as to facilitate the later surgical removal [12].

Left untreated, large pseudotumours may ultimately lead to pathological long bone fractures [13]. Faced with this complication, Ishiguro *et al.* [13] advised radical excision of the pseudotumour followed by rigid fixation of the bone whenever practical. Obviously, such limb salvaging surgery following a pathological fracture secondary to a pseudotumour is preferable to amputation. In children, surgical excision or amputation may be indicated in the light of failure of conservative management. Occasionally, though, amputation cannot be avoided and Heim *et al.* [14] reported the case of a young adult who presented with two separate pseudotumours in a single lower limb which was only cured by above-knee amputation.

Surgery for extensive pseudotumours of the ilium is not without its potential complications. Heeg *et al.* [15] described a patient with an extensive haemophilic pseudotumour of the ilium who went on to develop a chronic fistula 6 months following *en bloc* resection. This then required two further procedures and only a pedicled rectus abdominis flap was successful in eradicating the fistula.

Likewise, the presence of inhibitors poses a new set of problems, but Maliekel *et al.* [16] reported a case of an elderly woman with inhibitor formation, who required wide excision of a large haemophilic pseudotumour adjacent to the gluteus maximus. Haemostasis in this case was successfully achieved using recombinant factor VIIa. There was no recurrence at 18-month follow-up.

It is self-evident that factor VIII levels must be carefully monitored in patients undergoing surgery and this of course requires close liaison with the haematologist. It is recommended that factor VIII levels should be maintained at 100% for the first 3 days following operation, then 50% in the first 2 weeks. In the subsequent 6 weeks, patients are maintained on a level of 30–50%, depending on their response.

Percutaneous aspiration

In advanced or potentially inoperable pseudotumours there is a role for percutaneous aspiration with a large-bore trocar and under control of an image intensifier. Following aspiration of the contents, the cavity may be filled with either fibrin glue [17] or cancellous bone graft [18,19], depending on the size of the cavity. There have been encouraging reports that this may slow or even halt the condition. The procedure has three main advantages: it is easy, straightforward and relatively noninvasive, it is cheap and it does not require lengthy hospitalization.

SUMMARY

The management of the patient with a haemophilic pseudotumour is complex. It is hoped that with the advent of widespread maintenance therapy, pseudotumours will be less common in the future. It is important that they are diagnosed early, and prevention of muscular haematomas is key to reducing their incidence. Distal pseudotumours should be treated in the first instance with factor replacement and immobilization with a cast. Surgical excision may be indicated when conservative management fails to prevent progression. Occasionally, amputation may become necessary. Untreated, proximal pseudotumours will ultimately destroy soft tissues, erode bone and may produce neurovascular complications. Surgical excision is the treatment of choice but should only be carried out in major haemophilia centres.

REFERENCES

1 Heim M, Rodriguez-Merchan EC, Horoszowski H. Orthopedic complications and management of hemophilia. *Int J Pediatr Hematol Oncol* 1994; **1**: 545–51.

2 Heim M, Martinowitz U, Horoszowski H. The short foot syndrome: an unfortunate consequence of neglected raised intracompartmental pressure in a severely hemophilic child. A case report. *Angiology* 1986; **37**: 128–31.

3 Cohen MS, Garfin SR, Hargens AR *et al.* Acute compartment syndrome: effect of dermotomy on fascial decompression in the leg. *J Bone Joint Surg (Br)* 1991; **73B**: 287–90.

4 Rodriguez-Merchan EC, Villar A, Magallon M, De Orbe A. Spontaneous infection of soft tissue haematomas in two HIV seropositive haemophilia patients. *Haemophilia* 1995; **1**: 137–9.

5 Fernandez de Valderrama JA, Matthews JM. The haemophilic pseudotumour or haemophilic subperiosteal haematoma. *J Bone Joint Surg (Br)* 1965; **47B**: 256–65.

6 Koepke JA, Browner TW. Chondrosarcoma mimicking pseudotumour of haemophilia. *Arch Pathol* 1965; **80**: 655–8.

7 Ahlberg AKM. On the natural history of hemophilic pseudotumor. *J Bone Joint Surg (Am)* 1975; **57A**: 1133–6.

8 Gilbert MS. The hemophilic pseudotumor. *Prog Clin Biol Res* 1990; **324**: 263–8.

9 Chen YF. Bilateral hemophilic pseudotumors of the calcaneus and cuboid treated by irradiation. *J Bone Joint Surg (Am)* 1965; **47A**: 517–21.

10 Duthie RB, Matthews JM, Rizza CR *et al*. Haemophilic cysts and pseudotumours. In: Duthie RB, ed. *The Management of Musculo-Skeletal Problems in the Haemophilias*. Oxford: Blackwell Scientific Publications, 1972.

11 Rodriguez-Merchan EC. The haemophilic pseudotumour. *Int Orthop* 1995; **19**: 255–60.

12 Sevilla J, Alvarez MT, Hernandez D *et al*. Therapeutic embolization and surgical excision of hemophilic pseudotumor. *Haemophilia* 1999; **5**: 360–3.

13 Ishiguro N, Iwahori Y, Kato T *et al*. The surgical treatment of a haemophilic pseudotumour in an extremity: a report of three cases with pathological fractures. *Haemophilia* 1998; **4**: 126–31.

14 Heim M, Horoszowski H, Schulman S *et al*. Multifocal pseudotumour in a single limb. *Haemophilia* 1997; **3**: 50–3.

15 Heeg M, Smit WM, Van der Meer J, Van Horn JR. Excision of a haemophilic pseudotumour of the ilium, complicated by fistulisation. *Haemophilia* 1998; **4**: 123–35.

16 Maliekel K, Rana N, Green D. Recombinant factor VIIa in the management of a pseudotumour in acquired haemophilia. *Haemophilia* 1997; **3**: 54–8.

17 Fernandez-Palazzi F, Rivas S, Rupcich M. Experience with fibrin seal in the management of haemophilic cysts and pseudotumours. *Proceedings: Management of Musculoskeletal Problems in Haemophilia*. Denver, Colorado, USA: National Hemophilia Foundation, 1985.

18 Caviglia HA. Haemophilic pseudotumour treated by bone graft. Presented at the *International Symposium on Musculoskeletal Problems in Haemophilia*, Castellfranco Veneto, Italy, 1993.

19 Sagarra M, Lucas M, de la Torre E *et al*. Successful surgical treatment of haemophilic pseudotumour, filling the defect with hydroxiapatite. *Haemophilia* 2000; **6**: 55–6.

CHAPTER 14

Surgical Management of the Adult Haemophilic Blood Cyst (Pseudotumour)

M S GILBERT

INTRODUCTION

The adult haemophilic blood cyst (pseudotumour) develops following haemorrhage into large muscles in proximity to bone [1]. Most haematomas resorb without encystic encapsulation but, in some, resorption is incomplete and the haematoma encapsulates. Over a long period of time the cyst enlarges. It may become multilocular and neighbouring or 'daughter' cysts may develop. If left untreated, the cystic mass will displace muscle and destroy bone. Areas of bone adjacent to the cyst wall will be eroded and at the ends of periosteal elevation will result in areas of new bone formation. The cyst, as it enlarges, will displace or possibly surround adjacent neurovascular structures. Erosion through skin and vascular erosion resulting in haemorrhage have been reported [2]. These lesions are usually painless and the onset of pain may indicate either a haematogenous infection or a pathological fracture which may result in loss of life or limb. Because of the adverse natural history, the time-honoured approach to these cysts, if possible, has been surgical resection. Newer approaches to these lesions are being evaluated, but in this chapter I will discuss the surgical techniques that have been used by the author.

The majority of haemophilic bone cysts seen in the adult haemophiliac occur in approximation to the large bones of the proximal skeleton. The vast majority occur in proximity to the pelvis, femur and proximal tibia. The techniques for evaluation and surgery of the pelvic and long bone cysts differ and will be discussed separately. The treatment of massive lesions of the pelvis will be discussed in Chapter 16.

LESIONS IN PROXIMITY TO THE LONG BONES

The radiographic picture of lesions in proximity to long bones is characteristic in that there is a large, soft-tissue mass with areas of adjacent bone destruction (Fig. 14.1). The bone loss may be extensive, involving diaphysis and metaphysis and even destroying adjacent bones by crossing the joints. Periosteal elevation with new bone formation can be seen at the periphery of these lesions. The appearance of large bone

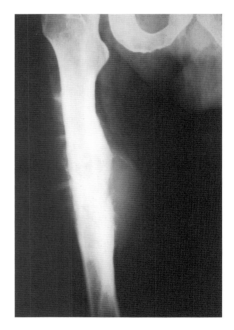

Fig. 14.1 Radiograph of large haemophilic blood cyst of the femur.

spicules surrounding the soft-tissue mass is probably secondary to this phenomenon. Calcification and ossification within the soft-tissue mass are frequently noted [1–3].

Computed tomography (CT) will demonstrate the fibrous wall and outlines the areas of loculation and daughter cysts. The CT scan is the best study for detailing the extent of bone destruction. The displacement of large neurovascular structures can also be seen on the CT scan. Magnetic resonance imaging (MRI) does not demonstrate the details of bone destruction as clearly as does the CT scan, but it can better evaluate the neurovascular structures, and the ability to obtain multiplanar cuts is very useful. In dealing with large lesions, frequently both studies are required. If there is any question about the course of the major vascular structures, angiography should be performed prior to surgery. It should be noted that the author has evaluated many angiographic studies both prior to surgery and, in one post-surgical limb, following amputation for an infected lesion. The author has yet to see a major vessel that could be considered a 'feeder vessel' to these lesions and therefore he has no experience with selective embolization to control bleeding during the surgical procedure.

The surgical approach to these lesions must be individualized. The aim should be complete resection of the lesion, stabilization of the bone, bone grafting if required, haemostasis and closure of the dead space. Prosthetic replacement for massive bone lesions can be considered. The author has no experience with their use in haemophilic patients, and potential problems include poor bone stock for prosthetic fixation and poor muscle mass for coverage of the prosthesis.

The surgical incision has to be planned to allow access to the neurovascular structures, removal of the lesion and fixation of bone. Tourniquets are not used. The dissection is best started in healthy tissue proximal to the lesion, where the neurovascular structures can be identified and retracted. The course of these structures should be traced through and distal to the lesion or to a point where they are known to be out of the surgical field. This usually does not represent a problem at the femur, but in lesions of the proximal tibia the dissection may be difficult. A separate incision may have to be made anteriorly to bone-graft the cystic lesion within the bone. It must be stated, again, that frequently the neurovascular bundle may be within the soft-tissue mass and this is usually due to the multilocular nature of the lesion (Fig. 14.2a) which results in the structures being surrounded.

Following the neurovascular dissection, the blood cyst itself can be surgically removed (Fig. 14.2b). It usually is within a muscle mass, having thinned and displaced involved muscle fibres. As much muscle as possible should be preserved. These multiple layers of thinned muscle fibres can, at times, appear to form a false capsule. An attempt should be made to stay on the fibrous capsule and this may require that the surgeon frequently evaluates and changes his plane of dissection. At the musculotendinous junction the plane of dissection becomes indistinct. The wall of the cyst merges with the tendon and may continue into the tendon in a fusiform manner. The cyst may have to be amputated in this area and, after the tendon is cleaned of fibrous and haemorrhagic tissue, any defect can be closed longitudinally.

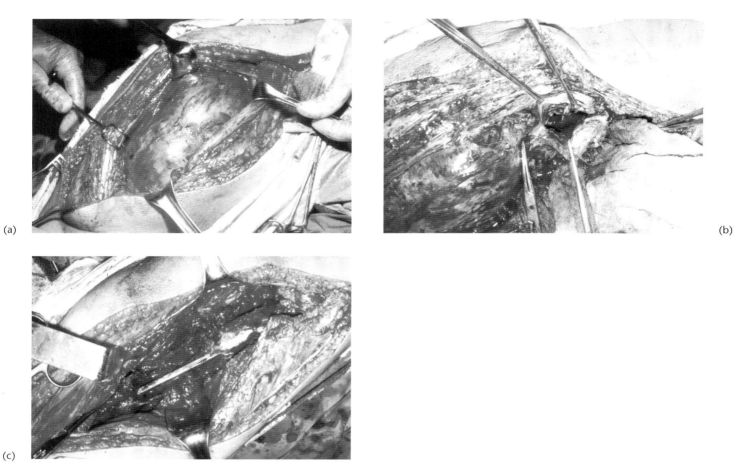

(a)

(b)

(c)

Fig. 14.2 (a) Multilocular cyst noted at surgery; (b) the cyst wall opened before resection; (c) erosion of femur noted after resection of cyst. Intramedullary fixation in place.

A portion of muscle wall will be directly adjacent to the bone where it has caused pressure necrosis. The wall usually can be removed easily either with cautery dissection or with the use of large curettes. Bleeding from the bone can be controlled by the use of fibrin glue, which also can be used on other large bleeding surfaces prior to closure.

Bone fixation and stabilization is an important part of the preoperative planning. Intramedullary fixation has been most often used (Fig. 14.2c), supplemented by bone grafting if required. It should be noted that the large denuded bone surfaces seem to result in abundant new bone formation, and nonunion has not been seen in the author's patients.

At this point, meticulous haemostasis should be obtained. Coverage of the remaining bone should then be addressed, using a muscle flap if necessary. A suction drain is always used and a bulky pressure dressing applied. The use of plaster and the weight-bearing status must be individualized depending upon the lesion itself and the extent of arthropathy in other joints.

There is a significant amount of haemorrhage during and following these procedures. It is recommended that the factor levels be maintained at 100% for at least 1 week following the procedure, with lesser levels for at least 2 weeks. The use of prophylactic antibiotics, a cell saver and the planning of transfusion requirements should be carefully considered by the haemophilia team prior to undertaking surgery.

These procedures are demanding and may last in excess of 6 hours. To deal with the real problem of surgical fatigue, a team of two experienced surgeons is recommended, enabling one to take a break. One surgeon should be familiar with vascular exposure and repair and, in fact, a vascular surgeon may be considered as the second surgeon.

LESIONS OF THE PELVIS

Haemophilic blood cysts of the pelvis develop following haemorrhage into either the iliacus or psoas muscles. The radiographic picture differs from those previously described in that the soft-tissue mass and the extent of pelvic bone destruction, most of which occurs in the iliac wing, may be difficult to appreciate on plain X-ray films. Periosteal elevation and calcification within these lesions are much less common. CT and MRI scans are considerably more useful than plain X-rays and may be sufficient to evaluate displacement of the large vessels. Angiography was utilized in the past but in the later cases has not been found to be of value. An intravenous pyelogram should be performed if there is any concern about displacement of the ureters.

This procedure is usually done in connection with a general surgeon. The surgical approach to the pelvic blood cyst is different from that for the extremities. Before starting the procedure, a ureteral catheter is placed so that the ureter can be more easily identified during surgery. The patient is placed on his or her back with the affected side of the pelvis on two sandbags with the lower limb draped free. A flank incision, starting at the proximal aspect of the mass and approximately 3 cm above the iliac crest is made, extending distally to the inguinal ligament and then continuing distally in order to expose the femoral vessels and nerve. These structures are identified and marked with vascular tapes. The flank muscles are then divided and the cysts can be identified. If possible, the dissection is kept within the retroperitoneum. The dissection is carried anteriorly and medially, but the mass of the cyst may limit this dissection. If so, the cyst can be opened and evacuated. The contents usually consist of various amounts of gritty coagulum and dark bloodstained fluid. At this point, it is important to identify the course of the femoral nerve; in one case it was noted to run directly through the centre of the cyst. The femoral nerve should be dissected from distal to proximal until it dips posterior to the cyst. It is not necessary to attempt removal of the cyst *en masse*. Rather, sections of the wall should be carefully removed. As the dissection is carried medially, care should be taken to identify the iliac vessels and the ureter. The wall is frequently in close proximity to these structures; in one case a tear in the iliac vein required vascular repair. It is wiser to leave a small cuff of the cyst wall attached to these vessels or to the ureter.

When the dissection is completed, the cyst wall can then be dissected off the inner ileum. The cyst may have eroded through the wing, leaving only a thin rim at the iliac crest. This rim of bone may have to be removed so that the cavity itself can be closed. Closing this defect is problematic and an attempt to either fill it with mobilized omentum or a muscle flap should be made. Fibrin glue should be used to control oozing from the exposed bone and tissue surfaces. The skin is then closed over a large closed suction drain and a pressure dressing applied.

In some lesions, the cyst may extend distally below the inguinal ligament or into the gluteal area. In these cases, an extension of the anterior incision or a separate incision in the buttock may be required.

RECURRENCE

Recurrent cysts have been seen and can be the result of incomplete resection, failure to identify small daughter cysts or postoperative haematomas that develop and repeat the pathological process that caused the primary cyst. The author has noted three recurrent tumours in 19 operations. The recurrences were found 1–4 years following the first procedures. Once noted, these recurrences should be resected, bearing in mind that the dissection through fibrous tissue may be difficult. However, if the important neurovascular structures were identified during the first procedure, it may be possible to plan the approach so that they need not be exposed. It is tempting to delay the repeat surgery, but it should be done early to avoid the need for an extensive reconstructive procedure.

CONCLUSION

These procedures are fraught with difficulty and carry a high complication rate including vascular and neurological damage, haemorrhage and infection [4]. Careful preoperative planning is required and the operations should only be performed at haemophilia centres where the haematologist, orthopaedic surgeon, physiotherapist and other members of the team have collaborated and participated previously in less demanding haemophilia surgery.

REFERENCES

1 Fernandez de Valderrama JA, Matthews JM. The haemophilic pseudotumor or haemophilic subperiosteal haematoma. *J Bone Joint Surg (Br)* 1965; **47B**: 256–65.

2 Gilbert MS. In: Brikhous KM, Hemker HC, eds. *Handbook of Hemophilia*. Amsterdam: Excerpta Medica, 1975: 435–46.

3 Brant EE, Jordan HH. Radiological aspects of hemophilic pseudotumors in bone. *Am J Roentgenol Med* 1972; **1150**: 525–39.

4 Heaton DC, Robertson RW, Rothwell AG. Iliopsoas haemophilic pseudotumours with bowel fistulisation. *Haemophilia* 2000; **6**: 41–3.

CHAPTER 15

Percutaneous Treatment of Haemophilic Pseudotumours

H A CAVIGLIA, F FERNANDEZ-PALAZZI, G GALATRO, R PEREZ-BIANCO AND M S GILBERT

INTRODUCTION

The haemophilic pseudotumour is really an encapsulated haematoma, which has a tendency to progress and produce clinical symptoms in relation to its anatomical location. Therefore, it is a clinical entity rather than a specific pathological lesion. Two kinds of pseudotumours exist: true pseudotumours affecting bone structure and false pseudotumours that are blood collections located in muscles which do not affect bone structure. Haemophilic pseudotumour is an infrequent complication since it occurs in 1% of severe haemophiliacs [1]. Nevertheless, when patients do not receive adequate treatment for their haemorrhage episodes, its incidence increases, and it may even appear in patients with only moderate haemophilia [2].

Once established, the pseudotumour tends to spread, leading to bone or soft-tissue lesions, and even neurovascular complications due to vessel and nerve compression. The clinical behaviour of the pseudotumour varies between adults and children. Children often present with cysts at distal bone locations and respond to replacement therapy with VIII and IX factor. In adults, however, the cyst is frequently to be found at a proximal bone location and does not respond to replacement therapy. Resection of the pseudotumour and its pseudocapsule used to be the conventional treatment. Occasionally, depending on the magnitude of the lesion, amputation was resorted to as the only means of eradicating the lesion [3].

In 1982, Fernandez-Palazzi *et al.* pioneered a new technique for treating early cysts. The procedure consisted of locating the cyst by means of an image intensifier, puncture with a trocar, and finally, aspiration of the cavity content and filling the cavity with fibrin seal [4]. In 1990, the Mariano R. Castex Investigations Institute of the National Academy of Medicine decided upon treatment of larger cysts and pseudotumours with aspiration and posterior filling of the cavity with bone graft in true tumours and with Spongostan® or fibrin seal in false ones [5].

This treatment is non-aggressive and may be chosen for patients with factor VIII inhibitor. To treat this lesion appropriately, a complete evaluation of the patient and preoperative replacement therapy are necessary, followed by a non-traumatic surgical technique and adequate post-operative care. It is essential for the specialists who deal with this pathology to understand that the only way to achieve a successful result is to provide multidisciplinary treatment through the combined team effort of haematologist, orthopaedic surgeon, immunologist, nurses, physiotherapists, psychologist and social worker.

PREOPERATIVE EVALUATION

The haematologist should perform preoperative corrective tests with factors VIII and IX to define the most adequate doses and to detect whether an inhibitor is present. The latter case implies an alternative strategy in the replacement therapy (for example, factor VII).

An overall evaluation of the patient needs to be made to obtain adequate information concerning the limb alignment and the degree of proximal and distal articular compromise caused by the pseudotumours. The orthopaedic surgeon has a number of means at his or her disposal for evaluating the type and characteristics of the pseudotumours.

Radiology

Radiographs enable us to find out whether the tumour involves bone (true pseudotumour) or not (false pseudotumour). When bone is compromised, X-rays will help reveal the location of the pseudotumour (diaphysis, metaphysis, epiphysis), its size, the degree of cortical destruction (thinning, erosion or pathological fracture) and the presence of regional osteoporosis. Radiography will also inform us about proximal and distal joints that may be compromised.

Ultrasound

Ultrasound is a suitable method for diagnosing tumours of soft tissue. It provides information about size in the three spatial planes, location, characteristics and associated vascular compression, and will show whether there are one or more cavities and if there are connections between them.

Computed tomography scan

The CT scan can be extremely useful in true pseudotumours, since it provides exact information on their location, number of cavities and their possible interconnections. It also shows the degree of cortical involvement and the spread of the pseudotumour towards soft tissue (Fig. 15.1). The three-dimensional image provides clear information about the pseudotumour's characteristics, especially in complex locations such as the pelvis.

Magnetic resonance imaging

MRI is a very useful complementary diagnostic test. It provides information about the location, size and number of cavities of the pseudotu-

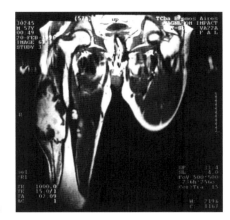
(a)

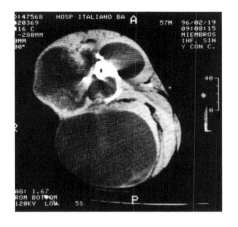
(b)

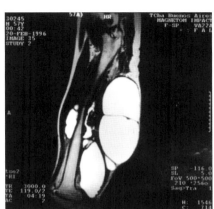
(c)

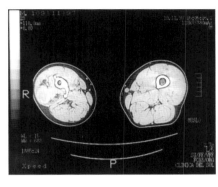
(d)

Fig. 15.1 (a–c) The extent of destruction caused by a haemophilic pseudotumour can best be assessed from different CT scans. (d) The same pseudotumour pictured in (a–c), after successful treatment.

mour, as well as the characteristics of the cavity contents (liquid or solid), on the extension to soft tissue and its degree of compromise. An adequate reconstruction will permit evaluation of the interconnections among the cavities.

Every patient's immunological status (presence of HIV or HIC) should be evaluated. When a patient presents with a CD4 count of < 400 cells/mm^3, the possibility of conservative treatment should be evaluated and factor VIII prophylaxis considered.

The nurse should evaluate the degree of cooperativeness of the patient and the presence of access routes for administering replacement therapy. The role of the physiotherapist is to evaluate the degree of musculoskeletal compromise and gain the cooperation of the patient in designing a suitable rehabilitation programme. The psychologist will determine the psychological profile of the patient and the need for pre-operative and postoperative assistance. The social worker will have to carry out the necessary measures so that the patient and his family have access to the treatment with no distinction of social assistance or place of residence.

PREOPERATIVE REPLACEMENT THERAPY

Every patient without inhibitor will require no less than 6 weeks of preoperative replacement therapy with a daily dose of 50–100 IU/kg of factor VIII or IX. The purpose of this treatment is to reduce the size of the pseudotumour before surgery and to determine the degree of aggressiveness of the lesion. Less aggressive pseudotumours respond to conservative treatment. A new MRI scan is carried out 6 weeks later and if the tumour has reduced 50% in size a new similar procedure must be repeated for another 6 weeks (Fig. 15.2).

If after a new MRI the lesion does not show changes, surgery is performed. In contrast, if the pseudotumour has reduced to 25% of its original size, the replacement therapy should be continued for another 6 weeks. Then a new MRI scan for control is indicated. If the tumour has disappeared, it is considered to be cured, but if the tumour is still present it should be treated surgically. Every pseudotumour treated with preoperative replacement therapy that does not reduce by 50% in size after 6 weeks, or to 25% after 12 weeks, or is still present after 18 weeks, should be surgically removed. Primary replacement therapy in children lasts 12 weeks, and after that the same algorithm of treatment continues (Fig. 15.3).

PREOPERATIVE PLANNING

Once the decision for surgery has been made, preoperative planning is undertaken by a multidisciplinary team. The haematologist will decide on the length of time for continuous infusion according to the pseudotumour type and the need for catheter implantation. When the patient requires replacement therapy for a period longer than 8 weeks, or does not present good venous access, the preoperative implantation of an infusion catheter is required. Factor VIII or IX is administered at a dosage of 50–100 IU/kg daily. The orthopaedic surgeon will evaluate the location of the pseudotumour, whether in bone or in soft tissue.

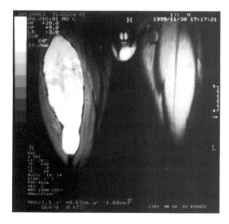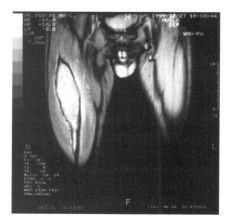

Fig. 15.2 (a) Pseudotumour in right thigh. (b) Pseudotumour reduced by more than 50% following replacement therapy.

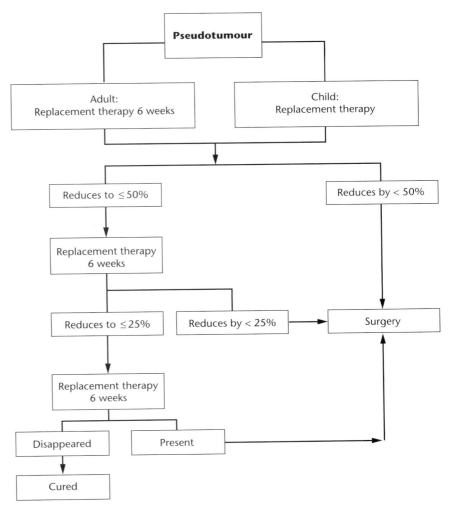

Fig. 15.3 Treatment algorithm with primary replacement therapy for 12 weeks in children and 6 weeks in adults.

Pseudotumour in soft tissue

In the presence of a tumour in soft tissue, the existence of a single cavity or multiple ones and their content have to be verified. If the cavity is single and less than 3 cm in size, it is important to know the characteristic of the content. If the content is liquid, it will be aspirated with the guidance of ultrasound and the cavity filled with fibrin seal. In contrast, if it is dense the patient will be treated surgically: a small incision, opening, washing, removal of solid contents by means of a curette and posterior filling with fibrin seal.

In the case of single cavities > 3 cm, a small incision is made to introduce a laparoscopic cannula, the cavity will be washed and filled with Spongostan under video control. In superficial tumours access is percutaneous, but when tumours are deep access must take account of important vessels. When solid material is present, the location has to be identified to enable removal with a curette under laparoscopic control. With multiple cavities without clear communication, they will be evacuated separately using ultrasound control. There will be as many approaches as there are cavities.

Figure 15.4 is an algorithm for the treatment of soft-tissue pseudotumours. The purpose of the curette is to remove the solid content that comes off with washing, taking care not to damage the inner wall of the pseudotumour as this may cause bleeding.

Pseudotumour in bone

The location, size and degree of cortical compromise of a pseudotumour in bone will be evaluated to confirm the true loss of bone stock. When the pseudotumour is diaphyseal or diaphy-metaphyseal it generally consists of a single cavity. In contrast, with a pseudotumour that is epiphyseal or epiphy-metaphyseal (in cancellous bone) the cavities are multiple. The number of cavities should be determined, as on the whole the number of approaches equals the number of cavities, except when a CT or MRI scan shows extended communication between them. Lack of aspiration of one cavity may lead to only partial cure of the lesion. It is very important to clarify the cortical damage. In diaphyseal or diaphy-metaphyseal areas with damage of the cortex, or in the presence of pathological fracture, additional intramedullary fixation with a locking nail is necessary. Patients with very large epiphyseal or epiphy-metaphyseal pseudotumours with cortical erosion will require postoperative orthosis.

Approach

When the pseudotumour is large, with cortical erosion and extending to the skin, a small incision (5 cm) can be made and then the laparoscope cannula can be introduced in the side of the lesion. If the pseudotumour does not extend to the skin, a careful approach must be made to avoid injury to important vessels. Where the cortex is thick, a pin

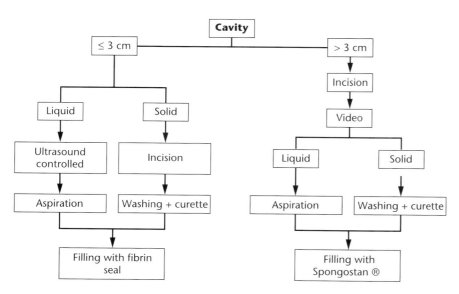

Fig. 15.4 Treatment algorithm for soft-tissue pseudotumours.

has to be inserted by means of the image intensifier, and then a cannulated drill will permit the introduction of the video cannula.

Cavity content and cavity filling

If the cavity content is liquid it is easy to aspirate, but solid contents cannot be evacuated by aspiration but will need to be washed out and removed with curettes. Cavities of < 3 cm may be filled with fibrin seal; larger cavities should be filled with lyophilized bone graft or bone substitute such as coralline hydroxyapatite. The filling procedure is performed by manually pressing the graft into the cavity (bone packing). Figure 15.5 is an algorithm for the treatment of osseous pseudotumours.

SURGICAL PROCEDURE

Each patient should receive thromboembolic prophylaxis and antibiotic prophylaxis with cephalosporin, 1 g preoperatively and a similar dose 6 hours later. No tourniquet is used to control intracavitary bleeding. Incisions are small and used exclusively for the placement of the cannula inside the pseudotumour. Washing and aspiration are done through the same incision. In the soft-tissue pseudotumour, evacuation of the

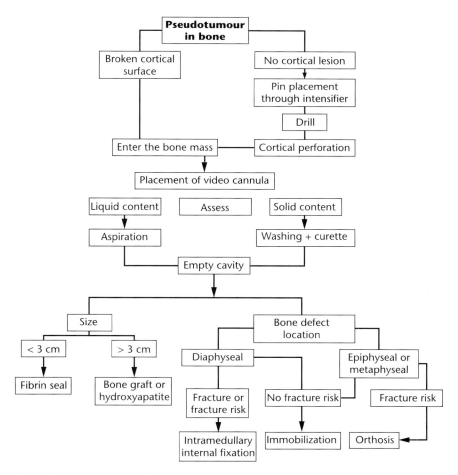

Fig. 15.5 Treatment algorithm for osseous pseudotumours.

cavity and filling are carried out assisted by ultrasound, while in the true pseudotumour this is performed with an image intensifier and video assistance. The availability of a CT scanner in the operating room facilitates control of evacuation and the filling of the cavity. When intramedullary fixation is necessary the steps are: cavity aspiration, placing of the locking nail and filling of the cavity. The wound is closed with separate nylon stitches. In patients with >3 cm cavities a suction drain should be in position for 24 hours.

Postoperative replacement therapy depends on the size of the pseudotumour, its location, the result of cavity filling and extent of postoperative bleeding. A compression bandage ought to be used in patients with pseudotumours of soft tissue for 3 days. On the third day, external elastic compression will be applied to avoid collection of liquid in the aspirated area. On the day after surgery, the patient can start to actively and passively exercise the areas unaffected by the pseudotumour. Rehabilitation of the affected area will depend upon the size and location of the lesion, postoperative immobilization, postoperative bleeding and any compromised proximal and distal joints. It is the job of the physiotherapist to evaluate all these variables to design the rehabilitation plan. The time for bone healing depends on the size of the lesion. In our own experience the average for pseudotumours is 8 months, with a quicker recovery in children.

CONCLUSION

Although this relatively non-invasive treatment represents an advance in the treatment of this pathology, we believe that efforts should be made towards its prevention. Every patient should receive adequate treatment of their bleeding episodes through education and the elimination of the geographical and/or social barriers that prevent the patient from having access to proper care. As has been said by Tezanos-Pinto *et al.*, 'the best treatment for pseudotumours is prevention by means of early replacement therapy for bleeding episodes' [6].

REFERENCES

1   Gunning AJ. The surgery of haemophilic cysts. In: Biggs R, Macfarlane RG, eds. *Treatment of Haemophilia and Other Coagulation Disorders*. Oxford: Blackwell, 1966.

2   Fernandez-Palazzi F, Rivas S, de Bosch NB *et al.* Percutaneous treatment of haemophilic cysts and pseudotumors. In: Lusher JM, Kessler CM, eds. *Hemophilia and Von Willebrand's disease in the 1990s.* Amsterdam: Excerpta Medica, 1991: 157–64.

3   Gilbert MS. The Hemophilic Pseudotumor In: Kasper CK, ed. *Recent Advances in Hemophilia Care*. New York: Liss Inc, 1990: 257–62.

4   Fernandez-Palazzi F, Rivas-Hernandez S, Rupeich M. Experience with "fibrin seal" in the management of hemophilic cysts and pseudotumors. In: Wiedel JD, Gilbert MS, eds. *Management of Musculoskeletal Problems in Hemophilia*. New York: National Hemophilia Foundation, 1986: 42–6.

5   Caviglia H. An alternative to surgical resection of the pseudo-tumour. *Haemophilia* 1996; **2** (Suppl. 1): 5.

6   Tezanos-Pinto M, Nieto R, Perez-Bianco R. Hemophilic pseudotumor: a report of 25 cases. In: Lusher JM, Kessler CM, eds. *Hemophilia and Von Willebrand's Disease in the 1990s.* Amsterdam: Excerpta Medica, 1991: 165–78.

CHAPTER 16

The Management of Giant Haemophilic Pseudotumours

M HEIM, J LUBOSHITZ, Y AMIT AND U MARTINOWITZ

INTRODUCTION

Earlier chapters have dealt with the detailed surgical treatment and percutaneous management of pseudotumours and this chapter aims at dealing with the problems caused by giant pseudotumours. The aetiology of pseudotumours is poorly understood [1]. The incidence in the western world has been calculated as between 1% and 2%. Their anatomical distribution identifies areas of predilection and its destructive sequelae have been described in many small series [2,3] and case reports [4–6]. The vast majority of reported cases originate in areas of the world where adequate coagulation factor replacement is scarce, and many patients suffering from a pseudotumour have an antibody to the clotting factor. However, there is a lack of evidence-based information to link lack of factor replacement to the development of pseudotumours. The intention of this chapter is not to discuss the aetiology but rather to look at methods of management of massive pseudotumours.

PRESENTATION

These tumours are slow growing, expansile (Fig. 16.1a) and locally destructive. The tumour's expansive nature results in the erosion and final destruction of rigid structures (such as the iliac bone) (Fig. 16.1b) and displacement of mobile structures, for example, kidney and bowel. Fortunately, these pathological pseudotumours do not metastasize, but multiple lesions have been reported [1]. The size of the pseudotumour causes many symptoms and pain may be so severe that patients lose their independence, become bedridden and require analgesia which may even include narcotic medications. Patients' ability to walk may be affected not only through pain but also because of neurological motor weakness caused by nerve compression. The pseudotumour may also compress the ureter, bladder and/or blood vessels (Fig. 16.1c). This chapter outlines a systematic approach to dealing with the many facets of the comprehensive management of large pseudotumours.

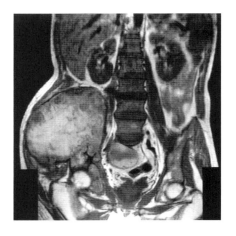
(a)

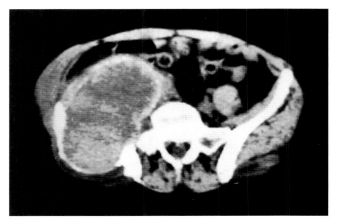
(b)

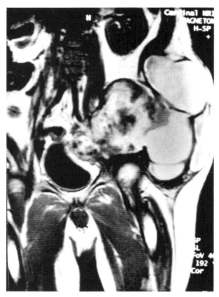
(c)

Fig. 16.1 (a) MRI demonstrating a huge pseudotumour filling the right side of the abdomen; note distended abdominal wall, absence of iliopsoas shadow and missing ileum. (b) CT scan showing transected view of pseudotumour which extends from the abdominal wall almost to the midline. Compare the normal shape of the left ileum with destruction of the right ileum. (c) Longitudinal MRI demonstrates the pressure exerted by the pseudotumour on the bladder: also note the relationship between the tumour and the external iliac artery.

MANAGEMENT

The exact location of the mass needs to be accurately assessed in order to plan the most appropriate surgical approach. Computed tomography scans and magnetic resonance imaging investigations add significant information regarding the structure of the tumour and its involvement with the surrounding tissues and organs. Further examinations such as arteriograms, venograms, intravenous pyelograms and barium bowel studies may be necessary in order to assess the precise relationship of major blood vessels, ureters and other organs with the pseudotumour.

The contents of a pseudotumour are usually blood clots and necrotic tissues that are all avascular. The tumour may incorporate major blood vessels that complicate the surgical extraction. The capsule of the pseudotumour has a rich blood supply and this is most probably the reason for massive bleeding during tumour resection. Embolization of the pseudotumour's feeding arteries has been reported [7,8] and may be beneficial prior to surgery. This procedure can result in the reduction of the tumour's size and can also assist in preventing blood loss at surgery. The embolization should be performed close to the date of the surgery to avoid revascularization, which can occur within a few weeks.

Once all this information has been gathered, a multidisciplinary surgical team (for example, orthopaedic, general and vascular surgeons, urologist) needs to meet with the haematologist, physical medicine specialist and radiologist in order to discuss and set the boundaries of expectations. When dealing with giant pseudotumours, palliation of symptoms and improving the quality of life is generally a more realistic goal than total eradication of the tumour. The combined team should set priorities regarding procedures which are essential as opposed to those that are desirable, and decide whether the procedure can be undertaken in a single multidisciplinary session or whether surgery should be staged.

Treatment options

Embolization

Pseudotumours are avascular internally but have a very rich blood supply in the capsule. This is most probably the reason for the repeated haemorrhages inside the capsule, which result in the expansion of the mass. The rich vascular supply of the capsule is the cause of excessive bleeding during and after surgery, and this vascular supply usually originates from more than a single artery. Embolization alone has only a temporary effect, as canalization occurs within a few weeks. In view of its temporary effect embolization should be performed, as a preparatory procedure, about 2 weeks prior to surgery. This time lapse will allow for mass shrinkage but is insufficient for vessel restoration.

Irradiation

With regard to irradiation of the pseudotumour, the limited data suggest that this treatment modality may be beneficial for unresectable lesions [4,5]. The rationale for this treatment is the direct injury to the blood vessels feeding the pseudotumour and disruption to the endothelial proliferation of the pseudotumour's wall. Irradiation *prior* to surgery is not, in our opinion, recommended, as the ensuing fibrosis will make surgery more difficult. Once the pseudotumour has been excised, focal irradiation to any remaining capsule may be beneficial. The quantity of radiation delivered has been reported in the range 600–2350 Gy with delivery by multiple small dose (200 Gy) treatments. It was noted that radiotherapy was more effective when used in younger patients [5]. Two of our patients with huge pelvic pseudotumours received radiotherapy, one after repeated evacuation and the other after partial resection. We believe that the radiotherapy together with continuous infusion of factor replacement for long periods, maintaining factor levels above 10%, may halt the process.

Chemical and radioactive materials

While joint cavities have been injected by chemical and radioactive materials in order to destroy the synovium, the interior of a pseudotumour is not comparable. Theoretically, this injection may have a similar effect by irradiating the capsular blood vessels. This may be effective in small pseudotumours [9], but has not been described in large pseudotumours. The interior of a large pseudotumour is usually divided into compartments that would prevent the spread of the injected material. Should some of the capsular blood vessels become affected, revascularization may follow shortly. The puncture of the pseudotumour with its necrotic contents and poor internal vascularization carries a considerable risk of infection and the formation of a chronic fistula.

Percutaneous evacuation

Percutaneous evacuation of the contents of the pseudotumour may be difficult for the structural reasons described above. Furthermore, the capsule will continue to bleed and the pseudotumour will reconstitute. The high risk of introducing an infection and causing a permanent fistula versus the low expected benefit makes this procedure questionable. There may be some value in this treatment modality for small localized lesions where the empty space may be packed with fibrin glue. A combined approach was used in one of our patients with a giant pelvic pseudotumour. The patient underwent repeated evacuation of the mass and the dead space was filled with fibrin glue and the area irradiated. He received a continuous infusion of factor VIII for 2 years in order to prevent rebleeding inside the capsule. This treatment resulted in the shrinking of the pseudotumour mass and substantial improvement in the patient's condition, although he has a persistent fistula and recurrent infections. A more detailed description is presented in the Haemophilia Forum website.

Surgical principles

The surgical principles were described by Gilbert [10], who noted that if removal of the capsule could endanger a vital structure it is better left intact. Surgery is the most effective treatment and should be performed upon diagnosis when the pseudotumour is still small and relatively easily resected. In many instances, it is tempting to try prophylactic replacement therapy, hoping that the pseudotumour will not evolve or will even resolve. Such treatment has been found to be ineffective [3]. Complete resection when possible *is* a curative modality. Dissection of the mass should be carried out circumferentially as far as possible. When it is impossible to excise the entire wall, then as much as possible should be excised [10]. Fibrin glue should be used to obliterate the cavity in small cysts and in large pseudotumours fibrin glue should be used as an adjuvant [11]. Many methods have been employed to eliminate the dead space and they include the use of the omentum [12], muscles [13], dexon mash [7] and bone grafting [6].

The spraying of fibrin glue onto large raw areas is in our opinion mandatory, for it is effective in preventing immediate bleeding from the raw areas and minimizes the postoperative risk of haemorrhage. In one of our patients a mass the size of a football was removed from the pelvic area. No intraoperative blood transfusion was necessary and the postoperative blood loss was only 45 mL.

Our centre has been involved in the treatment of two patients who owing to their large tumours were doomed to be bedridden. After partial tumour resection in one, and drainage with cyst filling with glue, irradiation and prolonged continuous infusion in the other, the first patient returned to working and walking and the other was able to sit in a wheelchair. In another patient, only about one-third of the mass could be removed and at follow-up, a month later, the tumour had enlarged beyond its original size.

One of the major problems with surgery in patients with massive pseudotumours is that one knows the starting point but one is never sure of where and when the procedure will end. The decision to operate should not be taken lightly, for the complications include fistula formation, regrowth of the pseudotumour, sepsis, bleeding and death.

Haematological evaluation is carried out preoperatively. Pharmacokinetic evaluation is carried out according to Morfini *et al.* [14]. This is essential for the planning of replacement therapy and is especially important in countries with limited resources where the overall factor requirements for the surgery and the postoperative period have to be known in advance in order to secure sufficient supplies of concentrate. Preoperative pharmacokinetic evaluation is especially important in patients with inhibitors owing to the large variations in the pharmacokinetic parameters of recombinant factor VIIa between patients and even in the same patient during different periods of treatment [15].

Factor replacement therapy

Based on our experience with numerous surgical procedures, we follow the following protocol for factor replacement. A bolus dose calculated from the pharmacokinetic evaluation is intended to raise the circulating factor level to 80–100% just prior to surgery. In addition, a preoperative bolus of antifibrinolytic agent (tranexamic acid 15–25 mg/kg) is given routinely in our centre for all surgical procedures in persons with haemophilia. In addition to the bolus, patients receive about 20 mg/kg three times daily for 2–3 weeks. Although the benefit of this treatment has not been proven in the prevention of rebleeding, the rationale of blocking or reducing clot degradation together with the very low risk of thromboembolic complications makes this treatment desirable.

Continuous infusion of coagulation concentrates has been proven in a prospective study to be safer than 12-hourly doses, with significantly lower risks of dangerous drops in factor levels, lower postoperative blood loss and a lower risk of a major postoperative bleed. Continuous factor infusion saves at least 36% of factor concentrate requirements and theoretically even higher savings have been achieved [16]. Since 1990, this protocol has been followed in our centre and we feel it is desirable in operations with a high risk of major postoperative complications; as with pseudotumour resection. The rate of infusion is calculated from a steady-state equation using the clearance from the preoperative pharmacokinetic evaluation [17].

Rate of infusion = clearance × desired level
(IU/kg/h)   (mL/kg/h) (IU/mL)

Because of the known phenomenon of the gradual decline in the rate of clearance in the first week of continuous infusion [17] the daily circulating factor levels are measured. The new clearance is then calculated and the dose adjusted according to the equation. This reduction in clearance rate is the source of further saving of factor concentrate.

Our target factor levels for pseudotumour surgery are 80% for the first 3 days, 60% until day 10, and thereafter 50% until day 21. Where only partial resection of the pseudotumour is possible, factor levels are retained, by continuous infusion, at a minimum of 10% for prolonged periods. One of our patients received a continuous infusion of factor for 2 years and during this time numerous attempts were made to halt the continuous infusion and treat with prophylactic bolus injections, but each time the patient bled. During a surgical procedure one patient developed massive uncontrolled intraoperative bleeding from a large cavity in the ileum where the pseudotumour capsule persisted. The patient's factor VIII level was 80% and an additional bolus of factor VIII was ineffective. A single dose of 90 mg/kg of recombinant factor VIIa immediately halted the bleeding. Sufficient crossmatched blood and replacement products should be held in stock, especially for patients with inhibitors. Intra- and postoperative disseminated intravascular coagulation may be encountered in patients who have received large quantities of blood replacement.

Care of the patient

The management of patients with massive pseudotumours, where the aim of treatment is improvement of the quality of life and not total eradication of the tumour, requires that the patient and his family have an understanding of the treatment goals. It is essential that psychological counselling be available prior to, during and after the surgical procedure. Long-term follow-up is essential as instances of tumour regrowth have been reported. Should further surgery be necessary, the timing of this secondary procedure is significant, particularly if the initial surgery dealt mainly with tumour debulking. The additional fibrosis resulting from previous surgery compounded with the fibrosis within and of the pseudotumour wall makes the differentiation and separation of tissues complicated and vital structures may be inadvertently damaged.

This chapter has dealt with massive intra- and retroperitoneal pseudotumours, but these masses may also appear within a limb, causing extensive destruction to the musculoskeletal system. Limb salvage should always be seen in the light of the ultimate expected function. If by excision of the tumour a functional limb can be achieved, even if a brace is required, then the limb should be saved, but where salvage is likely to lead to severe functional compromise it is more advisable to amputate the limb and provide the patient with a prosthesis [18].

SUMMARY

Our report is based upon our limited experience and hence it would not be appropriate for us to suggest strict guidelines for the management of giant pseudotumours. It is our belief that pseudotumours should be excised in order to prevent them from reaching inoperable dimensions. The surgical procedure should be meticulously planned by a multidisciplinary team and as much as possible of the tumour resected. The intraoperative raw areas should be sprayed with fibrin glue and the remaining capsule should be irradiated. In order to decrease the chances of postoperative bleeding, factor replacement should be delivered by continuous infusion.

REFERENCES

1 Heim M, Horoszowski H, Schulman S et al. Multifocal pseudotumour in a single limb. Haemophilia 1997; 3: 50–3.

2 Ahlberg AKM. On the natural history of hemophilic pseudotumor. J Bone Joint Surg (Am) 1975; 57A: 1133–5.

3 Magallon M, Monteagudo J, Altisent C et al. Hemophilic pseudotumor: multicenter experience over a 25-year period. Am J Hematol 1994; 45: 103–8.

4 Meyers L, Hakami N. Pseudotumor of hemophilia in the orbit: the role of radiotherapy in management. Am J Hematol 1985; 19: 99–104.

5 Castaneda V, Parmley R, Bozzini M, Feldmeier J. Radiotherapy of pseudotumors of bone in hemophiliacs with circulating inhibitors to Factor VIII. Am J Hematol 1991; 36: 55–9.

6 Iwata H, Oishi Y, Itoh A et al. Surgical excision of hemophilic pseudotumor of the ileum. Clin Orthop 1992; 284: 234–8.

7 Sevilla J, Alvarez MT, Hernandez D et al. Therapeutic embolization and surgical excision of haemophilic pseudotumour. Haemophilia 1999; 5: 360–3.

8 Pisco JM, Garcia VL, Martins JM, Mascarenhas AM. Hemophilic pseudotumor treated with transcatheter arterial embolization: case report. Angiology 1990; 41: 1070–4.

9 Fernandez-Palazzi F, Rivas S. The use of "fibrin seal" in surgery of coagulation diseases with special reference to cysts and pseudotumors. In: Dohring S, Schulitz KP, eds. Orthopedic Problems in Hemophilia. Munich: W Zuckshwerdt, 1986: 170–9.

10 Gilbert M. Pseudotumors (hemophilic blood cysts) In: Forbes CD, Aledort LM, Madhok R, eds. Hemophilia. London: Chapman & Hall, 1997: 123–30.

11 Fernandez-Palazzi F, Rivas S, Marulanda A, Boada A, de Saez AR, de Bosch NB. On two extensive surgeries of giant soft tissue haemophilic pseudotumors of the thigh (abstract). Presented at the World Federation of Hemophilia 5th Musculo-skeletal Congress, Sydney, Australia, April 1999.

12 Bellinazzo P, Silvello L, Caimi MT, Baudo F, De Cataldo F. Novel surgical approach to pseudotumour of ileum in haemophilia. Lancet 1989; 340: 1333–4.

13 Heeg M, Smit WM, Van Der Meer J, Van Horn JR. Excision of a haemophilic pseudotumour of the ileum, complicated by fistulation. Haemophilia 1998; 4: 132–5.

14 Morfini M, Lee M, Messori A. The design and analysis of half-life and recovery studies of factor VIII and factor IX. Thromb Haemost 1991; 61: 384–6.

15 Schulman S, Bech Jensen M, Varon D et al. Feasibility of using recombinant factor VIIa in continuous infusion. Thromb Haemost 1996; 75: 432-6.

16 Batorova A, Martinowitz U. Intermittent injections vs continuous infusion of FVIII in haemophilia patients undergoing major surgery (submitted for publication).

17 Martinowitz U, Schulman S, Gitel S, Horoszowski H, Heim M Varon D. Adjusted dose continuous infusion of factor VIII in patients with haemophilia A. Br J Haematol 1992; 82: 729–34.

18 Heim M, Azaria M, Heijnen L. Lower limb prosthetic considerations in persons with coagulopathies. Haemophilia 1997; 3: 87–9.

CHAPTER 17

Articular Contracture of the Knee

E C RODRIGUEZ-MERCHAN, M BLANCO, C LOPEZ-CABARCOS AND A VILLAR

INTRODUCTION

Treatment options are varied in the management of articular contractures of the knee in haemophiliacs, and decision-making is based on the degree of the contracture, its chronicity, the presence of articular subluxation, the patient's ability to participate in treatment and the available medical facilities.

Treatment should primarily be by physiotherapy, splintage and corrective devices, although the late or severe case may require surgical correction in the form of soft-tissue procedures. Soft-tissue correction of muscle shortening may be performed, such as hamstring release of the flexor muscles of the knee. Lower femoral osteotomy has been used for correction of flexion deformity at the knee joint, and mechanical distraction using external fixators for treatment of severe knee flexion contractures has been reported by Heim *et al.* with satisfactory results [1]. The main principle underlying the treatment of haemophilic contracture is the restoration of the patient's lifestyle and mobility, rather than anatomical or radiographic normality.

AETIOLOGY AND PATHOGENESIS OF KNEE FLEXION CONTRACTURE

Flexion deformity results from several causes. The painful knee will assume a flexed posture for comfort, particularly if a severe haemarthrosis is present, as this position allows for greater accommodation of fluid within the joint. Hamstring spasm is common, with the painful haemarthrosis causing the knee to be held in flexion to lessen the irritability in the muscle group. Although pure flexion contraction can exist alone, it is probably more common where there are other associated deformities.

Fixed flexion deformity may be complicated by posterior subluxation and external rotation of the tibia due to the pull of the hamstring muscles, tethering of the iliotibial band, shortening of the anterior cruciate ligament and contraction of the posterior capsule. These deforming forces can also produce a valgus deformity. A hip flexion contracture and/or an equinus foot deformity will also contribute to flexion deformity at the knee.

Flexion deformity of the knee is associated with both soft-tissue and bony changes. Although soft-tissue involvement is global, the fixed contractures that develop primarily involve contracture of the structures posterior to the axis of knee rotation. The posterior capsule is particularly contracted and adherent to the posterior femur and tibia. The posterior cruciate ligament can be contracted, together with the hamstring tendons, especially the semimembranosus. Proliferative posterior osteophytes can contribute to the flexion contracture because of the tethering effect.

The articular surface of the knee demonstrates severe destruction of the articular cartilage and compensatory changes produced by load-bearing on a flexed knee when walking. The posterior surfaces of the tibial plateau are generally depressed, causing an exaggerated posterior slope of the tibial articular surface and increased subchondral bone sclerosis. As the knee is extended during the stance phase of gait, a hingeing rather than the normal gliding motion occurs, causing anterior impingement of the tibia and femur. This leads to irreversible damage to the articular surface at the site of impingement. The distal femur may also demonstrate flattening along its posterior condylar margin. Asymmetric deformity will occur with fixed external rotation and valgus deformity.

To constitute a true fixed flexion contracture, the deformity must persist despite local or systemic analgesia to alleviate the pain. Persistent flexion contractures cause a significant ambulatory deficit, with patients unable to obtain full extension to achieve adequate relaxation of the quadriceps mechanism. Therefore, the correction of flexion deformity is a tremendous advantage during any total knee arthroplasty [2].

TREATMENT

Articular contractures in patients with haemophilia are the result of recurrent intra-articular and intramuscular bleeding episodes. Approximately 50% of people with severe haemophilia (factor VIII or IX level <2 IU/dL) have articular contractures >10°, which can be disabling, causing decreased mobility and functional impairment. The management of an articular contracture in a patient with haemophilia represents a major challenge, as the problems that arise are complex and require a range of knowledge, from an understanding of basic biological events to fine details of surgical technique [3]. The treatments available are physiotherapy, orthotics and corrective devices, and surgical procedures. End-stage arthropathy of the knee is the most frequent cause of severe pain and disability in haemophiliacs. Some patients have such severe arthropathy that a total joint arthroplasty is required.

Physiotherapy

The aim of physiotherapy is to maintain muscle power and a good range of joint movement. Patients with haemophilia have unique and complicated problems, and the assignment of a special physiotherapist to care for them is an invaluable aid. According to Buzzard [4] it is esential that those with haemophilia are taught the importance of physical fitness at an early age as a means of preventing articular contractures. Physiotherapy is of great importance in this field, especially in Third World countries where the supply of replacement products are scarce or non-existent.

Heijnen and De Kleijn [5] have reported that articular contractures are impairments that cannot be cured by means of physiotherapy because of the pathophysiology of the joints. Rehabilitation, however, tries to diminish the disabilities and prevent handicaps caused by the impairments. Physiotherapy aims at pain reduction by means of manual traction. In addition to manual traction, an intensive physiotherapy programme includes mobilization techniques, muscle strengthening exercises and stretching, joint stability training, postural and gait training, and functional training. The role of physiotherapy in the case of articular contractures is limited; so ideally, physiotherapy should be instituted before articular contractures are present.

Orthotics and corrective devices

Several specific devices have been used to overcome haemophilic contractures.

Serial casting and wedging, and extension/desubluxation orthoses (EDO)
The most basic of these is the serial application of plaster of Paris casts, which are changed approximately weekly as the deformity is gradually overcome, but such serial casting can be complicated by skin necrosis, joint cartilage compression and joint subluxation. For the non-operative treatment of flexion contracture of the haemophilic knee Fernandez-Palazzi and Battistella [6] have used serial casting and wedging in 58 patients, and extension/desubluxation orthoses in 13 patients. On average it was possible to achieve –5° of extension by 4 weeks, with only a little improvement in the following 4 weeks. The short- to medium-term results using either extension/desubluxation hinges or serial casting were similar. Both methods have been shown to result in significant improvement in joint contracture. An extension-only hinge device between cylinder casts on a thigh and calf is currently being used by Dr Teixeira in Belo Horizonte (Brazil) for the treatment of severe knee flexion contractures. He is also using the bidirectional EDO, and Dr Llinas in Bogotá (Colombia) has also begun to use it [C.K. Kasper, personal communication]. It is copied from the original used at the Orthopedic Hospital, Los Angeles with great success in the first 10–15 years of this centre at a time when Dr Kasper and her colleagues were still seeing many patients from the countryside with severe flexion contractures.

These non-invasive methods are generally successful in mild contractures, and are used as adjuncts after radical soft-tissue release, in order to stretch the tight neurovascular structures gradually. The amount of corrective force that may be applied with casts, splints and braces is limited by the inability of the skin to tolerate direct pressure. Additionally, these methods can cause articular subluxation.

Reversed slings and inflatable splints
Serial casting has been supplemented by the use of reversed dynamic slings and inflatable splints (Flowtron Machine, Huntleigh Medical, Luton, England). Reversed dynamic slings require admission to hospital and close supervision, whereas Flowtron is easy to use and suitable for home treatment [7].

SURGICAL PROCEDURES

Late or severe cases may require surgical correction in the form of soft tissue procedures, osteotomies or mechanical distraction using external fixators.

Soft-tissue procedures

In this situation, the chronically contracted vessels and nerves prevent full correction. Rodriguez-Merchan *et al.* [8] and Wallny *et al.* [9] have demonstrated that hamstring release and dorsal capsulotomy in fixed knee flexion contracture is beneficial, if strict criteria are adhered to [8] (Fig. 17.1). This technique is particularly recommended for early forms of arthropathy. However, the soft-tissue procedures are often insufficient to gain full correction.

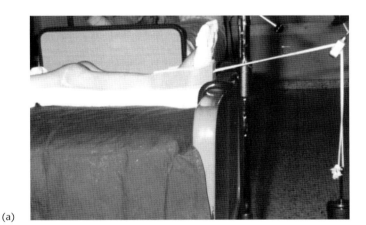

(a)

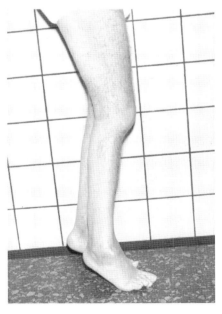

(b)

Fig. 17.1 A 30° flexion contracture of the right knee in a 14-year-old boy who was treated by hamstring release and posterior capsulotomy. (a) Preoperative soft traction commonly used in these cases; (b) standing: note the knee flexion contracture associated with equinus deformity. (*Continued.*)

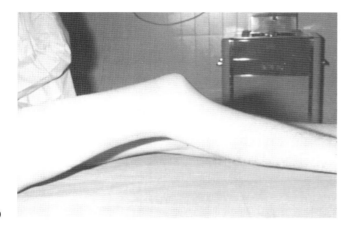

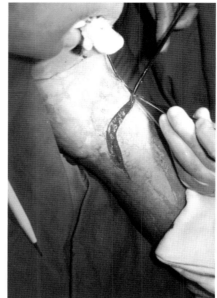

(c)

(d)

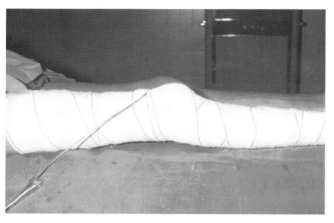

(e)

Fig. 17.1 (*Continued.*) (c) Supine: the degree of flexion contracture can be seen; (d) a posterior surgical approach is commonly used; (e) after surgery the involved knee is in full extension.

Osteotomies

The experience of Caviglia *et al.* [10] has shown how osteotomy performed for flexion contracture brings to the patient a better quality of life, scarcely impinging on the range of motion but placing it on a more useful level in which there is a low incidence of complications. However, supracondylar extension osteotomy of the femur creates a secondary deformity (angulation and shortening) instead of correcting the deformity, and may lead to abnormal joint-loading forces when the patient walks.

Mechanical distraction using external fixators

Russian investigators have developed external fixators to produce gradual joint distraction and to allow ambulatory treatment [11]. These fixators represent a more efficient way of applying forces to the skeletal deformity. Advantages of these techniques include versatility and minimized risk of neurovascular complications. Problems encountered include a rebound phenomenon after frame removal, with loss of the temporarily increased total arc of motion [12].

Experimental evidence suggests that low-load prolonged stretch is preferred to high-load brief intermittent stretch in the elongation of collagen. There are still two unanswered questions: Why does the muscle stretch? How can the rebound phenomenon be minimized? A combination of continued clinical and basic research will, it is hoped, provide answers to these questions. The results obtained with mechanical distraction by external fixators warrant its wider application.

Correction of fixed contractures during total knee arthroplasty

For a fixed deformity to pose a significant surgical challenge, the deformity must usually exceed 30°. The insertion of a semiconstrained knee replacement requires a thorough understanding of the relationship between component and overall alignment and stability through flexion and extension. Small flexion contractures can be reduced by removal of posterior osteophytes, elevation of the posterior capsule, and a few millimetres of extra distal femoral bone resection. Correction by bone resection alone unbalances the collateral ligaments so that stability in extension is provided by the tight posterior capsule [13].

The procedure should be performed under tourniquet control. Preoperative antibiotic prophylaxis is indicated and appropriate factor concentrate should be given immediately preoperatively to achieve at least 100% level at the time of surgery. A straight longitudinal midline incision is recommended, followed by a medial parapatellar arthrotomy. In addition to the intra-articular supracondylar fibrosis, a common finding is a significant extensor mechanism contracture, which makes exposure very difficult.

A quadricepsplasty may be required for exposure. This can be done using the inverted V incision with the apex in the quadriceps tendon, the quadriceps snip or a distal tibial tubercle osteotomy. A synovectomy should be performed following the exposure if synovial hypertrophy exists. The medial collateral ligament is approached as in any primary total knee replacement. Distally, the superficial fibres of the medial collateral ligament can be elevated from the bony surface of the tibia quite easily. The medial collateral ligament dissection has to be carried posteriorly as far as the semimembranosus attachment on the posterior tibia. This manoeuvre, and the excision of the anterior cruciate ligament (if still present), will allow for translocation of the tibia anteriorly.

Lateral release
The anterior cruciate ligament is excised and a lateral release is performed, prior to any bone resection. The anatomical elements of a lateral release are the lateral capsule, lateral ligament, arcuate ligament, popliteus tendon, lateral femoral periosteum, distal iliotibial tract and adjacent lateral intramuscular septum. In addition, associated flexion contracture requires posterior capsulotomy. The first stage of a lateral release is the separation of the iliotibial band from its insertion to the tibia, including Gerdy's tubercle, and separation of the capsular attachments from the lateral margin of the tibia.

Further stages of a lateral release include raising a flap from the lateral femoral condyle to a point 75 mm proximal to the joint. The periosteum is incised transversely. The lateral intramuscular septum and proximal iliotibial tract are divided transversely at the same level. The remaining distal attachment of the lateral intramuscular septum is divided vertically and separated from the femur [14]. Such an extensive release, although likely to correct almost any deformity, may leave a posterolateral instability in flexion that can lead to subluxation. Extensive stripping of the lateral femoral condyle reduces its vascularity. After the fixed valgus deformity is corrected with lateral soft-tissue release, attention is paid to the correction of the flexion contracture [15].

Posterior capsulotomy

Posterior capsulotomy is the preferred method for severe contractures. The shortened posterior capsule is first separated from the collateral structures by making vertical incisions at the medial and lateral corners and the posterior capsule is divided transversely close to the femoral attachment. Resection of the posterior cruciate ligament is most likely necessary and aids in the division of the midline fibres. The dissection should be done with the knee flexed, applying distal traction on the capsule. In almost all cases, the posterior cruciate ligament has to be sacrificed because of its shortening during the prolonged flexed position. This can be most easily accomplished in the area of the intercondylar notch proximally on the femur, giving additional access to the posterior soft-tissue structures of the femur.

All posterior osteophytes and loose bodies can be removed from the posterior condyles of the femur with a right-angled curette. On removing the osteophytes, the posterior capsule attachment on the femur can be easily seen; now, from both medial and lateral approaches, it can be stripped in the coronal plane in 90° of flexion to protect the posterior vessels. If it is still not possible to obtain full extension after stripping the posterior capsule from the femur, the proximal heads of the gastrocnemius complex on the femur can also be stripped far proximally on the femur. Posterior capsular release should be done after the bone cuts, because until they are made posterior visualization is poor and impeded by the posterior femoral condyles [16].

Bony approach

Bone cuts of the distal femur and proximal tibia should initially be conservative. After the capsulotomy, the components are inserted and the knee brought into as much extension as possible. If extension is still not complete, further bone can be removed from the distal femur. The distal femur is best approached following intramedullary instrumentation. The ultimate limit of resection is the soft-tissue attachment of the posterior cruciate and collateral ligaments, although, in most cases of severe deformity, the posterior cruciate ligament will need to be sacrificed.

Excessive femoral resection will also move the joint line proximally, negatively affecting extension stability and patello-femoral forces. Following adequate femoral resection, the proximal tibia can then be approached. It is also important not to excise excessive tibial bone because of two separate factors [2]: first, flexion stability is lost with excessive tibial loss and, second, tibial bone stock becomes worse due to the inverted 'cone' effect of the proximal tibia in metaphyseal bone.

All posterior osteophytes and loose bodies must be removed from the posterior condyles of the femur with a right-angled curette. There is no necessity for an incision through the posterior capsule, which may jeopardize the posterior neurovascular structures. The patella should be routinely resurfaced with a polyethylene component, unless there has previously been a patellectomy. A lateral retinacular release is required in most haemophilic knees to permit proper tracking of the patella and 90° of knee flexion. The tourniquet is deflated after the placement of the implants. After wound closure, a bulky compressive knee dressing with plaster splints is placed and maintained postoperatively for 5 to 7 days, followed by active physiotherapy.

It is wise to splint the knee in extension after correcting severe contractures, but the limb must be carefully observed for signs of peroneal and posterior nerve palsies. Peroneal nerve palsy should be treated by prompt removal of the dressing and flexion of the operative knee to 20–30°. In patients who have absent nerve function not responding in the immediate postoperative period, long-term follow-up has shown complete motor recovery is rarely achieved.

SUMMARY

Treatment of knee contractures in patients with haemophilia should be primarily by physiotherapy, splintage and corrective devices. The late or severe case may require surgical correction in the form of soft-tissue procedures (hamstring release of the flexor muscles of the knee). Lower femoral osteotomy has been used for correction of flexion deformity at the knee joint, and satisfactory results have been reported for mechanical distraction using external fixators for treatment of severe knee flexion contractures. Restoration of the patient's lifestyle and mobility, rather than anatomical or radiographic normality, is the main aim of treatment of haemophilic contracture [17].

REFERENCES

1 Heim M, Horoszowski H, Varon D, Schulman S, Martinowitz U. The fixed flexed and subluxed knee in the haemophilic child: what should be done?. *Haemophilia* 1996; **1**: 47–50.

2 Colwell CW Jr. Fixed flexion contracture. In: Fu FH, Harner CD, Vince KG, eds. *Knee Surgery*, Vol. 2. Baltimore: Williams & Wilkins, 1994: 1391–7.

3 Atkins RM, Henderson MA, Duthie RB. Joint contractures in the hemophilias. *Clin Orthop* 1987; **219**: 97–106.

4 Buzzard BM. Physiotherapy for the prevention of articular contraction in haemophilia. *Haemophilia* 1999; **5** (Suppl. 1): 10–15.

5 Heijnen L, De Kleijn P. Physiotherapy for the treatment of articular contractures in haemophilia. *Haemophilia* 1999; **5** (Suppl. 1): 16–99.

6 Fernandez-Palazzi F, Battistella LR. Non-operative treatment of flexion contracture of the knee in haemophilia. *Haemophilia* 1999; **5** (Suppl. 1): 20–4.

7 Nelson IW, Atkins RM, Allen AL. The management of knee flexion contractures in haemophilia: brief report. *J Bone Joint Surg (Br)* 1989; **71B**: 327–8.

8 Rodriguez-Merchan EC, Magallon M, Galindo E, Lopez-Cabarcos C. Hamstring release for fixed knee flexion contracture in hemophilia. *Clin Orthop* 1997; **343**: 63–7.

9 Wallny T, Eickhoff HH, Raderschadt G, Brackmann HH. Hamstring release and posterior capsulotomy for fixed knee flexion contracture in haemophiliacs. *Haemophilia* 1999; **5** (Suppl. 1): 25–7.

10 Caviglia HA, Perez-Bianco R, Galatro G, Duhalde C, Tezanos-Pinto M. Extensor supracondylar osteotomy as treatment for flexed haemophilic knee. *Haemophilia* 1999; **5** (Suppl. 1): 28–32.

11 Volkov MV, Oganesyan OV. Restoration of function in the knee and elbow with a hinge-distractor apparatus. *J Bone Joint Surg (Am)* 1975; **57A**: 591–600.

12 Herzenberg JE, Davis JR, Paley D, Bhave A. Mechanical

distraction for treatment of severe knee flexion contractures. *Clin Orthop* 1994; **301**: 80–8.

13 Lachiewicz PF. Management of the knee in hemophilia. In: Insall JN, ed. *Surgery of the Knee*, 2nd edn. New York: Churchill Livingstone, 1993: 1149–69.

14 Insall JN. Surgical techniques and instrumentation in total knee arthroplasty. In: Insall JN, ed. *Surgery of the Knee*, 2nd edn. New York: Churchill Livingstone, 1993: 739–804.

15 Ranawat CS. Total-condylar knee arthroplasty for valgus and combined valgus-flexion deformity of the knee. In: Ranawat CS, ed. *Total-Condylar Knee Arthroplasty. Technique, Results, and Complications*. New York: Springer, 1985: 31–40.

16 Sculco TP. Technique of correction of flexion contracture during total knee arthroplasty. In: Ranawat CS, ed. *Total-Condylar Knee Arthroplasty. Technique, Results, and Complications*. New York: Springer, 1985: 51–3.

17 Rodriguez-Merchan EC. Therapeutic options in the management of articular contractures in haemophiliacs. *Haemophilia* 1999; **5** (Suppl. 1): 5–9.

CHAPTER 18

Arthroscopy in Haemophilia

H H EICKHOFF AND J D WIEDEL

INTRODUCTION

Haemophilic arthropathy produces a wide range of pathological and radiological signs [1–3]. According to Hofmann [4], 35% of all joint bleeding episodes affect the knee, followed by the ankle joint (27.5%) and the elbow joint (25%). After the age of 30 years, 90% of the knee joints in patients with haemophilia have sustained severe destruction. Open synovectomy of the knee after arthrotomy in patients with haemophilia was first described by Storti *et al.* in 1969 [5], while more recently arthroscopic synovectomy has been used to treat haemophilic knee joints [6–8]. Kim *et al.* [9] and Wiedel [10] reported on the first experiences with arthroscopic synovectomy of the knee at the World Federation of Hemophilia Congress in Stockholm, Sweden, in 1983 and both authors later published their results [11,12]. Luck and Kasper [13] performed the procedure in nine cases with severe arthropathy and stressed the advantages of arthroscopy in comparison with arthrotomy. Arthroscopy, as a relatively low-risk technique, can be used to achieve good results for haemophilic ankle arthropathy as well [14].

TECHNIQUE

Knee joint

A closed-circuit video system, a 30° standard arthroscope and the usual arthroscopic hand instruments are needed. The procedure has to be carried out under general anaesthesia with the patient supine. A leg holder or a lateral post is used and a tourniquet is essential. Joint distension is maintained by electrolyte or non-electrolyte solution, depending on the type of the electrosurgical equipment (monopolar or bipolar). The authors use a pressure and flow controlled irrigation pump. In severe arthropathy, adhesions are a major problem because of the impaired distension of the joint cavity and orientation. Therefore, at the beginning of the operation the movement of the arthroscope is difficult and vision is reduced. In such cases and in every synovectomy, a shaving device is needed. For haemostasis and tissue ablation, electrosurgical instruments are necessary. Multiple procedures can be performed during each arthroscopic assessment (i.e. lavage, plica resection, resection of adhesions, meniscal resection, cartilage shaving, synovectomy). To perform a synovectomy, in addition to the two anterior standard portals, two suprapatellar and two posterior portals are essential. Portals are changed in order to reach all regions of the joint. At the end of the operation, an intra-articular drain is mandatory for at least 2 days. Before releasing the tourniquet a compression bandage is applied.

Ankle joint

The same arthroscopic equipment as described above is needed. Three arthroscopic portals are established (anteromedial, anterolateral and posterolateral). After incising the skin, the subcutaneous tissue is bluntly dissected in order to avoid nerve damage. Transillumination is required for establishing the second portal. In addition, an ankle distraction device has to be applied in most cases of severe haemophilic arthropathy because of the rigid capsule. Medial pin placement in the tibia and talus allows dorsiflexion of the foot while maintaining parallel separation of the joint surfaces. The proximal pin is placed in the medial side of the tibia approximately 4 cm above the joint line, entering one cortex only, parallel to the joint line. The distal pin is driven from medial to lateral into the body of the talus, beginning from a skin puncture placed just inferior and slightly anterior to the palpable tip of the medial malleolus.

This medial entry point places the pin near the central rotation axis of the talar dome. Using the distractor, the joint surfaces are separated about 7 mm under direct arthroscopic visualization.

A normal 30° arthroscope is used. With an electric shaver system a synovectomy or débridement is performed beginning in the anterior compartment. Portals are changed in order to reach all areas. A special chisel and a grasper are useful for removing a large anterior tibial osteophyte.

For synovectomy of the posterior compartment the arthroscope is guided posteriorly. The shaver is placed through the posterolateral portal. When synovectomy is completed, the distractor is removed and a drain is placed through one of the anterior portals. All incisions are closed with single stitches and a simple dressing is applied.

POSTOPERATIVE TREATMENT

Active physiotherapy has to begin immediately. After knee arthroscopies, continuous passive motion on a machine and electrostimulation of the muscles is applied additionally.

FACTOR REPLACEMENT

Preoperatively, factor replacement was administered to produce a concentration of 30–40%. Immediately before surgery, factor activity was raised to 80–100% by giving approximately 30–40 IU/kg of body weight. Postoperatively a coagulation test was performed and, if required, factor was given again. Until the 4th postoperative day factor concentration was kept at 60%, and until the 14th day a factor concentration of 50% was maintained. During the following period of intensive physiotherapy the factor concentration was kept at 20%. After rehabilitation, a return to normal concentrations was allowed.

RESULTS

Knee joint

Medium-term results are available for 20 arthroscopic operations in 19 patients [8] whose mean age was 30 years (range 14–53 years). In 18 patients the preoperative factor activity was less than 1%. The radiographs showed a high degree of joint destruction in all cases. The 10 patients who underwent arthroscopic total synovectomy (all late synovectomies) were considered separately. The mean follow-up time for all patients was 5 years (range 4–7 years), and for the synovectomy group alone 5 years (range 4–6 years). Comparative criteria preoperatively and postoperatively were pain, the amount of extension deficiency and the subjective judgement of the patient.

Pain
Intensity of pain was graded as severe, moderate, mild or none. Comparison of preoperative and postoperative grades showed significant pain reduction for all patients and for the synovectomy group alone (Table 18.1). The two patients with severe pain preoperatively had advanced arthropathy with acute bleeding. After lavage of the joint, these two patients underwent synovectomy.

Extension deficiency
To judge the range of movement of the affected joint, the ability to straighten the leg was examined and was expressed by extension deficiency or lag. The individual changes are shown for each patient (Table 18.2).

Subjective judgement
The results of the operation as judged subjectively by the patients are shown in Table 18.3 (significant improvement, moderate improvement, no improvement or deterioration). In 18 of 20 cases, there was a significant or moderate improvement. There was no deterioration in subjective assessment. In the two patients in the synovectomy group who

Table 18.1 Pain: preoperative and postoperative comparison.

Pain	Total ($n=20$)		Synovectomy group ($n=10$)	
	Preoperative	Postoperative	Preoperative	Postoperative
Severe	2	0	2	0
Moderate	10	1	6	1
Mild	7	13	1	8
None	1	6	1	1

Table 18.2 Extension deficiency (in degrees of extension lag): preoperative and postoperative comparison.

Case	Nonsynovectomy group ($n = 10$)		Synovectomy group ($n=10$)	
	Preoperative	Postoperative	Preoperative	Postoperative
1	0	0	0	5
2	0	0	5	5
3	0	0	5	5
4	0	0	10	0
5	0	0	10	5
6	0	0	10	5
7	10	5	10	10
8	10	10	20	5
9	10	10	25	10
10	20	10	30	0

Table 18.3 Subjective judgement of the operative result.

Subjective judgement	Total ($n=20$)	Synovectomy group ($n=10$)
Significant improvement	13	8
Moderate improvement	5	0
No improvement	2	2
Deterioration	0	0

experienced no improvement, the disappointing result was because of persistent pain.

Complications and reoperations

In six cases (one lateral release and five synovectomies), bleeding was a minor problem after the operation and was treated successfully by drainage, factor substitution, compression and cold packs.

An infection developed in one knee (*Staphylococcus epidermidis*) after synovectomy. Eleven days after the first operation, the patient underwent an arthroscopic revision with the use of an irrigation drainage system postoperatively. Continuous passive motion was begun immediately postoperatively and antibiotics were given. The final result was good and the follow-up showed a significant improvement. An extension deficiency of 10° preoperatively improved to 5° initially postoperatively but eventually returned to 10° again.

Long-term results are available in nine knees in nine patients [15] who underwent arthroscopic synovectomy between 1980 and 1985 for chronic haemophilic arthropathy involving the knee. The age at the time of surgery ranged from 8 to 36 years with an average of 16 years. The evaluation of these patients at 10–15 years' follow-up was based upon the objective criteria of recurrent haemarthroses, joint motion and radiographic evaluations (Table 18.4). The results clearly demonstrated that the patients maintained good functional status and had a decreased frequency of bleeding episodes. There was, however, evidence of progression of the haemophilic arthropathy. The loss of range of

Table 18.4 Long-term results of arthroscopic synovectomy in haemophilic knees.

Case	X-ray stage		Recurrent bleedings	Extension lag (°)		Follow-up time (yr)
	Preop.	Follow-up		Preop.	Follow-up	
1	IV	IV	None	5	5	15
2	II	V	After injury	0	20	15
3	IV	V	None	5	10	15
4	III	IV	None after 2nd procedure*	0	15	14
5	III	III	None	0	0	14
6	II	IV	None	0	0	12
7	III	III	None	0	0	11
8	II	III	None	20	0	10
9	IV	IV	Occasional	20	10	10

*Posteromedial synovectomy performed 10 months after initial procedure.

motion occurred both in flexion and extension and was limited to the final 10° but not to an extent that created functional impairment. The loss of motion was no more than expected from a slowly progressive intra-articular degenerative condition. The radiographic changes confirmed this progressive condition. The longer the follow-up, the greater the changes, which were demonstrated in all of the knees. Some of the knees did not change the stage of involvement, but there were progressive bony changes. The cartilage space was well maintained. This study showed clearly that arthroscopic synovectomy was successful in controlling the recurrent haemarthrosis and probably retarded the progression of the haemophilic arthropathy.

Ankle joint

Eickhoff *et al.* studied four patients [14], all of whom had a factor activity level less than 1%. In one case, a synovectomy alone and in another case a synovectomy and additionally an osteophyte resection at the ventral tibia were performed arthroscopically. In the case of a 37-year-old patient with von Willebrand's disease with severe arthropathy of the right side (Pettersson score 12), an arthrodesis, performed arthroscopically, was needed. With an electric shaver system a débridement was carried out. Care was taken to maintain the bony contour of the talar dome and the tibial plafond. Once viable cancellous bone is visualized surrounding the fusion area, the distraction device is released, and the surfaces are reduced. Under control of an image intensifier an internal fixation was obtained with two 6.5-mm cancellous screws (fibulotalar and tibiotalar) placed percutaneously. The patient is free of pain and very satisfied with the result.

An arthroscopic lavage was performed in a 4-year-old boy with a haematologically infected haemarthrosis of the left ankle joint. The joint infection was cured with additional antibiotics and 4 years after operation there was neither pain nor swelling. Unfortunately, there was a significant reduction in the range of movement in the affected joint (dorsal extension/plantar flexion: right 15/0/50, left 5/0/45).

DISCUSSION

In cases of haemophilic arthropathy, arthroscopy of the knee and ankle can be performed with satisfactory results. In particular, wound healing problems are avoidable using an arthroscopic technique because there is less soft-tissue damage. However, an arthroscopic operation in hae-mophilia is a demanding procedure and the surgeon should be skilled and should be experienced in the treatment of haemophilic muscu-loskeletal problems. The indications, the technique and the result are dependent on the stage of the arthropathy and the presenting prob-lems [16].

A major joint bleeding episode often leads to a persistent synovitis. Intra-articular blood clots are only slowly resorbed. Arthroscopic lavage allows several litres of fluid to pass through the joint, washing out clots. In addition, blood clots can be removed directly using a motorized shav-er.

In chronic or recurrent synovitis, synovectomy should be performed. The authors' experience is based on late synovectomies. Limbird and Dennis [17], who published five cases, stated that after arthroscopy there is less reduction of the range of movement. Our results confirm this finding. A study by Triantafyllou *et al.* [18] compared eight open syn-ovectomies with five arthroscopic synovectomies of the knee. The re-sults clearly demonstrated the benefit of arthroscopic synovectomy as regards postoperative rehabilitation and maintaining good functional range of motion.

Previous authors have performed late synovectomies [5,7,9,10,13,17–20]. Although there is a reduction in bleeding episodes, there is no sig-nificant improvement in the long-term prognosis in the presence of severe arthropathy [15,20]. Partial synovectomies or resection of the hypertrophic medial plica have a similar outcome. Permanent irrita-tion causes a local synovitis with a higher incidence of bleeding. As in the patient without haemophilia, mechanical problems can be solved successfully by arthroscopic resection.

The operation can be completed by meniscal resections, cartilage shaving, removal of loose bodies or complete débridement. The patient with haemophilia often has features suggestive of meniscal lesions, but very rarely are relevant lesions found intraoperatively. Cartilage shav-ing is indicated only if there are cartilage flaps or ulcers with loose bor-ders. As little resection as possible should be performed. Inhibitory antibodies to factor replacement are a contraindication for arthroscopy in haemophilic patients. Arthroscopy in these patients should be per-formed only in collaboration with an experienced haematology depart-ment [21]. In severe arthropathy, the use of the arthroscope should be limited, and if definite problems are encountered the procedure should be converted to open surgery immediately [22,23].

SUMMARY

Arthroscopy of the haemophilic knee and ankle can be performed with satisfactory results. The arthroscopic technique has proven to be very successful in significantly reducing the frequency of haemarthroses as well as maintaining good joint function over the long term. The indications, technique and result are dependent on the stage of the arthropathy and the presenting problems. Although the joint condition does progress over time, very few patients who undergo this procedure require any additional surgical management over a long period. The arthroscopic operation in haemophilia is a demanding procedure and the surgeon should be skilled and should have experience of the treatment of haemophilic musculoskeletal problems. Arthroscopic procedure in hemophiliacs should be done only in collaboration with an experienced haematology department.

REFERENCES

1 Arnold WD, Hilgartner MW. Hemophilic arthropathy. Current concepts of pathogenesis and management. *J Bone Joint Surg (Am)* 1997; **59A**: 287–305.

2 Stein H, Duthie RB. The pathogenesis of chronic haemophilic arthropathy. *J Bone Joint Surg (Br)* 1981; **63B**: 601–9.

3 Storti E, Magrini U, Castello A, Pandolfi M. The histochemistry of fibrinolysis in haemophilic synovial membranes. *Acta Haematol (Basel)* 1973; **49**: 142–53.

4 Hofmann P. Orthopaedische Probleme der plasmatischen Gerinnungsstoerungen. In: Witt AN, Rettig H, Schlegel KF, eds. *Orthopaedie in Praxis und Klinik*, Band VII, Teil 1. Stuttgart, New York: Georg Thieme, 1987: 16.1–16.56.

5 Storti E, Traldi A, Tosatti E, Davoli PG. Synovectomy, a new approach to haemophilic arthropathy. *Acta Haematol (Basel)* 1969; **41**: 193–205.

6 Casscells CD. Commentary: The argument for early arthroscopic synovectomy in patients with severe hemophilia. *Arthroscopy* 1987; **3**: 78–9.

7 Eickhoff HH, Koch W, Brackmann HH. Arthroskopische Behandlung der haemophilen Kniegelenkarthropathie. *Orthop Praxis* 1994; **8**: 477–82.

8 Eickhoff HH, Koch W, Raderschadt G, Brackmann HH. Arthroscopy for chronic hemophilic synovitis of the knee. *Clin Orthop* 1997; **343**: 58–62.

9 Kim HC, Klein K, Hirsch S *et al*. Arthroscopic synovectomy in the treatment of hemophilic synovitis. *Scand J Haematol* 1984; **33**: 271–9.

10 Wiedel JD. Arthroscopic synovectomy in hemophilic arthropathy of the knee. *Scand J Haematol* 1984; **33** (Suppl. 40): 263–70.

11 Klein KS, Aland CM, Kim HC, Eisele J, Saidi P. Long term follow-up of arthroscopic synovectomy for chronic hemophilic synovitis. *Arthroscopy* 1987; **3**: 231–6.

12 Wiedel JD. Arthroscopic synovectomy for chronic hemophilic synovitis of the knee. *Arthroscopy* 1985; **1**: 205–9.

13 Luck JV, Kasper CK. Surgical managment of advanced hemophilic arthropathy: an overview of 20 years' experience. *Clin Orthop* 1989; **242**: 60–82.

14 Eickhoff HH, Koch W, Seuser A *et al*. Orthopädische Therapie der hämophilen Synovitis und Arthropathie unter besonderer Berücksichtigung des oberen Sprunggelenkes. In: Scharrer I, Schramm W, eds. *28. Hämophilie-Symposium Hamburg 1997*. Berlin, Heidelberg, New York, Tokyo: Springer, 1998: 32–41.

15 Wiedel JD. Arthroscopic synovectomy of the knee in hemophilia: 10- to 15-year followup. *Clin Orthop* 1996; **328**: 46–53.

16 Eickhoff HH, Raderschadt G, Koch W, Brackmann HH. Control of the synovium in haemophilila. *Haemophilia* 1998; **4**: 511–13.

17 Limbird TJ, Dennis SC. Synovectomy and continuous passive motion (cpm) in hemophiliac patients. *Arthroscopy* 1987; **3**: 74–7.

18 Triantafyllou S, Hanks G, Handal J, Greer III R. Open and arthroscopic synovectomy in hemophilic arthropathy of the knee. *Clin Orthop* 1992; **283**: 196–204.

19 Eickhoff HH, Koch W, Brackmann HH. Arthroskopische Behandlung der haemophilen Kniegelenkarthropathie. *Arthroskopie* 1992; **5**: 267–71.

20 Montane I, McCollough NC, Chun-Yet Lian E. Synovectomy of the knee for hemophilic arthropathy. *J Bone Joint Surg (Am)* 1986; **68A**: 210–16.

21 Brackmann HH, Hofmann P, Hammerstein U *et al*. 6-Jahresergebnisse einer kontrollierten Dauerbehandlung der schweren Haemophilie A an 122 Kindern und Jugendlichen unter Zugrundelegung des klinisch-orthopaedischen und radiologischen Scores. In: Wenzel E, Hellstern P, Morgenstern E, Köhler M, von Blohn G, eds. *Rationelle Therapie und Diagnose von haemorraghischen und thrombophilen Diathesen*. Stuttgart, New York: Schattauer, 1985: 3.71–3.74.

22 Rodriguez-Merchan EC, Galindo E, Ladreda JMM, Pardo JA. Surgical synovectomy in haemophilic arthropathy of the knee. *Int Orthop* 1994; **18**: 38–41.

23 Rodriguez-Merchan EC, Magallon M, Galindo E. Joint debridement for haemophilic arthropathy of the knee. *Int Orthop* 1994; **18**: 135–8.

CHAPTER 19

Surgical Complications in the HIV-positive Haemophilia Patient

J L HICKS AND W J RIBBANS

INTRODUCTION

Surgical procedures in patients with haemophilia are usually undertaken in specialist centres, where the specific risks are understood. The primary aim is to prevent bleeding complications, but secondary aims address the risks of other complications, such as those associated with severe soft-tissue contractures, bone loss and immune compromise [1,2]. Surgery in HIV-positive haemophilic patients requires additional evaluation, as the pattern of immunosuppression, co-morbidity and therapeutic regimen further affects the risk profile. The extent of the problem of HIV infection varies geographically, and the prevalence of HIV infection in many haemophilic populations is naturally declining with time. However, this decline is slowing as a result of effective anti-retroviral treatment regimens which are able to suppress HIV infection and thus prolong life. As a result, we are seeing increasing numbers of HIV-positive haemophilic patients in whom elective orthopaedic procedures may be indicated, and small numbers in whom surgery is required following trauma. In this chapter, we address the potential complications arising from any surgery in such patients; complications associated with specific procedures are dealt with in the relevant chapters.

INFECTIOUS COMPLICATIONS

Postoperative infection is the most significant additional risk applicable to haemophiliacs who are HIV-positive, although HIV-negative haemophiliacs are already more prone to such infections than the normal population (see below). Much of the work published on infection following orthopaedic procedures relates to joint replacement, and we will consider this first.

Arthroplasty

In a review of the medical literature conducted in 1998, 45 publications presenting the results of total joint replacement in patients with haemophilia, reporting 715 procedures, were identified. Of these procedures, 663 (93%) were primary arthroplasties; the remainder were revisions. Of the primary procedures, 70% were knee replacements, 25% hip replacements, 1.4% shoulders, 3.4% elbows and 0.6% ankle replacements. The average age of patients at the time of surgery was 39.1 years, with average duration of follow-up 4.2 years (range 0–23 years). Of the 311 patients in whom the type of haemophilia was stated, the distribution was 91% haemophilia A, 7% haemophilia B and 2% von Willebrand's disease.

In 145 (20%) patients, a positive diagnosis of HIV infection was made either before surgery or during the follow-up period. In the remainder of cases, the HIV status was not given (the majority), or stated as HIV-negative (this group subsequently referred to as 'HIV-negative'). Average CD4 count preoperatively was 220 cells/mm^3 (range 100–380), but CD4 counts were stated for only 10 of 145 procedures. Overall, infection was reported as a complication in 7.2% of the primary arthroplasties. For specific joints, infection rates were 6.7% of knee replacements, 8.5% of hips and 14% of elbow replacements. In patients specified as HIV-positive, the infection rate was 11.7%. Average elapsed time to the diagnosis of infection was 27 months (range 1–60 months) in the 'HIV-negative' group, and 67 months (range 0–252 months) in the HIV-positive group. Overall average time to infection was 51 months. Only a single case of infection was reported in the 11 studies completed before 1979 [3], which may reflect lower infection rates prior to HIV.

Organisms isolated in the 'HIV-negative' group were predominantly *Staphylococcus epidermidis*, *Staphylococcus aureus* and *Pseudomonas aeruginosa*. One organism, *Staphylococcus aureus*, predominated in the HIV-positive group, although many different infecting organisms have been reported, including one report of *Candida parapsilosis* infection [4].

A multicentre study into infection rates following arthroplasty in HIV-positive haemophiliacs has been undertaken, with contributions from eight centres in the UK, US and Australia. One hundred and two arthroplasties in 73 HIV-positive patients were identified. The distribution of joints was similar to that published in the literature – 73.6% knee replacements, 25.3% hip replacements and 1% shoulder replacements. There were 91 primary arthroplasties and 11 were revision procedures. The average age was 39 years (range 22–60 years), and average duration of follow-up was 5.7 years (range 0–20.8 years). In 92% of patients a diagnosis of haemophilia A was given, with 3% having haemophilia B, and the diagnosis was not stated in 5%. Most (88%) had less than 1% factor VIII or factor IX activity, 4% had 1–5% activity, with 1% having 5–10% and 1% having 10–50% activity; the rest not stated.

The patient was diagnosed HIV-positive prior to surgery in 52% of the procedures and in 36% the diagnosis was made after the operation; for 12% the date of diagnosis was uncertain. Following primary procedures the deep sepsis rate was 18.7% (17 out of 91 procedures), and following revision procedures it was 36.3% overall; 43% (3 of 7) when revised for sepsis and 25% (1 of 4) when revised for other causes. The mean time to the diagnosis of sepsis following primary procedures was 47 months (range 2–190 months) postoperatively.

In a separate study, Ragni *et al.* [5] studied a subset of HIV-positive patients in whom the CD4 count was below 200 cells/mm^3 and found an incidence of nine immediate and early infections following 34 total joint arthroplasties (26.1%), although they excluded a further four infections which occurred 2–10 years later following unspecified orthopaedic procedures. These figures should be compared with quoted infection rates of up to 1.5% following arthroplasty in the normal population, which are considered acceptable [6]. The mean time before deep sepsis was diagnosed, in both the literature and in the multicentre study, was 5 years, representing a high proportion of 'late' infections. This follows the tendency of HIV-positive patients, particularly as immuno-suppression increases, to develop distant foci of sepsis which can seed to an implant at any time.

Preoperative CD4 counts were available for 49% of procedures with a mean CD4 count of 390 cells/mm^3 (range 30–1300). Of the 81 procedures where infection did not develop, 42 (52%) had CD4 counts measured preoperatively, with a mean value of 400 cells/mm^3 (range 90–1210). In the 21 procedures which were complicated by infection, eight (38%) had known preoperative CD4 counts, with a mean value of 310 cells/mm^3 (range 30–1300). The mean logarithmic CD4 count was significantly lower in the infected group (–22.42 vs. –21.78, t-test, $P < 0.01$). Where organisms were grown (7 out of 21 infected cases), in five cases these were Gram-positive cocci, and in the other cases diphtheroids and *Klebsiella* species were isolated.

Other procedures

The literature available on infection following other orthopaedic procedures consists mainly of isolated case reports, but HIV-positive individuals are certainly more prone to develop sepsis following such procedures. Even without surgery, it appears that the joints of HIV-positive patients are more subject to infection than those of seronegative haemophiliacs; septic arthritis in native haemophilic joints was extremely rare prior to the appearance of HIV, and although less than 50 cases have been reported, the risk appears to increase several-fold with HIV infection [7]. The spectrum of infecting organisms includes *Salmonella* and fungal species, rarely found in HIV-seronegative individuals.

GENERAL COMPLICATIONS ASSOCIATED WITH HIV INFECTION

Although we have been concerned primarily with complications arising as a result of surgery, any physician caring for patients with HIV must be aware of the range of clinical events which are associated with HIV infection, independently of whether surgery has been performed. These include pneumonias, particularly with *Pneumocystis carinii* and mycobacteria such as *M. avium-intracellulare* and *M. tuberculosis,* diarrhoea, neurological diseases including subacute encephalitis (manifesting as dementia) and peripheral neuropathy, and certain malignancies. The first presentation of these may be around the time of surgery, or during follow-up, and the surgeon should remain alert to these possible diagnoses. They are generally associated with advanced disease, but not exclusively.

Co-morbidity

Many patients who became infected with hepatitis B and/or hepatitis C have become chronic carriers. Although in the acute stages of infection there may be extrahepatic manifestations including arthropathy, in the chronic stages the pathology appears confined to the liver except in end-stage disease. It is the risk to healthcare workers that is particularly important, and only those with proven immunity to hepatitis B should come into contact with carriers, as this disease is far more infectious than HIV.

HIV disease progression

The extent to which surgical procedures may influence HIV progression has been studied by several authors [8,9]. No significant difference in CD4 cell count or in clinical disease progression, including the development of AIDS, has been demonstrated in HIV-positive patients undergoing both orthopaedic and non-orthopaedic surgical procedures, when compared with patients not undergoing such procedures.

Pharmacological factors

In addition to complications associated with haemophilia treatments already discussed, patients with HIV infection taking anti-retroviral drugs may be subject to further risks of complications. A new class of agent, the HIV protease inhibitors, has recently been introduced, and their action may complement the existing reverse transcriptase inhibitors in controlling the effect of HIV. There have been reports of patients who take protease inhibitors developing bleeding problems, apparently despite adequate factor replacement [10]. Affected patients develop unusual bleeds, particularly into the soft tissues, which may require very high doses of factor VIII to control. Surgeons should therefore be aware of potential problems in patients taking this class of drug, which includes Indinavir and Ritonavir, although reports so far published seem to indicate that bleeding problems occur only within the first week or so of taking the drug. The surgeon should, however, consider the possibility of this cause of unexpected bleeding after any duration of treatment. Patients usually take protease inhibitors in combination with two other drugs (generally reverse transcriptase inhibitors), and there is scope for adjusting the combination where there is real concern over the risk of bleeding.

Psychological factors

Haemophilic individuals with asymptomatic HIV infection show no additional physical disabilities when compared with HIV-negative haemophiliacs, but they are more likely to have psychological and social morbidity [11] which can affect both sides of the risk–benefit equation, in a way that varies in each patient. The patient's counsellor(s) should be consulted wherever possible, as they can provide invaluable insight which surgeons may not perceive in discussion with the patient alone.

As it is now clear that long-term survival is a reality for a significant proportion of the HIV-positive population, affected individuals have had to reassess their life goals, and their needs must be reflected in the treatment options offered to them [12].

Risks to the surgeon and other healthcare workers

In any invasive procedure performed on an HIV-positive patient, the risks to surgeons and other staff, although very small, are significant. Therefore, reasonable precautions must be taken to prevent the surgical team from coming into contact with blood and other body fluids during and after the procedure. Wearing of waterproof gowns/suit, visors and waterproof footwear in the operating room are minimum requirements, and many surgeons use Kevlar gloves to prevent needlestick injury. It is important to have an experienced operating team who are able to use correct instrument handling techniques. Postoperatively, meticulous sharps-handling techniques must again be employed, with careful disposal of soiled dressings and so on. There is a theoretical risk of disease transmission through the use of therapy adjuncts such as continuous passive motion machines, and therefore these should not be shared between patients.

Avoiding complications

Careful selection of patients, and counselling, are essential to minimize the incidence and effects of complications. By close liaison with treating physicians, the surgeon can ensure that HIV suppression is optimized before surgery. Both CD4 cell count and viral load can be used to assess the effectiveness of combination therapy in suppressing the disease [13]. Our own study used CD4 count as a marker of HIV progression, but increasingly, viral load is used to monitor and adjust the therapeutic regimen. Although studies based on viral load measurements are at present relatively short-term, it is logical to recommend that the ideal time for surgery is when the plasma viral load is undetectable on standard assays. There are still patients who develop clinical events despite undetectable viral loads, and in some patients the correlation between increasing viral load and falling CD4 count is weak, so in addition the CD4 cell count should be considered.

In our study, patients with low CD4 counts preoperatively were more likely to develop deep sepsis. The average preoperative CD4 count was less than 200 cells/mm^3 in five of eight (62.5%) of the infected group, compared with 7 of 42 (16.7%) in the uninfected group, and there was a significant difference between the mean logarithmic CD4 counts of the two groups. We do not, however, suggest that the value of 200 cells/mm^3 is used as a threshold for a decision as to whether to operate, as at the time of our study HIV suppression therapy was less effective and, particularly in the cases of late infection, a falling CD4 count at a time long after surgery is more likely than the preoperative CD4 count to have been the critical factor in the development of infection. It follows that, in order to prevent late infection in patients with prosthetic implants, ongoing monitoring of disease progression should perhaps be more close than in patients having other types of surgery, although even in these individuals the timing of surgery should be carefully selected. More intense treatment is associated with an increased tendency to develop resistance to therapeutic agents, and this must be balanced against the risk of prosthetic infection.

Where multiple joints are involved and multiple procedures are being considered, where appropriate these may be performed simultaneously so that HIV suppression and factor VIII administration can be optimized [14] without apparent risk of causing disease progression. Prevention of infection at the time of surgery is as for any orthopaedic procedure, and for arthroplasty includes laminar-flow operating theatres, antibiotic prophylaxis with a broad-spectrum agent such as a third generation cephalosporin for 24 hours (and continued if bleeding problems occur), and meticulous surgical technique. The British Orthopaedic Association published detailed guidelines in 1999.

Liaison within the multidisciplinary team at all stages of planning surgery, perioperatively and during follow-up, is crucial in order for the patient to obtain maximum benefit from surgery. It is important, therefore, that members of the team, in addition to the surgeons themselves, are aware of the symptoms and signs of complications, and it is the surgeon's responsibility to ensure that they are educated appropriately. During follow-up, a high index of suspicion for infection must be maintained, and early investigation, with early and thorough surgical intervention for sepsis, should be instituted.

TREATMENT OF INFECTION

Prompt treatment of both local and distant sepsis should prevent translocation of bacteria onto the implant as, once established in a biofilm on the implant surface, eradication is difficult without removal of the implant. Long-term suppression with antibiotics is an option mostly reserved for less fit patients in whom the risks of further surgery are too great, but some fitter patients may elect this option to avoid the trauma of further surgery for their own reasons.

From published literature, the treatment given was specified for 43 infected primary joint replacements; in 33% antibiotics alone were used, whereas in 67% antibiotics were used in conjunction with various surgical procedures ranging from arthroscopic débridement to amputation of the limb. In half of the cases where antibiotics alone were used, the infection was successfully eradicated, compared with eradication in 83% of all surgical procedures. Where the initial treatment failed, 55% continued treatment with long-term antibiotics alone, in 36% the prosthesis was removed, and in 9% (one case) the limb was amputated.

The results of treatment in cases where sepsis developed in patients in the multicentre study are summarized in Fig. 19.1. These cases comprise all 17 primary procedures which developed sepsis, and the single case revised in the absence of proven sepsis, which subsequently became infected. Compared with the results reported in the literature review, these initial treatments were much less successful, with eradication of infection reported in only 22% overall, and antibiotics alone resulting in resolution in only one out of eleven cases (9.1%). Where initial

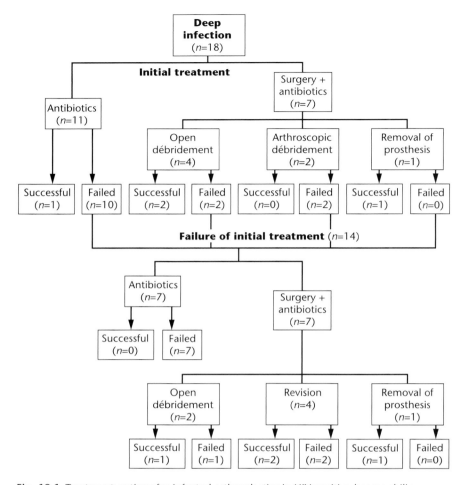

Fig. 19.1 Treatment options for infected arthroplasties in HIV-positive haemophilic patients.

treatment failed, 50% were placed on long-term antibiotics and continued to be symptomatic, thus representing overall treatment failure. In the remaining seven cases, further surgery was performed, which resulted in the successful eradication of infection in four cases (57%).

The question of how to manage deep infection once it develops is a controversial one, and depends on the condition of the patient, the quality of bone stock, the state of other joints and other factors. Antibiotics alone may suppress the appearance of deep infection but, except at a very early stage, are unlikely to eradicate it. This situation may be acceptable for some individuals, but if the aim is for a sterile joint, then surgery to remove all infected tissue is usually required. Figure 19.1 shows successful eradication of infection in only 37.5% patients undergoing open or arthroscopic débridement, compared with 100% where the implant was removed, and 50% where revision was undertaken.

In general terms, therefore, these data support the view that the more radical the procedure, the greater the chance of successful eradication of infection. A less extensive procedure may be chosen to preserve a 'precious' prosthesis, whereas infection around an implant in a fit patient with good bone stock may be treated with a two-stage revision or joint fusion.

Implant survival

Using the data from the multicentre study, analysis of overall patient survival, where the diagnosis of HIV infection had been made preoperatively, showed 55% survivorship at 10 years postoperatively. With current triple chemotherapy regimens, this figure is likely to be much higher in the future. Analysis of the sepsis-free survivorship of prostheses implanted in primary procedures showed 71.8% survivorship at 10 years and 54.9% 'aseptic survivorship' at 20 years.

SUMMARY

HIV poses an additional challenge to surgeons already dealing with the complex issues surrounding surgery in haemophilia. Infection risks are significantly higher, but with careful planning and an awareness of these risks, a successful result should be achieved in the majority of cases. This involves a multidisciplinary approach at all stages. Prompt and adequate intervention appropriate to the patient is necessary in those patients who do develop sepsis. Complications may arise not just from the disease itself, but from its treatment and its effect on the patient's psychological and social state; as in all areas of medicine, it is essential to treat the whole patient. Despite the increased risks involved, as long as these risks are understood by all concerned, surgery in HIV-positive haemophilic individuals can achieve very beneficial results.

REFERENCES

1 Kelley SS, Lachiewicz PF, Gilbert MS, Bolander ME, Jankiewicz JJ. Hip arthroplasty in hemophilic arthropathy. *J Bone Joint Surg (Am)* 1995; **77A**: 828–34.

2 Lachiewicz PF, Inglis AE, Insall JN, Sculco TP, Hilgartner MW, Bussel JB. Total knee arthroplasty in hemophilia. *J Bone Joint Surg (Am)* 1985; **67A**: 1361–6.

3 Luck JV Jr, Kasper CK. Surgical management of advanced hemophilic arthropathy: an overview of 20 years' experience. *Clin Orthop* 1989; **242**: 60–82.

4 Tunkel AR, Wispelwey B. *Candida* prosthetic arthritis: report of a case treated with fluconazole and review of the literature. *Am J Med* 1993; **94**: 100–3.

5 Ragni MV, Crossett LS, Herndon JH. Postoperative infection following orthopaedic surgery in human immunodeficiency virus-infected hemophiliacs with CD4 counts ≤200/mm³. *J Arthroplasty* 1995; **10**: 716–21.

6 Fender D, Harper WM, Gregg PJ. Outcome of Charnley total hip replacement across a single health region in England. *J Bone Joint Surg (Br)* 1999; **81B**: 577–81.

7 Barzilai A, Varon D, Martinowitz U, Heim M, Schulman S. Characteristics of septic arthritis in human immunodeficiency virus-infected haemophiliacs versus other risk groups. *Rheumatology (Oxford)* 1999; **38**: 139–42.

8 Astermark J, Löfqvist T, Schulman S, Stigendal L, Lethagen S. Major surgery seems not to influence HIV disease progression in haemophilia patients. *Br J Haematol* 1998; **103**: 10–14.

9 Phillips AM, Sabin C, Ribbans WJ, Lee CA. Surgery in hemophilic patients with human immunodeficiency virus. *Clin Orthop* 1997; **343**: 81–7.

10 Yee TT, Amrolia PJ, Lee CA, Mir N, Giangrande PLF. Protease inhibitors and unusual bleeding in haemophiliacs. *Haemophilia* 1997; **3**: 220–1.

11 Tanaka S, Hachisuka K, Okazaki T, Shirahata A, Ogata H. Health status and satisfaction of asymptomatic HIV-positive haemophiliacs in Kyushu, Japan. *Haemophilia* 1999; **5**: 56–62.

12 Taylor G. The emerging needs of persons living with haemophilia and HIV/AIDS in British Columbia. *Haemophilia* 1999; **5**: 1–8.

13 Gazzard BG, Moyle GJ. 1998 revision to the British HIV Association guidelines for antiretroviral treatment of HIV seropositive individuals. *Lancet* 1998; **352**: 314–16.

14 Arnold WA, Post M, Larsen L, Rhodes J, Kasper C. Surgery in hemophilia. In: McCullough N III, ed. *Comprehensive Management of Musculoskeletal Disorders in Hemophilia*. Washington: National Academy of Sciences, 1973: 181–4.

CHAPTER 20

Orthopaedic Surgery in Haemophilic Patients with Inhibitors: A Review of the Literature

E C RODRIGUEZ-MERCHAN AND H DE LA CORTE

INTRODUCTION

The development of an inhibitor against factor VIII or factor IX is the most common and most serious complication of replacement therapy in patients with haemophilia A or B, resulting from the exclusive use of virus-inactivated, plasma-derived concentrates or recombinant products. When present, the inhibitor inactivates the biological activity of infused factor (F) VIII or IX, making the patient refractory to treatment. Moreover, even when the inhibitor titre is low, allowing some partial efficacy, the titre will increase within a few days of the use of FVIII- or FIX-containing products, making the treatment rapidly ineffective. The management of bleeding episodes and the cover of surgical procedures in haemophilic patients with inhibitors is particularly difficult [1] and, until recently, elective orthopaedic surgical procedures were never or only rarely proposed for patients with inhibitors, in most cases despite the desperate need for them, as their existing bleeding episodes such as haemarthroses have often not been optimally treated.

Haemophilic patients with inhibitors

Between 10% and 30% of patients with severe haemophilia A, and 2–5% of patients with severe haemophilia B or mild/moderate haemophilia A, develop an inhibitor against FVIII or FIX after treatment with either plasma-derived or recombinant products. Inhibitor detection using the Bethesda assay, measured in Bethesda units (BU), is part of the regular follow-up for all haemophilic patients treated with such products. After the development of the inhibitor, the inhibitor titre decreases if no FVIII- or FIX-containing products are used for a long period so that the inhibitor may become undetectable. However, the inhibitor usually reappears after a new challenge with FVIII- or FIX-containing products (anamnestic response).

Two approaches for the management of patients with inhibitors have been proposed. Immune tolerance induction using high dose FVIII or FIX daily or twice daily for a period of a few months to several years may completely eliminate the inhibitor, allowing the patient to again be treated efficiently with FVIII or FIX [2,3]. However, immune tolerance induction fails in around 20% of cases and is not proposed for all patients due to the high probability of failure or adverse events. Furthermore, this procedure is very costly. The other possibility is to treat bleeding episodes with prothrombin complex concentrates (PCC), activated prothrombin complex concentrates (APCC; Autoplex™, Feiba™) [4–6] or, more recently, with recombinant-activated factor VIIa (rFVIIa; NovoSeven™) [7–10]. In case of failure of APCC or rFVIIa in life- or limb-threatening bleeds or as first-line treatment for major bleeds, high-dose human [11] or porcine FVIII [12] or human FIX may be efficacious if the inhibitor is low or is lowered using plasmapheresis [13] or protein A immunoadsorption [14]. However, the anamnestic rise of the inhibitor will render treatment with FVIII or FIX ineffective within a few days, making the patient resistant to rescue with FVIII or FIX for months or even years.

SURGICAL PROCEDURES IN PATIENTS WITH HIGH RESPONDING INHIBITORS

Before the availability of rFVIIa, surgical procedures in patients with inhibitors were rarely performed due to the difficulty in obtaining effective haemostasis so that, in most cases, only emergency procedures were performed. These procedures usually used high-dose human FVIII [4,11,16], porcine FVIII [14,15] or high-dose FIX. The use of FVIII, FIX or porcine FVIII is only possible when the inhibitor titre is low (< 5 BU) and the anamnestic response allows a window of only 4–10 days of efficient treatment. This is barely sufficient for major surgical procedures, thereby making alternative treatment such as APCC [4,16] or rFVIIa necessary to cover the second postoperative week. Moreover, the increase in inhibitor titre, as a result of the use of FVIII or FIX, means that there is a risk of no alternative treatment being available should a life- or limb-threatening bleed occur in the following months or years.

APCC has been used in some cases to cover emergency surgical procedures [4,5,17] or to treat intra- or perioperative bleeding [6] and, more rarely, to cover elective surgical procedures [16], although efficacy was not always optimal in the postoperative period [16,17]. Furthermore, APCCs are plasma-derived coagulation factor concentrates that contain some FVIII and FIX and may, therefore, provoke an anamnestic rise in inhibitor in up to 30% of patients [4,11,16]. The use of repeated injections over 8–15 days has been reported to increase the risk of side-effects such as thrombosis, myocardial infarction [16] and intravascular coagulation [16,17].

Recombinant factor VIIa was first reported as effective in elective orthopaedic surgery in 1988 [7], and since then a large body of experience has accumulated in the use of rFVIIa as cover for emergency or elective surgical procedures [8,9,18–27]. As rFVIIa is a recombinant product with no human derivatives, the product contains no trace of FVIII or FIX and is therefore without risk of anamnestic response by the inhibitor.

ELECTIVE ORTHOPAEDIC SURGERY IN PATIENTS WITH HIGH RESPONDING INHIBITORS BEFORE RECOMBINANT FACTOR VIIa

Some elective orthopaedic surgical procedures have been described using human FVIII with or without previous lowering of the inhibitor titre by plasmapheresis or protein A immunoadsorption [4,11,16]. However, even if the inhibitor titre allows an effective level of circulating FVIII and the treatment allows coverage of the surgical procedure, the anamnestic rise of the inhibitor induces an increased risk of rebleeding in the second postoperative week [4,16]. Consequently, the number of elective orthopaedic procedures reported are few. Porcine FVIII was used to cover 19 orthopaedic procedures ranging from minor procedures (knee joint aspiration) to major surgery in haemophilia A patients with inhibitors. Eleven major surgical procedures (three knee arthroplasties, one hip arthroplasty, three osteotomy/osteosynthesis, one synovectomy, one elbow disarticulation and one pseudotumour resection) were performed in patients with low anti-porcine FVIII titre with good to excellent results in nine and fair results in two. However, the inhibitor titre against human factor VIII, in addition to that against porcine FVIII, increased in some cases.

Major elective orthopaedic surgical procedures have rarely been reported using APCCs, despite these products being available for more than 20 years and the pressing need for orthopaedic surgery in patients with inhibitors. A data search found three major elective orthopaedic surgeries using APCC (one knee arthroplasty, one knee synovectomy and one bilateral knee arthroplasty). The results of the first two procedures were reported as excellent, but there was excessive bleeding after the knee arthroplasty and a cutaneomuscular plasty was required.

ELECTIVE ORTHOPAEDIC SURGERY IN PATIENTS WITH HIGH RESPONDING INHIBITORS USING RECOMBINANT FACTOR VIIa

The first elective orthopaedic surgery performed under cover of rFVIIa was a surgical knee synovectomy on a patient with severe haemophilia A and a high inhibitor titre, carried out under general anaesthesia and without a tourniquet [7]. Haemostasis was achieved using local fibrin glue and general antifibrinolytic drugs, but without electrocoagulation. The result was excellent with no abnormal bleeding during or after surgery and with no adverse events. This patient was the first ever treated with rFVIIa. Subsequently, two open surgical synovectomies (knee and ankle) were performed [18] with rFVIIa, antifibrinolytic drugs and local glue with an excellent outcome. A complex orthopaedic surgical procedure (knee synovectomy, hamstring release, posterior capsulotomy, proximal and distal realignment of the extensor mechanism, and supracondylar extension–varus osteotomy stabilized with a blade-plate sliding screw) was performed in a young haemophiliac with inhibitors to correct a 90° flexion contracture of the right knee associated with a valgus deformity, which had left him unable to walk and confined to a wheelchair [19]. The procedure lasted 3 hours, 160 minutes of which were under ischaemia. Pre-, peri- and postoperative periods were covered only with rFVIIa and antifibrinolytic drugs. The result was excellent with no bleeding complications. After these first three cases [7,18,19], the dose of 90 µg/kg body weight of rFVIIa every 2 hours for 24–48 hours was recommended for surgical procedures.

Since these first reports on single elective orthopaedic surgical procedures, eight publications [20–27] reported personal experiences or data collection on elective orthopaedic surgical procedures using only rFVIIa (Table 20.1). A total of 32 major surgical procedures were reported, including knee arthroplasty ($n = 8$), hip arthroplasty ($n = 5$), ankle arthroplasty ($n = 2$), removal of infected hip arthroplasty ($n = 1$), knee arthrodesis ($n = 1$), amputation of lower limb ($n = 1$), pseudotumour removal ($n = 2$), surgical joint synovectomy ($n = 7$), osteotomy or osteosynthesis for fracture ($n = 5$), as well as two minor procedures (knee manipulation with release of adhesion and revision of wound haematoma).

Most of the procedures were performed using the standard treatment regimen (90 µg/kg body weight of rFVIIa every 2 hours for 24–48 hours) [18–20] with an increasing dosing interval after the first 2 days (as recommended by the European approval for NovoSeven™). Some procedures were performed using continuous infusion of rFVIIa [21,22,24]. In most, but not all cases, oral antifibrinolytic drugs were also used in combination with rFVIIa.

Clinical tolerance was outstanding and efficacy was excellent in most cases. Moderate bleeding complications were observed in two patients treated with continuous infusion of rFVIIa; these took the form of postoperative haematoma and wound haematoma revision after a knee arthroplasty and excessive bleeding for 3 days after a hip arthroplasty [21,22]. Some moderate bleeding complications were also observed in the prospective randomized trial of two doses of rFVIIa. This study compared the standard regimen (90 µg/kg every 2 hours) to a lower dose regimen (35 µg/kg every 2 hours) [23]. A haemarthrosis was observed at postoperative day 7 following knee arthroplasty in a patient treated according to the standard regimen. Postoperative bleeding was observed in three patients treated with the low-dose regimen (bleeding in early postoperative period in two patients, moderate bleeding at day 19 in the third). Rescue was performed with APCC in the first case (postoperative haemarthrosis at day 7), with human or porcine FVIII in the two cases with early postoperative bleeding, and with antifibrinolytic drug in the last case.

Recombinant FVIIa has made major elective orthopaedic surgery possible in patients with high-titre inhibitors. Most of these procedures would not have been possible without rFVIIa, as it would have been difficult to overcome the inhibitor even with high doses of human or porcine FVIII or FIX. The reported experience with APCC, for example, is minimal despite APCCs being available for more than 20 years. There were no reported serious adverse events with rFVIIa in this data search, except for one episode of disseminated intravascular coagulation in a patient who had an excision of an infected pseudotumour and was treated with rFVIIa by continuous infusion [22].

This large series of major elective orthopaedic surgical procedures [7,18–27] is the largest ever reported in haemophilic patients with inhibitors, despite the long-standing existence of other treatment modalities such as high-dose human FVIII, porcine FVIII and APCC. This means

Table 20.1 Elective orthopaedic surgical procedures performed with rFVIIa as first-line therapy.

Reference	Orthopaedic surgery
Hedner *et al.* 1988 [7]	Knee joint synovectomy
Schulman *et al.* 1994 [18]	Knee and ankle joint synovectomies
O'Marcaigh *et al.* 1994 [19]	Knee joint synovectomy, osteotomy and other orthopaedic procedures*
Ingerslev *et al.* 1996 [20] (Compassionate Use Programme, October 1991–September 1994)	Knee joint arthroplasty Bilateral knee joint arthroplasty Knee joint arthroplasty and osteotomy Knee joint synovectomy Knee joint synovectomy Surgical removal of haemophilic pseudotumour Amputation of lower limb
Schulman *et al.* 1996 [21]	Knee joint arthroplasty[1] Revision of a wound haematoma[2]
Schulman *et al.* 1998 [22] (International Registry on continuous infusion of rFVIIa)	*Knee joint arthroplasty[1]* Knee joint arthroplasty Knee joint arthroplasty *Hip joint arthroplasty[3]* *Hip joint arthroplasty[4]* *Removal of infected hip arthroplasty[5]* Knee arthrodesis Excision of infected pseudotumour *Revision of wound haematoma[2]*
Shapiro *et al.* 1998 [23] (Prospective, randomized trial comparing two doses of rFVIIa, July 1995–July 1996)	Knee joint arthroplasty Hip joint arthroplasty Hip joint arthroplasty Synovectomy and radial head excision Synovectomy and capsulotomy Synovectomy Synovectomy Synovectomy Knee joint manipulation with release of adhesions Femoral bone graft
Vermylen and Peerlinck 1998 [24]	Hip joint arthroplasty[3] Bilateral ankle joint arthroplasty Removal of infected hip joint arthroplasty[5]
Mauser-Bunschoten *et al.* 1998 [25]	*Hip joint arthroplasty[3]* *Removal of infected hip joint arthroplasty[5]*
Goudemand 1999 [26]	Hip arthroplasty[4] Hip arthroplasty Osteosynthesis Osteosynthesis Osteosynthesis
Scharrer 1999 [27]	Reposition of a fracture and extension of the right leg Removal of the material used for the extension

*See text.
[1]Numbers refer to the same case reported by different authors.
Italicized text refers to publication by a non-primary physician.

that rFVIIa is a novel and real alternative for major elective orthopaedic surgery in inhibitor patients. The standard regimen is 90 μg/kg body weight every 2 hours for the first 48 hours with increasing interval between doses after this first postoperative period. Lower doses are much less efficient [23] and administration by continuous infusion is not yet approved for rFVIIa, as a few bleeds and one episode of disseminated intravascular coagulation have been reported with continuous infusion of rFVIIa [21,22].

CONCLUSION

Haemophilic patients with inhibitors frequently need elective orthopaedic surgery as a result of the high frequency of severe chronic arthropathies, but this surgery is denied them because of the lack of coverage for surgical procedures with acceptable efficacy and safety. A review of the literature on inhibitors has shown that, with the availability of rFVIIa, haemophilic patients with high inhibitor titres requiring elective orthopaedic surgery can undergo such surgery with a high expectation of success. Recombinant FVIIa appears to be an efficient haemostatic product for surgery in patients suffering from haemophilia A and B with inhibitors. Such a product makes elective orthopaedic surgery a viable option, leading to an improved quality of life for persons with haemophilia. Thorough analysis of each case as part of a multidisciplinary team will allow us to perform elective orthopaedic procedures in patients with inhibitors.

REFERENCES

1 The United States Pharmacopeial Convention, Inc. Hemophilia Management. *Transf Med Rev* 1998; **12**: 128–40.

2 Brackmann HH, Gormsen J. Massive factor VIII infusion in a haemophilia with factor VIII inhibitor: high response. *Lancet* 1977; **2**: 933.

3 Brackmann HH, Oldenburg J, Schwaab R. Immune tolerance for the treatment of factor VIII inhibitors. Twenty years "Bonn Protocol". *Vox Sang* 1996; **70** (Suppl. 1): 30–5.

4 Abildgaard CF, Penner JA, Watson-Williams EJ. Anti-inhibitor coagulant complex (Autoplex) for treatment of factor inhibitors in hemophilia. *Blood* 1980; **56**: 978–84.

5 Hilgartner MW, Knatterud GL and the Feiba study group. The use of Factor Eight Inhibitor By-passing Activity (Feiba Immuno) product for treatment of bleeding episodes in hemophiliacs with inhibitors. *Blood* 1983; **61**: 36–40.

6 Hilgartner M, Aledort L, Andes A, Gill J and the members of the Feiba study group. Efficacy and safety of vapor-heated anti-inhibitor coagulant complex in hemophilia patients. *Transfusion* 1990; **30**: 626–30.

7 Hedner U, Glazer S, Pinkel K *et al.* Successful use of recombinant factor VIIa in a patient with severe haemophilia A during synovectomy. *Lancet* 1988; **2**: 1193.

8 Hedner U, Glazer S, Falch J. Recombinant activated factor VII in the treatment of bleeding episodes in patients with inherited and acquired bleeding disorders. *Transf Med Rev* 1993; **7**: 78–83.

9 Hedner U, Ingerslev J. Clinical use of recombinant FVIIa (rFVIIa) *Transfus Sci* 1998; **19**: 163–76.

10 Roberts HR. Clinical experience with activated factor VII: focus on safety. *Blood Coag Fibrinol* 1998; **9** (Suppl. 1): S115–18.

11 White GC, Taylor RE, Blatt PM, Roberts HR. Treatment with a high titer anti-factor VIII antibody by continuous factor VIII administration: Report of a case. *Blood* 1983; **62**: 141–5.

12 A Multicenter US experience. The use of porcine factor VIII concentrate (Hyate:C) in the treatment of patients with inhibitor antibodies to factor VIII. *Arch Intern Med* 1989; **149**: 1381–5.

13 Bona RD, Pasquale DN, Kalish RI, Witter BA. Porcine factor VIII and plasmapheresis in the management of hemophilic patients with inhibitors. *Am J Hematol* 1986; **21**: 201–7.

14 Nilsson IM, Berntorp E, Freiburghaus C. Treatment of patients with factor VIII and IX inhibitors. *Thromb Haemost* 1993; **70**: 56–9.

15 Lozier JN, Santagostino E, Kasper CK, Teitel JM, Hay CRM. Use of porcine factor VIII for surgical procedures in haemophilia A patients with inhibitors. *Sem Hematol* 1993; **30** (Suppl. 1): 10–21.

16 Négrier C, Goudemand J, Sultan Y *et al.* Multicenter retrospective study on the utilization of Feiba in France in patients with factor VIII or factor IX inhibitors. *Thromb Haemost* 1997; **77**: 1113–19.

17 Heisel MA, Gomperts ED, Gordon McComb J, Hilgartner

M. Use of activated prothrombin complex concentrate over multiple surgical episodes in a hemophilic child with an inhibitor. *J Pediat* 1983; **102**: 951–4.

18 Schulman S, Lindstedt M, Alberts KA, Agren PH. Recombinant factor VIIa in a multiple surgery (letter). *Thromb Haemost* 1994; **41**: 154.

19 O'Marcaigh AS, Schmalz BJ, Shaughnessy WJ, Gilchrist GS. Successful hemostasis during a major orthopedic operation by using recombinant activated factor VII in a patient with severe hemophilia A and a potent inhibitor. *Mayo Clin Proc* 1994; **69**: 641–4.

20 Ingerslev J, Freidman D, Gastineau D *et al*. Major surgery in haemophilic patients with inhibitors using recombinant factor VIIa. *Haemostasis* 1996; **26** (Suppl. 1): 118–23.

21 Schulman S, Bech Jensen M, Varon D *et al*. Feasibility of using recombinant factor VIIa in continuous infusion. *Thromb Haemost* 1996; **75**: 432–6.

22 Schulman S, d'Oiron R, Martinowitz U *et al*. Experiences with continuous infusion of recombinant activated factor VII. *Blood Coag Fibrinol* 1998; **9** (Suppl. 1): S97–S101.

23 Shapiro AD, Gilchrist GS, Hoots WK, Cooper HA, Gastineau DA. Prospective, randomised trial of two doses of rFVIIa (NovoSeven) in haemophilia patients with inhibitors undergoing surgery. *Thromb Haemost* 1998; **80**: 773–8.

24 Vermylen J, Peerlinck K. Optimal care of inhibitor patients during surgery. *Eur J Haematol* 1998; **61** (Suppl. 63): 15–17.

25 Mauser-Bunschoten EP, de Goede-Bolder A, Wielenga JJ *et al*. Continuous infusion of recombinant factor VIIa in patients with haemophilia and inhibitors: experience in the Netherlands and Belgium. *Netherlands J Med* 1998; **53**: 249–55.

26 Goudemand J. Treatment of patients with inhibitors: cost issues. *Haemophilia* 1999; **5**: 397–401.

27 Scharrer I on behalf of the German NovoSeven Study Group. Recombinant factor VIIa for patients with inhibitors to factor VIII or IX or factor VII deficiency. *Haemophilia* 1999; **5**: 253–9.

CHAPTER 21

Fractures

M QUINTANA JR, M QUINTANA SR AND E C RODRIGUEZ-MERCHAN

INTRODUCTION

The lack of studies regarding fractures in patients suffering from haemophilia has allowed room for controversy. Some authors believe that fractures in the haemophilic population are infrequent [1–9] due to the fact that understanding the gravity of their illness leads individuals with haemophilia to reduce the activities which involve risk to their physical well-being. Abreu *et al.* are opposed to this argument [10,11]. They consider that the frequency of fractures suffered by haemophiliacs is higher than in the general population as a result of the loss of movement caused by haemophilic arthropathy in the bones, reduced torsion strength and flexibility, poor muscular function, osteoporosis, and the high number of traumas suffered by them because preventive treatment enables them to play sports and engage in other daily activities (leading to accidents at work, traffic accidents and so on).

In our previous study [12] we found that, of fractures in the haemophilic population, only 5% can be considered similar to those in the general population. Thanks to the increased freedom offered by preventive treatment haemophilic patients no longer need to restrict their activities. They can expose themselves to risk (sport, traffic accidents, accidents at work and so on) in a similar way to the normal population. In fact, in our study the average age of the haemophilic population that has suffered fractures was 26.8 years, a young population. This, compared with the previous musculoskeletal situation of the haemophilic patient, summarized by limitation of the joints and osteoporosis as a result of repeated haemorrhages, and the haematological change manifested in the severity of haemophilia, did not affect the higher incidence of apparent fractures. In general, this reinforces the idea that fractures in the haemophilic population are more prevalent than in the general population.

AETIOLOGY

Some theories consider fractures in the haemophilic population to be pathological in that they are the result of a trauma, sometimes slight, due to the reasons expressed above and mainly in cases of haemophilic pseudotumours of the femur. In general, skeletal injuries can occur as a result of a serious, naturally spontaneous trauma or an accident in the workplace, although in the haemophilic patient fracture can result from only modest trauma. Three groups of fractures can be distinguished in haemophilic patients:

1 Those that result from serious trauma.

2 Those that result from a trauma whose severity is difficult to quantify. In this case, haemophilia is the most significant factor because haemophilic arthropathy favours osteoporosis and a higher propensity for the bones to be fragile.

3 Those that are produced in skeletal areas with profound structural changes in bone section, such as subperiosteal haemorrhages or intraosseous changes (haemophilic pseudotumour), or with serious osteoporosis where the action causing trauma is so slight that it can pass unnoticed by the patient.

To summarize this theory, the fact that in haemophilic patients the fractures are usually found at the metaphyseal level of the large bones, in the proximity of the joint with arthropathy with loss of joint function, muscular hypotrophy and osteoporosis, has led authors such as Nilsson and Blombach [13] and Abreu et al. [10,11] to conclude that these injuries are similar to pathological fractures. Trueta [14] considers haemophilic fractures to be like pathological ones because the structural changes in the bones are a result of osteoporosis, making fractures more likely.

In contradiction to this, after carrying out an analytical study of fractures in haemophilic patients, Boni [1] refers to analysis of the bone before trauma, concluding that one can only speak of pathological fracture in particular cases. These will be the fractures that are produced in skeletal areas with deep structural changes of the bone structure, such as subperiosteal haemorrhages or intraosseous changes (haemophilic pseudotumour), or with serious osteoporosis, where the traumatic action is so slight that it can pass unnoticed by the patient. In our earlier study [12], it was found that the majority of fractures in the haemophilic population were the result of a high-impact trauma, and only in certain cases could they be considered to be pathological fractures.

Localization

In reviewing the international literature, it appears that fractures of the femur are the most frequent and represent up to 50% of all statistics [1,3,4,12]. Having accepted that fractures in haemophilic patients can result from slight traumas [1–3,7], and even including those where the patient is unaware of the fracture, fractures are usually located at the metaphyseal level of the large bones in the proximity of a joint with arthropathy, lack of function, muscular hypotrophy and osteoporosis. These two factors – limited mobility of the joint and osteoporosis – contribute to a poor response to stresses, especially in the knee, which cannot absorb all of the force which is transmitted to the supracondylar area of the femur, resulting in a spiroid fracture in the central region.

Clinical symptoms

Our own finding concurred with the majority of authors [1,3,10,11,14–16] in that the clinical symptoms of haemophilic patients sustaining a bone fracture were comparable to those found in other patients who have suffered a trauma with changes in the continuity of the bone section. However, for the first group the consequences of haematoma formation and its volume are strictly linked to the seriousness of the haemophilia itself and the degree of trauma.

TREATMENT

When dealing with injuries to the bones of haemophilic patients, one must take into account the need to immediately institute haematological and orthopaedic treatment in a coordinated way. The immediate objective must be to obtain a good haemostasis to help coagulation in the centre of the fracture. Coagulation is the essential element for the formation of bone callus. It prevents enlargement of the haematoma at the fracture site which can cause serious complications such as necrosis of the soft tissue with exposure of the centre of the fracture and its fistulization, formation of a haemophilic pseudotumour, delayed union or nonunion. The haemorrhage generally responds to early administration of an adequate dose of factor in such a way as to obtain minimal plasmatic activity of around 30–40%, continuing for at least 3–4 days after reduction of the fracture associated with the administration of ε-aminocaproic acid or equivalent doses of tranexamic acid for at least 30 days after reduction of the fracture [15].

According to Boni and Ceciliani [3], the administration of non-fibrinolytic drugs is of great importance because of the following.

1 At the beginning of treatment it helps maintain coagulation.

2 It limits the fibrinolytic action which continues in the haemophiliac due to high concentrations of plasminogen activator and the major liberation of proteolytic enzymes that could limit, retard or even prevent the consolidation process.

3 It stimulates the action of plasma and blood derivatives.

4 It reduces the possibility of the haemophilic patient producing inhibitors to factors VIII and IX. While this possibility always exists, it is not clear how it can be prevented.

5 The necessity of administering concentrations of red blood cells in those cases where it will be necessary to normalize haemoglobin and haematocrit (particularly in fractures with a haematoma that provokes a post-traumatic anaemia) must be reiterated.

Having obtained haemostasis, we can establish the orthopaedic indications of the fracture, which are no different to the general principles that regulate the treatment of traumatic skeletal injuries in the non-haemophilic population.

Reduction of the fracture can be obtained by either a bloodless method (by external manoeuvres or by transskeletal traction of any limb) or by surgical methods to reduce the fragments of the fracture and obtain bone fixation. In all cases, one has to look for the best functional result possible, and for this a good anatomical reduction of the fracture is fundamental. If it is not possible to achieve this through non-operative methods, it will be necessary to use an open treatment with reduction and bone fixation by plates, screws or pins depending on the characteristics of the fracture (Fig. 21.1).

The correct treatment, either haematological or orthopaedic, allows a rapid consolidation, although the bone callus, in particular periosteum, is not excessively abundant. The formation of periosteal callus and its distribution [6,7,14] is related to the type of factor, as well as the displacement of the fragments, the amount of coagulation and, obviously, the quality of the fracture reduction. Boni and Ceciliani [3] found a scarce formation of periosteal callus in fractures treated early and anatomically reduced, while on the other hand they discovered the abundant formation of periosteal callus in fractures reduced with a slight displacement.

Therefore, radiological aspect at the time of assessment of consolidation of the fracture, together with sound clinical judgement, is very important for haemophilic patients. Good alignment of the fragments, even when there is a slight separation between the fragments, allows good consolidation to be obtained. An interesting aspect of fractures in haemophilic patients is the structural repair with good remodelling of the skeletal segment [6,7]. Other special aspects of the process of consolidation can be found in the importance of rehabilitation treatment in the healing of the fracture [1,15–18].

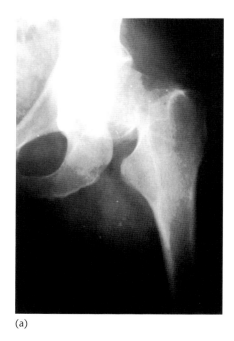
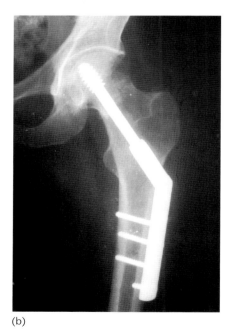
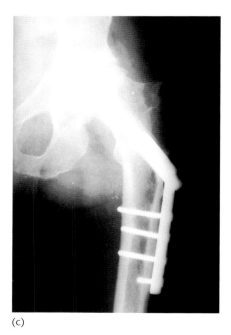

(a)　　　　　　　　　　　　　(b)　　　　　　　　　　　　　(c)

Fig. 21.1 Subcapital fracture of the left hip in a 28-year-old haemophilic patient after a casual fall. The fracture was fixed by means of an AO-ASIF DHS dynamic hip screw with a satisfactory result: (a) AP preoperative radiograph; (b) AP immediate postoperative view; (c) AP radiograph at 8 years' follow-up.

General principles

Three phases can be distinguished in the treatment of fractures in haemophilic patients.

1 Normalization of the coagulation process depends on obtaining rapid coagulation of the haematoma.

2 Continuation of the haemostatic treatment, administration of non-fibrinolytic drugs, and if necessary concentrated haemostatic drugs, in the days following reduction of the fracture, as appropriate to the severity of the haemophilia and the nature of the fracture produced.

3 Treatment of the fracture using closed or open methods, reducing it and approximating the bony ends to obtain good stability.

Medical treatment

Replacement therapy

The first objective of medical treatment is to control the haemorrhage by obtaining adequate haemostasis. This is achieved by replacement of the deficient factor, using concentrated factor obtained from frozen fresh plasma, the dose calculation being based on the weight of the patient and the amount (volume) of plasma. By definition, an international unit of FVIII or FIX is the quantity of activity that can be found in 1 mL of fresh plasma. To simplify the calculations, it can be assumed that there is an equilibrium between the circulating blood and the extracellular fluid, that a unit of factor for every kg of body weight will raise the level of plasma by a factor of 2% in the case of FVIII and by 1% in the case of FIX, and that the difference must be as great as the quantity of FIX passing through the extravascular space.

The calculation of the maintenance dose will depend on the level of plasma desired in the FVIII and the seriousness of the haemorrhage episode, the time needed for the replacement therapy, and the average life of the factor transfused. It is calculated with the evidence of transfusion in a series of decisions that can be made about the level of FVIII to establish how to reduce it after its administration. In a patient who is not bleeding, the average biological life of FVIII is 6–12 hours, while in FIX it is 8–18 hours. However, doses of FVIII can be repeated every 8 hours and FIX every 12 hours to maintain the desired levels in plasma, although generally the rhythm that can be maintained is every 12 hours in the first case and every 24 hours in the second.

Abilgaard [19] established that factor levels of 40–50% are sufficient to protect haemostasis for 24 hours. This treatment can be repeated every 24–48 hours if the haemorrhage is not controlled. However, just one dose, combined with immobility and non-weightbearing on the joint, can be sufficient to alleviate the pain and restore mobility. Levels of 30–40% are considered adequate. Basically, it is necessary to provide a covering of antihaemophilic factor transfusion to maintain levels of factor VIII or IX of 30–40% for 4–5 days, with complete immobilization of the fracture for up to 2 or 3 weeks. The treatment can continue for the time necessary to get consolidation of the fracture.

Analgesic treatment

Analgesics have played an important role in the treatment of patients with haemophilia. One of the difficulties is the different tolerance levels of patients. In addition, analgesics that produce secondary haemorrhages must be avoided. Analgesics that can be used with haemophiliacs are as follows.

1 Paracetamol (acetaminophen) does not seem to have a nephrotoxic effect. It does not affect anything in the intestinal walls, nor does it affect coagulation, and it is the preferred analgesic for patients with problem haemorrhages.

2 Dihydrocodeine is stronger than the aforementioned and is a good analgesic to use after a severe haemarthrosis or an intense muscular haemorrhage. It does not affect coagulation, or cause constipation like codeine.

3 Pentazocine is less likely to cause dependence than morphine derivatives. It is very effective for patients suffering chronic pain and severe haemorrhage.

4 Morphine and its derivatives are very strong analgesics and must be used with discretion because they can cause addiction and one of their side-effects is that they can depress breathing. Included in this group are pethidine, meperidine, dextromoramide, dipipanone and methadone.

Other analgesics such as mefenamic acid and acetylsalicylic acid and their derivatives must never be used as they cause gastrointestinal haemorrhages [15].

Anti-inflammatory drugs

Prednisone and prednisolone are steroidal hormones that are sometimes used to reduce inflammation in the joints after a haemorrhage, reducing the frequency and duration of the pain. Due to possible side-effects their use must be strictly controlled, although in practice they are seldom used [20].

However, some authors maintain that anti-inflammatory drugs such as phenylbutazone, indomethacin and oxyphenbutazone have adverse side-effects on the aggregation of the platelets and therefore their use is not recommended as they can cause problems of coagulation [21]. Others have used indomethacin without collateral side-effects [22].

Orthopaedic treatment

The advances in replacement therapy with plasma concentrates in haemophilic patients have favourably modified the prognosis of this illness [1]. The orthopaedic treatment of fractures in haemophilic patients who have received adequate replacement therapy is similar to that of non-haemophilic patients, and it is not necessary to modify the surgical techniques [10,15]. The orthopaedic non-operative treatment is focused on achieving complete immobilization of the fractured segment, initially with a padded splint, permitting a tight fit without risk of compression [15]. After 4–7 days of immobilization with the splint, when the inflammation should have reduced, immobilization can be achieved by fitting a plaster cast, similar to those used in non-haemophilic patients. Nevertheless, the casts must be closely monitored to avoid complications. During the acute phase, the patient should be treated not only with orthopaedic treatments such as immobilization, local compression and ice, but also by providing the appropriate factor, maintaining blood levels between 70% and 100%, and ensuring that the activity of the factor does not drop below 30% [11]. When the immobilized fracture is manipulated, for example, when changing or taking off the bandage, one must take the precaution of increasing the level of deficient factor by 10–15% to avoid new bleeding episodes. In cases where it is either not possible to use orthopaedic non-operative treatment or the treatment is unsuccessful, surgical orthopaedic treatment is recommended and must be guided by two fundamental principles [1,14–18,23–5]: firstly, to prevent deformities and restore functionality to the affected limb, and secondly, to control or reduce the haemorrhage produced at the local level.

The surgical techniques employed by the orthopaedic surgeon are similar to those used in the treatment of fractures of non-haemophilic patients, although the following should be noted: (1) the position of the joints in the affected limb; (2) the possibility of correcting a possible pre-existing residual deformity. The use of adequate replacement therapy during the surgical procedures is fundamental for their success, and therefore it is necessary to make an exact presurgical and postoperative diagnosis as well as carrying out routine investigation of the antibodies against deficient coagulation factors.

Although this treatment is being revised and new haematological treatments allow for the particular consideration of each case, the presence of antibodies (patients with inhibitors) is a relative contraindication for whatever type of intervention chosen [1,6–18]. This is due to destruction of the coagulation activity in the administered factors, which prevents adequate factor levels being attained. When it is necessary to surgically operate on fractures in haemophilic patients, the usual methods and techniques of orthopaedic surgery are used, treating the injury at once to avoid the possibility of further surgery. It is considered essential to carry out a careful tissue dissection using a clean bloodless area by using a pneumatic tourniquet with vascular ligature, ensuring that no dead spaces are left.

Whether or not to use electrocoagulation during surgery on these patients has been debated amongst those surgeons who operate on haemophilic individuals, because of the theoretical danger of new bleeding around 12 days, when the clot is shed. If this happens after 12 days, the patient is still under the postoperative transfusional covering when normal bleeding is highly unlikely. Also, assuming that the scab has been shed during that time, it would be rare for bleeding at this stage because the vascular focus will be closed and healed. Wounds or injuries to the soft tissues require surgical treatment similar to the non-haemophilic surgical technique, but the transfusional covering must be maintained from before the surgical procedure for up to 8–10 days, during which time healing takes place . The levels of factor should be above 30%, and then progressively reduced in the following 2–3 weeks. Open drainage and unnecessary transfusions must be avoided. In serious operations suction drainage should only be used for 24–48 hours.

Skeletal traction can be successful, although it should be avoided mainly because of the risk of cutaneous wounds. If this happens, the deficient coagulation factor should be administered for a longer period [16]. Surgical stabilization of fractures can be achieved with internal fixation [10]. Surgical reduction can be completed after carrying out an evaluation of the levels of coagulation factors and its correction. Hence, when the operation is initiated, the level of missing factor should be raised to between 70% and 100% [12]. Osteosynthesis *ad minimum* is not considered an indication in these patients because the patient does not benefit from the risks that surgery involves, as there is not sufficient stability and the fitting of a plaster cast is required.

The establishment of early replacement therapy and its correct use both in quantity and duration is the immediate objective when dealing with fractures in the haemophilic population. The correction of haemostatic defects allows optimum orthopaedic treatment of the fracture to be achieved. Traditional orthopaedic treatment of fractures in the haemophilic population, such as surgery, must not depart from the basic principles of the usual trauma techniques, with the therapeutic criteria being similar to those used for the general population.

Rehabilitation treatment

The patient can start active exercising as soon as possible, and need only stop when restoration is completed, with the aim of preventing muscular atrophy [26,27]. Contractures of the joints must be avoided and splints or orthoses [28] should be used. Rehabilitation treatment can be achieved through consecutive stages, passing from one to another depending on whether or not there is improvement. Movement is initiated with isometric exercises in such a way that muscular tone is improved and the strength reaches grade 3 (against resistance), removing the immobility [29]. Then hydrotherapy is used to increase mobility and improve muscular strength so that an improvement will always be objective, hence avoiding postoperative corrective surgery [29]. All types of physiotherapy measures (manual mobilization techniques, traction, functional training and so on) and all types of physiotechnical applications (icebags, ultrasound, intermittent short-wave diathermy and so on) can be used, but always under the protective shield of adequate doses of FVIII or FIX [30,31]. To summarize, rehabilitation is a cornerstone of treatment for haemophilic patients seeking favourable orthopaedic results (closed or open) through the maintenance of muscular function by limiting the period of immobility [18].

PROGRESSION

It has been observed in patients with a tendency to stressed bleeding that progression of healing of fractures tends to be similar to those of the non-haemophilic cases, with consolidation being obtained in the agreed time [1,15,18]. Fractures in haemophilic patients consolidate like other fractures inside the normal time frames and with the usual progression without complications [10,16,17]. Various authors differ in their view as to the type of bone callus that forms. According to Abreu *et al.,* it is a firm bone callus allowing early physiotherapy treatment to avoid aggravating the joint rigidity, osteoporosis and muscular atrophy which is present in haemophiliacs and increases with immobility [11]. Trueta holds the view that there is an acceleration of osteogenesis in haemophiliacs due to the consistency of the haematoma that would facilitate penetration of the vessels originating in the soft tissue that forms the callus [14].

CONCLUSION

A compartment syndrome may be present in significant haematomas [16]. It is necessary to maintain a high degree of vigilance and adopt appropriate and vigorous measures, such as opening the involved compartment in the forearm or the leg.

Even though our sample [12] was based on patients with heavy bleeding, variations between the type and number of complications in relation to the population in general have not been found, and it can be stated that if the fracture is correctly treated it will progress to consolidation in a similar time frame to those occurring in the general population.

REFERENCES

1 Boni M. Fracturas en los hemofílicos. In: *Libro de Resúmenes del Symposium Internacional sobre Hemofilia*. Cádiz, 13–15 December, 1979; 92.

2 Feil E, Bentley G, Rizza CR. Fracture management in patients with haemophilia. *J Bone Joint Surg (Br)* 1974; **56B**: 643–9.

3 Boni M, Ceciliani L. Le fratture negli emofilici. *Giornale Italiano di Ortopedia e Traumatologia* 1976; **2**: 197.

4 Biggs R. Thirty years of haemophilia treatment in Oxford. *Br J Haematol* 1967; **13**: 452.

5 Harrison JF. Haemophilic pseudotumor after fractures of the femur. *Br Med J* 1964; **1**: 554.

6 Monticelli G, Boni M. Il callo osseo normale e patologico. Fisiopatologia e Patologia del Callo Osseo. *Relazione al XL Congresso Societa Italiana di Ortopedia e Traumatologia*. Roma, 27–28 October, 1995.

7 Simonini D. Evoluzione del callo di frattura nell´emofilico. Atti Societa Emiliana, Romagnola, *Triveneta di Ortopedia e Traumatologia*, 1966, **11**: 233.

8 Jordan JJ. *Haemophilic Arthropathies*. Springfield, Illinois: Charles C Thomas, 1958.

9 Ikkala E. Haemophilia. *Scand J Clin Lab Invest* 1960; **12** (Suppl.): 46.

10 Abreu A. Tratamento ortopédico de urgencia no hemofílico. In: *Tratamiento Ortopédico de las Lesiones Hemofílicas del Aparato Locomotor*. New York: Schattauer Verlag, 1981: 105.

11 Abreu A, Elsade S, Seelig M. Tratamento ortopédico do hemofílico. *Pesq Med, Porto Alegre* 1973; **9**: 165.

12 Quintana M Jr, Rodriguez-Merchan EC, Magallon M. *Fracturas en el Paciente Hemofílico*. PhD thesis, Autonoma University, Madrid, Spain, April 1995.

13 Nilsson IM, Blombach B. Von Willebrand's disease in Sweden. *Acta Med Scand* 1959; **164**: 263.

14 Trueta J. The orthopedic management of patients with haemophilia and Christmas disease. Biggs R, MacFarlane RG, eds. *Treatment of Haemophilia and Other Coagulation Disorders*. Oxford: Blackwell, 1966: 279.

15 Fernandez-Palazzi F. Lesiones musculoesqueléticas en hemofílicos. In: *Tratamiento Ortopédico de las Lesiones Hemofílicas del Aparato Locomotor*. New York: Schattauer Verlag, 1981: 95.

16 Rubio-Fernandez I, Marques-Gassol F, Vila-Baucells M. Tratamiento de las fracturas en los pacientes hemofílicos. In: *Libro de Resúmenes del Symposium Internacional sobre Hemofilia*. Cádiz, 13–15 December, 1979; 201.

17 Eyster ME. Centers and the team approach. In: Hilgartner MW, ed. *Hemophilia in the Child and the Adult*. New York: Masson, 1982: 85.

18 Gilbert MS. Comprehensive care in hemophilia. Team approach. *Mt Sinai Med J* 1977; **44**: 313.

19 Abilgaard CF. Current concepts in the management of hemophilia. *Sem Hemat* 1975; **12**: 223.

20 Shanbrom E, Thelin GM. Experimental prophylaxis of severe hemophilia with factor VIII concentrate. *J Am Med A* 1969; **208**: 1853.

21 Heim M, Martinowitz U, Horoszowski H. Chronic post hemorrhagic arthritis. Conservative treatment. In: Döhring S, Schulitz KP, eds. *Orthopedic Problems in Hemophilia*. Munich: Zuckschwerdt, 1986: 93.

22 Arnold WD, Hilgartner MW. Hemophilic arthropathy. Current concepts of pathogenesis and management. *J Bone Joint Surg (Am)* 1977; **59A**: 287.

23 Duthie RB, Matthews JM, Rizza CR, Steel WM. Acute hemarthrosis. In: Duthie RB, ed. *The Management of Musculo-Skeletal Problems in Hemophilia*. Oxford: Blackwell, 1972: 29.

24 Hilgartner MW. *Hemofilia en el Niño y en el Adulto*, 2nd edn. Barcelona: Espax, 1985.

25 Duthie RB, Stein H. Ultrastructural changes in microprobe analysis of hemophilic joint tissues. *J Bone Joint Surg (Br)* 1977; **59B**: 118.

26 Boone DC. Common musculo-skeletal problems and their management. In: Boone DC, ed. *Comprehensive Management of Hemophilia*. Philadelphia: FA Davis, 1976: 53.

27 Duthie RB, Matthews J, Rizza CR, Steel W. The management of patients with hemophilia and Christmas disease and the principles of replacement therapy. In: Duthie RB, ed. *The Management of Musculo-Skeletal Problems in Hemophilia*. Oxford: Blackwell, 1972; 21.

28 Hofmann P, Menge M, Brackmann HH. Reconstructive surgery in the lower limb in hemophiliacs. *Israel J Med Sci* 1977; **13**: 988.

29 Heijnen L. Physiotherapy and rehabilitation. In: Döhring S, Schulitz KP, eds. *Orthopedic Problems in Hemophilia*. Munich: Zuckschwerdt, 1986: 194.

30 Hirschmann RJ, Itootiz SB, Shulman NR. Prophylactic treatment of factor VIII deficiency. *Blood* 1970; **36**: 189.

31 Kasper CK, Dietrich SL, Rappaport SI. Hemophilia prophylaxis with factor VIII concentrates. *Arch Int Med* 1970; **125**: 1004.

CHAPTER 22

Osteonecrosis of the Femoral Head

E C RODRIGUEZ-MERCHAN, A MARTINEZ-LLOREDA, M J SANJURJO AND V JIMENEZ-YUSTE

INTRODUCTION

While arthropathy is comparatively common in adults with haemophilia, osteonecrosis of the femoral head is rare. Osteonecrosis is usually caused by vascular compromise and may result in deformity and ultimately complete destruction of the hip joint. The femoral head is a common site for osteonecrosis because of the tenuous nature of its blood supply. Legg–Calvé–Perthes' disease (or simply Perthes' disease) is a well-known yet controversial paediatric hip disorder that is believed to represent idiopathic avascular necrosis (osteonecrosis) of the capital femoral epiphysis (Fig. 22.1). Of the 517 patients with moderate to severe haemophilia admitted to the Haemophilia Unit of La Paz University Hospital between 1980 and 1999, four had Perthes' disease. In addition, one man aged 18 years presented with avascular necrosis but did not have Perthes' disease.

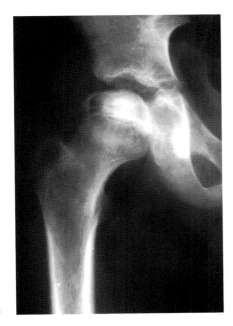

(a)

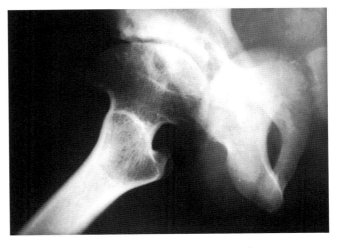

(b)

Fig. 22.1 Perthes' disease: (a) anteroposterior radiograph demonstrates partial head involvement in an 8-year-old patient with haemophilia; (b) radiograph of the same patient at 16 years of age demonstrates that rapid collapse of the femoral head resulted in a square shape to the femoral head.

PERTHES' DISEASE IN HAEMOPHILIC CHILDREN

The length of follow-up in the four patients with Perthes' disease described above ranged from 7 to 11 years (average 9.25 years). Our short-term results have been previously reported [1]. Primary treatment included adequate replacement therapy with concentrates of factor VIII (30 IU/kg per day) and bed rest for 1–2 weeks with the hip maintained at 45° of flexion by means of skin traction. The definitive treatment comprised ambulation-abduction bracing in three cases and proximal femoral varus osteotomy in the fourth.

As soon as the avascular process was noted, each patient was positioned so that no weight was borne on the involved hip. When the pain subsided, the patient was measured for an ambulatory containment orthosis. Patients were arbitrarily left in the containment orthosis, with full weight-bearing on the affected hip, for an average of 14 months. The main results of this study are summarized in Table 22.1.

On follow-up examination, no pain was reported but there was some degree of functional impairment. All patients could perform activities of daily living while maintaining a sedentary lifestyle. Thus, from a subjective point of view, the results were satisfactory. Follow-up radiographic examination revealed major collapse of the epiphysis in the anterior and superior quadrant in patient 1. Patient 2 showed squaring of the femoral head and patient 3 had an ovoid femoral head with mild acetabular dysplasia. Patient 4 showed a rapid collapse and resultant squaring of the femoral head.

With modern treatment and prophylaxis, haemophilic arthropathy of the hip has become a rare finding [2]. It has been reported that the use of Russell traction for 7 to 14 days decreases the intraosseous pressure significantly and increases the hip motion by a mean of 33.6° [3]. Wingstand et al. [4] reported that in some cases presenting with clinical symptoms of synovitis of the hip, a transient, spontaneously recovering ischaemia of the proximal femoral epiphysis occurs that is not followed by radiographic evidence of necrosis.

Table 22.1 Patients with Perthes' disease: main characteristics, data and results.

Patient	Age at detection (yrs)	Radiographic stage at detection	Primary treatment	Definitive treatment*	Follow-up (yrs)	Clinical result	Radiographic result
1	6	Early	Concentrates of factor VIII, bed rest, skin traction	Abduction orthosis (9)	11	Good	Poor
2	7	Late	Concentrates of factor VIII, bed rest, skin traction	Abduction orthosis (15)	7	Good	Poor
3	7	Late	Concentrates of factor VIII, bed rest, skin traction	Proximal femoral varus osteotomy	11	Good	Fair
4	8	Late	Concentrates of factor VIII, bed rest, skin traction	Abduction orthosis (12)	8	Good	Poor

*Number of months treatment in parentheses.

An intracapsular haematoma or effusion with an ensuing increase in intracapsular pressure could compromise blood flow through the proximal femoral epiphysis. Vegter [5] reported that in the presence of a synovial effusion in the hip, a position of extension and medial rotation causes an increase in intra-articular pressure which may compromise the blood supply to the capital epiphysis of the femur. Pettersson *et al.* [6] detected an intracapsular pressure of 273 mmHg in a haemophilic patient with the hip in extension and neutral rotation. However, Erken and Katz [7] reported that pressure tamponade in the irritable hip syndrome in haemophilic patients preceding Perthes' disease is probably not responsible for the condition.

The clinical picture of a fixed flexed hip associated with pain in a person with haemophilia is suggestive of a haemorrhage in that area. Sonography facilitates differentiation between a haemarthrosis, intraperitoneal haemorrhage, a subperiosteal bleed, a bleed into the soft tissue around the hip or a psoas haematoma. Where the use of narcotic drugs fails to alleviate pain, Pettersson *et al.* [6] and Heim *et al.* [8] recommend hip aspiration, which produces dramatic pain relief and early joint rehabilitation. However, in common with Heim *et al.*, we are not suggesting that every coxhaemarthrosis should be aspirated.

Early recognition of a change in the shape of the femoral head is important if it is to be corrected. In untreated patients lacking two or more of the radiologic head-at-risk signs during the active stages of the disease, no adverse outcomes have been demonstrated [9]. Therefore, the presence of two or more of these signs during the active phase of the disease is in itself an indication for treatment. Since it may take as long as 6 months to determine the extent of femoral head involvement in patients who present early in the disease process, non-operative methods may be used to improve the range of motion and to contain the femoral head within the acetabulum, thereby minimizing further deformity [10]. Thus, surgical intervention is indicated for many older children who have involvement of more than one-half of the femoral head, as well as for patients in whom non-operative efforts at containment have been unsuccessful.

OSTEONECROSIS OF THE FEMORAL HEAD IN HAEMOPHILIC ADULTS

Osteonecrosis is a disease of unknown pathogenesis that usually progresses to hip joint destruction, necessitating total hip arthroplasty. The pathology involves ischaemic events followed by death of bone and marrow elements. A process of repair is then initiated, but unless the lesion is small (less than 15% of the femoral head involved), this repair process is usually ineffective. The net result is weakening of subchondral bone with subsequent collapse of the articular surface [11].

An association between haemophilia and osteonecrosis of the femoral head has been reported previously [1,6,12–14]. Dye *et al.* [15] have illustrated the possibility that patients with haemophilia may develop osteonecrosis without coexisting haemophilic arthropathy. Between 1980 and 1999, we identified one 18-year-old male haemophilia patient with radiographic findings suggestive of osteonecrosis, but without unequivocal microscopic evidence of osteonecrosis. Recently, Dye *et al.* [15] have reported a case of bilateral osteonecrosis of the femoral head.

By using only clinical presentation and conventional radiographic information, early osteonecrosis may be very difficult to distinguish from haemarthrosis and haemophilic arthropathy. In case of doubt, magnetic resonance imaging may provide an additional diagnostic tool (Fig. 22.2). It is suggested that osteonecrosis should be included in the differential diagnosis of hip pathology in patients with haemophilia. Early recognition of osteonecrosis and its distinction from haemophilic arthropathy is important because there are surgical interventions for osteonecrosis which may preserve joint function and improve quality of life [16].

Because the results of hip arthroplasty in patients with osteonecrosis are relatively poor, much attention has been focused on modalities aimed at femoral head preservation. Ortiguera *et al.* [17] have recently published a matched comparison between total hip arthroplasties in osteonecrosis and those in osteoarthritis. All received cemented Charnley replacements and had a minimum follow-up of 10 years. Results of arthroplasty in both groups were comparable in patients over 50 years of age, although patients with osteonecrosis had an increased rate of dislocation. Patients with osteonecrosis who were younger than 50 years of age had a significantly higher rate of mechanical failure than those patients of a similar age with osteoarthritis. Cemented total hip arthroplasty should be recommended in this group with caution, if at all.

The surgical alternatives may include core decompression, osteotomy, non-vascularized and vascularized bone grafting, all of which may be enhanced with the use of growth and differentiation factors. At least three of these factors are potential candidates as therapeutic modalities: cytokines (such as interleukins, tumour necrosis factors, and signalling molecules such as fibroblast growth factors, platelet-derived growth factors, insulin-like growth factors, and transforming growth factor betas), bone morphogenetic proteins and angiographic factors [11].

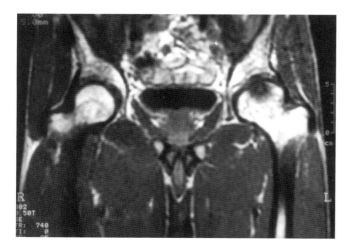

Fig. 22.2 Magnetic resonance imaging of an 18-year-old patient with haemophilia showing decreased signal intensity in the superior portion of the left femoral head (black area). These findings are consistent with osteonecrosis of the femoral head.

Recently, several investigators have attempted to mimic osteonecrosis in the femoral head of large mammals by combinations of devascularization, freezing, osteotomy of the femoral neck, or creation of a head defect. Results from some of these studies have confirmed the potential for growth and differentiation factors to effect more rapid healing and filling of defects with biomechanically competent and viable bone. The application of this therapy shows promise, and clinical studies on efficacy and safety are ongoing.

Core decompression for patients in stage I osteonecrosis of the femoral head is associated with an excellent result, no matter which failure endpoints are examined. The use of core decompression in patients with stage IIA and IIB osteonecrosisis is less reliable, as has been shown by Iorio et al. [18] in a series of 33 hips in 23 patients (followed for 5.3 years). A lower radiographic stage was associated with a better result. Patients who weighed less than 79.4 kg (175 lb) or whose bone stock was good (femoral index < 0.56) had significantly improved hip survival. When total hip arthroplasty was used as an endpoint, 90% of hips survived 1 year, 70% survived 2 years, and 61% survived 5 years.

SUMMARY

Early detection of hip haemarthrosis is paramount for the implementation of effective treatment. In cases where the use of narcotic drugs fails to alleviate pain, treatment will include factor replacement and hip joint aspiration. As soon as Perthes' disease is diagnosed, the patient should be placed in a non-weightbearing position on the affected hip. When the pain subsides, the patient should be measured for an ambulatory containment orthosis. Early recognition of osteonecrosis of the femoral head in the adult haemophilia patient is also important, because core decompression may preserve joint function. When osteonecrosis progresses to hip joint destruction, a total hip arthroplasty will be needed. Cemented total hip arthroplasty should be recommended with caution if at all.

REFERENCES

1 Rodriguez-Merchan EC, Ortega F, Galindo E, Magallon M, Lopez-Cabarcos C. Legg–Calvé–Perthes' disease in hemophilia. *Contemp Orthop* 1992; **25**: 472–9.

2 Pettersson H, Nilsson IM, Hedner U, Norehn K, Ahlberg A. Radiologic evaluation of prophylaxis of severe hemophilia. *Acta Pediatr Scand* 1981; **70**: 565–9.

3 Serlo W, Heikkinen E, Puranen J. Preoperative Russell traction in Legg–Calvé–Perthes' disease. *J Pediatr Orthop* 1987; **7**: 288–93.

4 Wingstand H, Bauer GC, Brismar J, Carlin NO, Pettersson H, Sunden G. Transient ischaemia of the proximal femoral epiphysis in the child: interpretation of bone scintimetry for diagnosis in hip pain. *Acta Orthop Scand* 1985; **56**: 197–201.

5 Vegter J. The influence of joint posture on intraarticular pressure: a study of transient synovitis and Perthes' disease. *J Bone Joint Surg (Am)* 1987; **69A**: 71–8.

6 Pettersson H, Wingstrand H, Thambert C, Nilsson IM, Jonsson K. Legg–Calvé–Perthes' disease in hemophilia: incidence and etiologic considerations. *J Pediatr Orthop* 1990; **10**: 28–32

7 Erken EHW, Katz K. Irritable hip and Perthes' disease. *J Pediatr Orthop* 1990; **10**: 322–7.

8 Heim M, Varon D, Strauss S, Martinowitz U. The management of a person with haemophilia who has a fixed flexed hip and intractable pain. *Haemophilia* 1998; **4**: 842–4.

9 Catterall A. Legg–Calvé–Perthes' disease. Pathology and classification. In: Fitzgerald RH, ed. *The Hip*. St. Louis: CV Mosby, 1985: 12–16.

10 MacEwen GD. Conservative treatment of Legg-Calvé-Perthes' condition. In: Fitzgerald RH, ed. *The Hip*. St

Louis: CV Mosby, 1985: 17–23.

11 Mont MA, Jones LC, Einhorn TA, Hungerford DS, Reddi AH. Osteonecrosis of the femoral head: potential treatment with growth and differential factors. *Clin Orthop* 1998; **355**S: 314–35.

12 Boettcher WG, Bonfiglio M, Hamilton HH, Sheets RF, Smith K. Non-traumatic necrosis of the femoral head. Part I. Relation of altered hemostasis to etiology. *J Bone Joint Surg (Br)* 1983; **65B**: 285–7.

13 Paton RW, Evans DIK. Silent avascular necrosis of the femoral head in haemophilia. *J Bone Joint Surg (Br)* 1988; **70B**: 737–9.

14 Winston ME. Haemophilic arthropathy of the hip. *J Bone Joint Surg* 1952; **36**: 412–20.

15 Dye CE, Frauenhoffer EE, Vrahas M. Osteonecrosis of the femoral head in haemophiliacs: not all joint disease is haemophilic arthropathy. *Haemophilia* 1997; **3**: 111–17.

16 Meyers MH. Osteonecrosis of the femoral head: pathogenesis and long-term results of treatment. *Clin Orthop* 1988; **231**: 51–61.

17 Ortiguera CJ, Pulliam IT, Cabanela ME. Total hip arthroplasty for osteonecrosis: matched-pair analysis of 188 hips with long-term follow-up. *J Arthroplasty* 1999; **14**: 21–8.

18 Iorio R, Haely WL, Abramowitz AJ, Pfeifer BA. Clinical outcome and survivorship analysis of core decompression for early osteonecrosis of the femoral head. *J Arthroplasty* 1998; **13**: 34–41.

3

Rehabilitation and Physiotherapy

CHAPTER 23
Rehabilitation

L HEIJNEN AND M T SOHAIL

INTRODUCTION

The general principles of rehabilitation are applicable when musculoskeletal problems in haemophilia arise. In this chapter, the concept of rehabilitation will be described using the definitions from the World Health Organization and the International Classification of Impairments, Disabilities and Handicaps (ICIDH). Practical aspects of rehabilitation in haemophilia will be mentioned, with suggestions for rehabilitation in the community. The need to measure the results of rehabilitation will be touched upon briefly; this has been described more extensively elsewhere by de Kleijn and von Meereren [1].

Definition

Rehabilitation of persons with haemophilia includes all measures aimed at reducing the impact of disabling and handicapping conditions and enabling the disabled and handicapped persons with haemophilia to achieve social integration [2].

DIAGNOSIS

The rehabilitation diagnosis includes three levels: organ level, person level and social level.

1 At the organ level the ICIDH speaks of 'impairment', which is any loss or abnormality of psychological, physiological or anatomical structure or function [3]. Post *et al.* [4] add 'somatic sensation', which includes feelings of pain, fatigue and so on, to organ level.

2 At the person level the ICIDH uses 'disability', which is any restriction or lack of ability to perform an activity in the manner or within the range considered normal for a human being. Post *et al.* add to this level 'perceived health' (general feelings of health, satisfaction with health).

3 At a social level the ICIDH speaks of 'handicap', which is a disadvantage for a given individual, resulting from an impairment or a disability, that limits or prevents the fulfilment of a role that is normal (depending on age, sex and social and cultural factors) for that individual. At this level Post adds 'life satisfaction' (satisfaction with role performance). In his proposal for an integrated conceptual framework for rehabilitation outcomes research, he states that the overall well-being which is perceived by a person, and which he names 'happiness', should also be taken into account.

The World Health Organization is currently working on a revision of the ICIDH [5]. This new version (ICIDH-2) still organizes information according to the same three dimensions: body (organ) level, individual (person) level and society (social) level. The body level is still concerned with the impairments mentioned above ('impairment' is regarded as a negative aspect; 'functional and structural integrity' is positive). At the level of the person as a whole, 'activity' is the positive description and the negative aspect is 'activity limitation', which is used instead of 'disability'. At the level of society the participation dimension classifies areas of life in which an individual is involved, has access to and/or for which there are societal opportunities or barriers: 'participation' is positive, 'participation restriction' the negative aspect.

The Beta-2 version of the ICIDH-2 has been released for field trials due to finish in July 2000. This last version will be tested and commented on throughout the world before it is finalized and submitted to the World Health Assembly in 2001. The ICIDH-2 classification can provide a scientific basis for understanding and studying the functional states associated with health conditions. Moreover, it establishes a common language for describing functional states associated with health conditions which will improve communications between healthcare workers, persons with disabilities and other sectors. When used, it permits comparison of data across countries, healthcare disciplines, services and time.

Treatment team

Based on the rehabilitation diagnosis an individually tailored complex plan of treatment can be defined. Only a multidisciplinary team of professionals who have their individual expertise and are able to communicate with each other can execute this plan. Ideally, a rehabilitation team specializing in haemophilia should have the following members: physiatrist (medical doctor, specialized in physical medicine and rehabilitation), orthopaedic surgeon, haematologist, nurse, physiotherapist, occupational therapist, social worker, psychologist, orthotist and orthopaedic shoemaker. In most comprehensive care centres that specialize in haemophilia and other clotting disorders, the majority of these professionals are available. Professionals such as the occupational therapist, orthotist or orthopaedic shoemaker may be posted from a general rehabilitation unit to the team. In the general rehabilitation setting a speech therapist will also be available, and instead of a haematologist a neurologist and/or rheumatologist may be a member of the team or available on a consultancy basis.

REHABILITATION IN HAEMOPHILIA

The clotting disorder which is present in haemophilia will lead to haemarthroses and muscle bleeds. These are diagnoses at organ level and will be treated as early as possible (at disease level) by intravenous administration of the appropriate clotting factor, ideally at home by the patient himself or by his parents or other family members. This should result in recovery of normal function of the joint and muscles involved. If the bleeding does not resolve completely within a short period of time, the remaining impairments will be diagnosed and advice will be given concerning further replacement therapy, rest, local application of ice or cold packs and splinting. The physiotherapist will advise and help the patient to perform exercises. The physiotherapist may also decide to use physiotherapeutic applications [6].

Following a severe haemarthrosis or muscle bleed, especially when clotting factor is not available, there may be lasting impairments such as contractures and loss of muscle strength which will cause disabilities. At this point, not only a diagnosis at organ level but also at person level should be made, because the limited joint and muscle function will result in practical problems for the patient. He may not be able to rise from his chair, visit the bathroom, climb stairs or travel to school or work. A plan to treat or compensate for these limitations of activity (disabilities) during the period in which reduction of contractures, improvement of the range of motion and muscle strength are worked at but not yet achieved, should be drawn up and executed. Walking adjuncts such as crutches or a wheelchair may be used to enable the patient to go to school or work. A temporary splint may be prescribed to support the leg and mobilize the patient while awaiting improvement of muscle strength by daily active exercises; or a heel raise can be provided while awaiting the reduction of an equinus foot after a calf bleed.

A severe muscle bleed with compression of a nerve or necrosis in a compartment may lead to permanent impairments which require a permanent brace and/or other adaptations to help the patient to lead an independent life and to prevent limitation of activity (disability) turning into restriction of participation (handicap). Worldwide, 80% of individuals with haemophilia have no access to adequate clotting factor. For them, recurrent haemarthroses in the major joints are inevitable. Developing strong muscles and good coordination is an advantage but cannot prevent all bleeding problems. At organ level a person with severe haemophilia without access to clotting factor is expected to have approximately five damaged joints by the age of 20.

It is important to realize that an impairment in one joint (for instance, a limited range of motion) can be compensated by adjacent joints, so that the impairment need not lead to limitation of activity (disability). Even multiple joint involvement in one limb may be compensated by the other limb, so that the patient is still able to climb stairs or wash and groom himself. But multiple joint involvement in more than one limb is bound to lead to disabilities. Whether a disability leads to a handicap depends on the social situation. For example, if someone can bend one or both knees less than 90°, he will be handicapped in societies where he is expected to squat on the floor, and he will not be able to ride an ordinary bicycle. The state of the art of rehabilitation in haemophilia has been described in 1989 [7] and in 1995 [8].

Rehabilitation in developing countries

Most developing countries have major social and health problems. Haemophilia is a rare disease. Persons with haemophilia should make use of already existing health and rehabilitation services, especially in situations where no comprehensive haemophilia care team is available. However, some developing countries that have no or few comprehensive care teams specializing in haemophilia also have almost no rehabilitation services. In others, institution-based services serve very few people. Larger countries have more developed services which are usually institution based, perhaps with outreach programmes. In other countries, community-based rehabilitation (CBR) may be available. If rehabilitation services are not available at all, we suggest that local haemophilia groups or even one family should start community-based rehabilitation with the help of any local professional and technician who may be available.

Hellander and colleagues' description [9] of CBR can be summarized as follows: the term CBR is used for situations where resources for rehabilitation are available in the community. The aim of the programme is to provide the service to those who need it, in their own community, utilizing their local resources, so that they do not have to travel too far for such help. There is a large-scale transfer of knowledge about disabilities and of the skills in rehabilitation to the people with disabilities, their families and the members of the community. This is done through local supervisors, community workers, persons with a disability and written information.

Incidence of disability

It is estimated that 2.5–3% of the population in developing countries is disabled and could benefit from rehabilitation. In some countries, a major part of the disabled population lives in rural areas: for instance, in India it is estimated that 78% of the generally disabled population lives in rural areas. The absolute number of persons with haemophilia with disabilities is low compared with the generally disabled population. However, for each person with haemophilia with impairments and limitation of activities rehabilitation is very important, especially if clotting factors are not available.

ORGANIZING COMMUNITY-BASED REHABILITATION (CBR)

On behalf of the World Health Organization, Hellander *et al.* [9] have written a manual for successful execution of CBR. The manual contains 34 modules, comprising four guides and 30 training packages. In the first place, there should be a local haemophilia supervisor who could be the community rehabilitation worker supervising the people in the rehabilitation programme. The local haemophilia supervisor should preferably be someone chosen by the local haemophilia society and should be familiar with the problems of haemophilia. If there is already a CBR programme, then the supervisor should work in close cooperation with the community rehabilitation committee. The National Haemophilia Federation or Society of the country concerned should develop educational materials to be distributed locally. These educational materials should give information concerning the clotting disorder and its inheritance and treatment of musculoskeletal problems if clotting factor is not available.

Guidelines explaining exercises to improve joint motion and muscle strength which can be performed by the person with haemophilia and taught by parents to their child with haemophilia are of the utmost importance. These guidelines should include discussion of physical activities and sports. The World Federation of Haemophilia provides information for both professionals and families which can be translated into the local language. Haemophilia societies and comprehensive care centres all over the world have developed their own material, which could also be translated and adapted to the local situation. Orthotics (splints and braces), shoe adaptations and walking aids should be available. Local materials and craftsmanship should be used as much as possible.

Service delivery system

It is not enough simply to formulate guidelines and distribute them; it is important that there are professionals or experienced volunteers to train and supervise local physiotherapists, nurses or other healthcare workers, and family members and the persons with haemophilia themselves. Children with haemophilia should be able to go to school, and teachers need to be informed about haemophilia so that schools can enable haemophilic children to participate safely in activities. Adult persons with haemophilia with musculoskeletal problems should not only be able to do exercises and be provided with orthotics or walking aids, but they should also have access to vocational services, assessment and job training. These services may not be available locally but at district or provincial level. Treatment of persons with haemophilia in developing countries will be described more extensively by the authors elsewhere [6].

PREVENTION OF DISABILITY

Physical activities and sports are important for all persons with haemophilia. A good physical condition and good motor coordination may prevent musculoskeletal problems and may speed recovery after joint and muscles bleeds. Persons with haemophilia should be encouraged to participate in activities which are normal for their age and peer groups. In *Go For It* [10] a number of sports are mentioned that most doctors consider safe for persons with haemophilia. These are badminton, bowls, cycling, dancing, fishing, frisbee, golf, hiking, sailing, snorkelling, swimming, table tennis, walking and yoga. Sports with high risk of trauma for all individuals are considered dangerous for persons with haemophilia. Another 54 sports are mentioned in which benefits may outweigh risks for the individual when supervised training is given and proper equipment used.

Participation in physical education at school and in many sports nowadays is normal for boys and adults with haemophilia living in countries where clotting factor is available and where persons with severe haemophilia are on home treatment, taking clotting factor prophylactically. If clotting factor is scarce, and only available for major bleeding incidents or not at all, sporting activities should be planned carefully. In these situations, however, sensible physical activities and sports should be emphasized even more, because strong muscles and good motor coordination will protect the joints.

MEASURING IMPAIRMENTS, DISABILITIES (ACTIVITY LIMITATIONS) AND HANDICAPS (PARTICIPATION RESTRICTIONS)

The pathology and impairments at organ level concerning haemarthroses, chronic synovitis and arthropathy of the haemophilic joint have been described extensively in the literature [11–13]. The range of motion of elbows, knees and ankles can be measured using a goniometer [14]. The joint damage visualized with plain radiographs can be scored according to Pettersson et al. [15]. However, Heijnen [16] found no correlation between limitation of range of motion in arthropathic elbows, knees and ankles and the Pettersson score. Johnson et al. [17] described the pattern of loss of motion in haemophilic joints. The descriptions of the pathology and impairments are so clear-cut that the ensuing disabilities and handicaps are easy to imagine. Few publications, however, describe the correlation between the level of impairment and disability.

Iwata et al. [18] described the consequences of limitation of joint movement for activities of daily living. They carried out a longitudinal study of 97 patients with haemophilia A and B. Analysis of ratings showed that flexion of the lower limbs tended to be limited. The functional limitation level differed significantly by age group. All but one of the study population were capable of all feeding activities and some grooming and dressing activities, 86% could tie or untie a necktie, 74% could go up and down stairs and 65% could ride a bicycle. However, even slight limitation of the flexion of knees and dorsiflexion of ankles resulted in disability because the Japanese patients had difficulties using Asian toilets (46%) and sitting in Japanese style (61%).

Heijnen et al. [19] compared the range of motion of elbows, knees and ankles of 155 patients with haemophilia A and B with normal values from the literature and with the description of range of motion necessary for the functional activities of daily living. Of the 155 patients, 34 had limitations of activity for both arms, 14 for one arm, and only 39 had a completely normal range of motion in both elbows. For 79 patients range of motion of both knees was near normal; 38 patients would not be able to ride an ordinary bicycle, while 16 patients were not able to climb a staircase normally because knee flexion was <60°. For 103 patients with limited dorsiflexion of the ankles squatting was difficult or impossible. Whether or not these limitations of activities cause handicap (restriction in participation) depends on the social circumstances. If a person does not need or want to ride a bicycle, has his living quarters on the ground floor and has access to his office by means of an elevator, he may not rate himself as handicapped.

Although the ICIDH-2 can provide a classification to describe the functional states associated with haemophilia, a simpler tool to measure disabilities (limitation of activities) and handicap (restriction of participation) is needed. Moreover, the perception of healthcare professionals and government officials as to the severity of the handicap of a person with haemophilia may differ from the person's own perception. A scale from the patient's perspective of the impact on participation and autonomy (handicap) (IPA) is being developed [20], which addresses the factors of autonomy indoors, family role, autonomy outdoors, social relations, work and education opportunities. The IPA is being designed as a generic measure to be used in combination with an appropriate disability (activity limitation) scale. More information concerning its validity and reliability will be needed before its usefulness in the haemophilic population can be assessed.

SUMMARY

The clotting defect in haemophilia can cause haemarthroses, chronic synovitis and arthropathy in shoulders, elbows, hips, knees and ankles at organ level. These complex impairments at organ level cause limitation of activity (disability) and restriction of participation (handicap). The rehabilitation diagnosis and the plan of treatment are based on these three levels. The multidisciplinary treatment aims at preventing limitation of activity and reducing restriction of participation. In countries where clotting factor is available for prophylactic treatment or treatment on demand in the home situation, prevention of musculoskeletal problems is possible.

The importance of good physical condition and motor coordination cannot be over-emphasized. Boys should participate in physical education at school, and all persons with haemophilia should be active in one or more sports all year around. In developing countries with little or no clotting factor available, rehabilitation should not only include physiotherapy, prescription of orthoses, walking aids and other adaptations, but also education of persons with haemophilia and their families. In these countries community-based rehabilitation (CBR) may be available. If this is not the case, the National Haemophilia Society should encourage local groups to take initiatives.

The concept of community-based rehabilitation (CBR) is very important in developing countries, where institution-based rehabilitation facilities and comprehensive care haemophilia centres are scare, communication is difficult and distances between the home of the person with haemophilia and those facilities available are great. The involvement of the local community and the education of the persons with haemophilia and their families are the first steps towards haemophilia comprehensive care. Tools to assess the needs of the individual person with haemophilia and to measure the long-term outcome of rehabilitation interventions are important. Measurements should be taken at organ, person and social level. The instruments should enable those involved in haemophilia care to share experiences and to compare treatment worldwide.

REFERENCES

1 de Kleijn P, von Meereren NLU. Use of a theoretical framework for health status in haemophilia care and research. In: Buzzard B, Beeton K, eds. *The Physiotherapy Management of Haemophilia*. Oxford: Blackwell Science, 2000.

2 WHO Expert Committee. *Disability Prevention and Rehabilitation*. Technical reports series 668. Geneva: WHO, 1981.

3 World Health Organization. *International Classification of Impairments, Disabilities and Handicaps*. Geneva: WHO, 1980.

4 Post WM, de Witte LP, Schrijvers AJP. Quality of life and the ICIDH: towards an integrated conceptual model for rehabilitation outcomes research. *Clin Rehab* 1999; **13**: 5–15.

5 WHO Collaborating Centre for the ICIDH in the Netherlands. *Newsletter* 5, 1999.

6 Buzzard B, Beeton K, eds. *The Physiotherapy Management of Haemophilia*. Oxford: Blackwell Science, 2000.

7 Battistella R, Heijnen L. *Rehabilitation in Haemophilia*. Brighton: Medifax International, 1989.

8 Heijnen L. *Recent Advances in Haemophilia*. Hove, East Sussex: Medical Education Network, 1995.

9 Hellander E, Mendis P, Nelson G, Goerdt A. *Training in the Community for Peoples with Disabilities*. Geneva: WHO, 1989.

10 Jones P, Buzzard B, Heijnen L. *Go For It: Guidance on Physical Activity and Sports for People with Haemophilia and Related Disorders*. World Federation of Haemophilia, 1998.

11 König F. Die Gelenkerkrankungen bei Blutern mit besonderer Berücksichtigung der Diagnose. *Klin Vorträge NF* 1982; **36**: 233–42.

12 Key AJ. Hemophilic arthritis. *Annals of Surgery* 1932; **95**: 198–225.

13 De Palma AF, Cotler J. Hemophilic arthropathy. *Clin Orthop* 1956; **8**: 163–90.

14 Rothstein JM, Miller PJ, Roettger RF: Goniometric reliability in a clinical setting: elbow and knee measurements. *Phys Ther* 1993 **63**: 1611–15.

15 Pettersson H, Ahlberg GA, Nilsson IM. A radiologic classification of hemophilic arthropathy. *Clin Orthop* 1980; **149**: 153–9.

16 Heijnen L. *Haemophilic arthropathy: a study of the joint status of haemophilic patients comparing prophylactic replacement therapy with treatment on demand*. Thesis. Dordrecht: ICG Printing BV, 1986.

17 Johnson RP, Vasudevan SV, Lazerson J. Arc-aggregation: a new method of range of motion analysis in hemophilia. *Arch Phys Rehabil* 1984; **65**: 584–7.

18 Iwata N, Hachisuka K, Tanaka S, Naka Y, Ogata H. Measuring activities of daily living among haemophiliacs. *Disabil Rehabil* 1996; **18**: 217–23.

19 Heijnen L, de Kleijn P, Heim M. Functional kinesiology in haemophilia, an area yet to be explored. *Haemophilia* 1998; **4**: 524–7.

20 Cardol M, de Haan RJ, van den Bos GAM, de Jong BA, de Groot JM. The development of handicap assessment questionnaire: the impact on participation and autonomy (IPA). *Clin Rehabil* 1999; **13**: 411–19.

CHAPTER 24

Physiotherapy Management of Haemophilia in Children

B M BUZZARD

INTRODUCTION

The role of the physiotherapist in the management of children with haemophilia has progressed rapidly in keeping with the improvements made with blood products in the developed world. Home therapy programmes and prophylaxis have enabled most children to develop normally with little or no abnormal joint or muscle pathology. Children with haemophilia are now integrated into mainstream schools and are participating in activities including sport along with their peers [1].

Unfortunately, despite replacement therapy there are still some children who present with joint or muscle problems related to bleeding episodes. There may be several reasons for this, such as poor compliance with prophylaxis, breakthrough bleeding, trauma or the development of inhibitors. Those children with severe haemophilia A and B learn to recognize bleeding episodes in their early years of life and seek treatment; however, we are now seeing increasing numbers of patients with mild haemophilia presenting with joint pathology [2]. Mild haemophilia often goes undiagnosed for a long time, especially if there is no previous family history, until the patient presents with a severe joint haemorrhage or haematoma which is often related to direct trauma. Those with mild haemophilia must not be forgotten as the consequences of bleeding episodes are equally damaging, whatever degree of severity of haemophilia is present. The need to educate all those involved with haemophilia is paramount.

PATTERNS OF BLEEDING

Each child develops at their own pace, usually through the same stages or milestones in about the same order. Children grow and learn continually, but often in an erratic pattern, some learning skills quickly while others do so more slowly. Babies grow at varying rates, and by 9 months they will be exploring everything within reach, able to roll easily from tummy to back and then back onto tummy and learn to sit without any support. It is at this stage that the baby with haemophilia may develop bruises as he rolls onto toys in his cot.

By 9–12 months, the child will be able to sit unsupported for quite some time, turn sideways without losing balance, and stretch out and pick up a toy from the floor. Progress then follows from rolling and crawling on all fours and then to pulling themselves up to stand against furniture. As the child's motor skills develop and he or she begins to crawl and walk, we often see bruises on the outer aspects of the arms and knees, and even knee and elbow bleeds. From 12 months, most babies will be walking, talking and starting to climb. At this age they will always be active and showing signs of independence. As the toddler gains his balance he will inevitably have numerous falls, with increased bruises to the head and buttocks.

The 2-year-old is an exciting combination of baby and toddler, who is constantly busy exploring the world around him and learning about it. Toddlers have spent the past few months practising and coordinating their body movements. Walking is nearly perfect and most are running safely. Falls are still common because they cannot avoid obstacles quickly. By the age of 3, most children can go up and down steps, ride a tricycle, kick or throw a ball, and pick up small objects with their forefingers and thumb. As the child continues to grow and develop, further joint bleeds may occur, especially in the weight-bearing joints, such as the ankle and knee. Bleeding episodes into the ankle joint may be related to the immaturity and relative instability of the ankle joint in growing children [3,4].

Once the child starts school, he will then be participating in sports. The child with haemophilia need not be restricted in his choice of activities provided prophylactic treatment is given if necessary and the child wears the correct equipment for the particular activity and he receives appropriate instruction [1–6].

Sport and exercise for those with haemophilia has been shown to be beneficial in the prevention of haematomas [7], however, all sporting activities are not without the risk of injury. It is part of the physiotherapist's role to advise, educate and treat patients with haemophilia on these aspects and to give them the necessary information to make informed choices and to weigh up the cost–benefit relationship [6,8,9].

Prophylaxis and home therapy programmes appear to be the key factor in prevention of haemophilic arthropathy, however, there is an ongoing debate as to when prophylaxis should be commenced. The Swedish experience has shown that patients who were started on primary prophylaxis between the ages of 1 and 2 years have shown excellent joint preservation [10].

Patterns of bleeding in children with bleeding disorders are difficult to predict. There has been little research into this area. Janco *et al.* [11] carried out a prospective study among boys with haemophilia over a 6-month period to describe the patterns of bleeding. Their results showed that most bleeding episodes occurred during weekdays, Monday to Friday, and that those with severe haemophilia had more joints involved and bled more frequently than those with moderate or mild haemophilia. They also described a high rate of bleeding episodes associated with direct trauma.

PHYSIOTHERAPY MANAGEMENT OF BLEEDING EPISODES

No physiotherapy intervention should begin without a full musculoskeletal assessment of the child. Physiotherapists are unique in their understanding of anatomy and physiology, and with this knowledge they are able to devise a treatment programme which will enable the person with haemophilia to recover from the sequence of haemorrhagic bleeding. Due to the rarity of haemophilia, it is essential that physiotherapy management is carried out by those who have knowledge of bleeding disorders, as damage or harm can result from inappropriate interventions. In the UK, the Haemophilia Chartered Physiotherapy Association (HCPA) has attempted to standardize a musculoskeletal assessment form which has been published in the *Haemophilia Standards of Care* [12,13]. By using data from previous bleeding episodes in the child, the physiotherapist may be in a position to devise a programme of prevention and education in order to halt the progress of the disease.

The overall aim of physiotherapy is to restore and improve muscle and joint function, relieve pain, give advice, treat the consequences of each bleeding episode and assess the individual needs of the patient for orthotic devices, if required.

Acute bleeds

Early recognition of bleeding episodes and factor replacement are the keys to successful treatment of joint bleeds. Babies and toddlers are not able to tell their parents if they are bleeding, but by careful observation the parent may notice that the child is not using a limb properly, or cries when an arm or leg is placed into a garment. He may also be holding a joint in a flexed position and there may be swelling and heat. The earlier treatment is administered the better. Physiotherapy intervention with very young children is often difficult, but if the joint bleed is severe it may be necessary to immobilize the joint with some form of splint or bandage. Resting the joint is also advised, but getting a young child to lie still may prove very difficult.

Most children in the developed countries are on prophylactic treatment from an early age following the first major joint bleed, which may be around the age of 2–3 years. The Swedish Centres of Malmö and Stockholm commence primary prophylaxis at 1 year old. Evidence shows that primary prophylaxis can prevent haemophilic arthropathy in boys with severe haemophilia A and B [14–17].

As the child grows older, he is more likely to recognize a bleed before major symptoms develop. Physiotherapy should be aimed at stopping the bleed and relieving pain and swelling. The affected joint should be rested in a position of comfort. If the knee or ankle joint is affected, it may be necessary to provide crutches for mobility until the bleed has resolved. Any splinting should be short-term (24–48 hours) in order to prevent muscle imbalance.

Once the bleeding has stopped, active exercise should be started consisting of static exercises, progressing to graduated activities until full function is restored as the bleed resolves. Most bleeds that are treated early will respond very quickly with physiotherapy in conjunction with replacement therapy (Fig. 24.1).

Parents and older children should also be taught the mnemonic RICE (rest, ice, compression and elevation). The application of ice at home can help to reduce swelling and pain and therefore aid the recovery process. Electrotherapy treatment has also been shown to be beneficial in the management of acute haemarthrosis (see later in this chapter).

Subacute phase

The bleeding episode becomes subacute once intra-articular or intra-muscular bleeding has stopped. The aim of treatment at this stage is to restore the joint range of motion and muscle power. The integrity of the joints are dependent upon the musculature supporting them. If the muscles remain weak, there is a danger of rebleeding. Exercise programmes should be devised for the child to perform at home, but they should be made interesting – swimming or hydrotherapy is a useful medium for increasing strength and mobility. Strength training programmes for children should be carefully monitored and supervised [18]. The child's musculoskeletal system should not be overloaded with maximum weights, and movements should be controlled, avoiding ballistic movements.

Despite early treatment, some children continue to have breakthrough bleeds which may target one particular joint or muscle group. A change in the prophylactic dosage may halt this process, however, some children go on to develop a joint synovitis. The ankle joint in children is prone to repeated bleeding because of the large amounts of synovium within the joint [4,19]. Treatment of chronic synovitis consists of prophylactic replacement therapy and an intensive course of physiotherapy [13,14]. Once a programme has been introduced to reduce synovial thickening, the child will need support and encouragement to complete the programme, which may last up to 18 months. Support from parents, siblings, peers and the physiotherapist will help during this process.

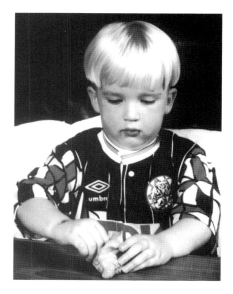

Fig. 24.1 Child exercising fingers and hands using plasticine.

CHRONIC ARTHROPATHY

This is characterized by joint change, soft-tissue contracture and deformity. Due to the introduction of home therapy programmes, we are fortunate not to see too many children suffering from chronic joint arthropathy, at least in the developed world. A single episode of bleeding into a joint is sufficient to start the process of joint destruction. Therefore, it is important that joint haemarthroses are prevented if possible, or treated early. Once the joint has developed arthropathy the aim of physiotherapy is to reduce pain, maintain range of motion and muscle power, and to increase independent function to normal or as near normal as possible.

Children tend to bleed into the ankle joint from an early age and from experience many adolescents and young adults have developed articular damage in one or both joints. The child may present with a painful, stiff joint. Radiological changes are present, often with the for-

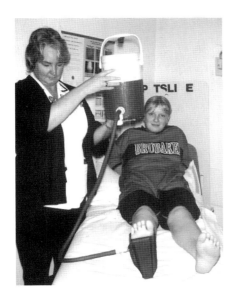

Fig. 24.2 Ice therapy using Cryocuff just after cheilectomy of an ankle joint.

mation of osteophytes on the distal tibia or talus. A painful, stiff arthritic ankle interferes with normal gait and can lead to impairment, disability and handicap. If both ankles are affected, as well as other joints in the foot and lower limb, then normal everyday activities may become difficult. In the past, the remedy for severe haemophilic arthropathy of the ankle lay in subtalar or ankle joint fusion.

However, it has been shown that cheilectomy can delay or prevent the need for such procedures [20,21]. The procedure is very simple and physiotherapy is commenced immediately under factor cover. On return from the operating room, active ankle exercises commence and ice therapy using Cryocuff is commenced (Fig. 24.2). The child can then weight-bear as tolerated 24–48 hours after the procedure. Hospital admission is required, but only for 3–4 days. Physiotherapy is then continued on an outpatient basis with a graded exercise programme to include range of motion exercises, strengthening and proprioception training [22].

INHIBITORS

Patients with severe haemophilia A or B develop inhibitors to factor VIII or IX. In retrospective studies, it has been shown that one-third will develop an inhibitor by the age of 4 years and 50% by the age of 9 [23,24]. The development of an inhibitor is a serious complication of haemophilia, which predisposes the patient to more frequent and prolonged bleeding episodes. The management of inhibitors is a complicated process and also expensive. Immune tolerance programmes have been introduced in a few centres in Europe, and the use of Porta-Caths in children for the administration of large doses of factor VIII or IX have been successful to a certain extent [25].

Physiotherapy management for children with inhibitors is of equal importance. It is essential that physiotherapy is only undertaken with knowledge of the underlying condition and the coagulation parameter being as optimal as possible. Physiotherapy intervention will need to be carefully monitored, and progressed at a slow rate. If a child presents with an acute joint haemarthrosis, a splint should be applied before factor replacement is given. This may well prevent the breakdown of the clotting process and allow bleeding to cease. Physiotherapy is not a contraindication for the child with an inhibitor as long as the child is monitored and assessed carefully by the physiotherapist.

SPORT

The benefits of sport and exercise for those with haemophilia have been well documented [1,6,8]. Every sport carries some risk, but it is necessary for the child and his parents to weigh up the risk–benefit of sports participation. Guidelines exist for those with haemophilia to refer to when choosing a sport or activity. The choice of sports varies from country to country and within countries. Some centre doctors may disagree with a person's choice of activity, but again it is up to the child and his family to make informed choices using the information available.

When sports injuries occur, the role of the physiotherapist is invaluable. Accurate assessment and diagnosis of the injury by an experienced physiotherapist will speed up the repair process. We are seeing increasing numbers of children with mild and moderate haemophilia presenting with sports injuries, especially involving the muscles of the thigh and calf. Physiotherapy treatment of sports injuries is also well documented [6,8]. Each patient's injury should be treated individually with appropriate techniques such as electrotherapy, stretches, strengthening exercises and sports retraining. If there is a definite link between a particular sporting activity and recurrent bleeding, a change of sport may be necessary.

ELECTROTHERAPY

The use of electrotherapy modalities in physiotherapy is well known and its popularity tends to ebb and flow, but it should be stressed that electrotherapy should only be used as an adjunct to exercise programmes. The human body is made up of millions of cells, each of which has a membrane potential. The endogenous electrical activity of the body arises from a variety of sources. Research has shown that by enhancing the endogenous electrical activity of damaged tissue the healing process can be stimulated and speeded up [26].

Pulsed short-wave diathermy (PSWD) is commonly used in the management of haemophilia. The primary effect of the pulsed magnetic field appears to be at the cell membrane level and is concerned with the transport of ions across the membrane. A cell involved in the inflammation process shows a reduced cell membrane potential, therefore disturbing the normal functionality of that cell. The altered potential affects ion transport across the membrane leading to an imbalance of ions, which in turn alters cellular osmotic pressure. This cell damage leads to pain and swelling in the tissue. By applying PSWD to the damaged tissues it restores the cell membrane potential to normal.

The general effects of PSWD on tissues are (1) to increase the number of white cells, histocytes and fibroblasts in the soft tissue, (2) to improve the rate of dispersion of oedema, (3) to encourage the reabsorption of the haemarthrosis, (4) to reduce inflammation and (5) to encourage collagen layering at an early stage. Using current research, it is suggested that the minimum energy required to achieve a therapeutic effect should be utilized. Guidelines issued by Haynes in 1984 [27] are still widely used by physiotherapists. For acute bleeds a mean power < 3 W should be used – the more acute the condition, the narrower the pulses. A dose of 2–5 W is suggested for subacute episodes using a wider pulse, and for chronic conditions a mean power of > 5 W is usually required to achieve a reasonable tissue response.

Ultrasound

Therapeutic ultrasound is also used in the treatment of haemophilia, but at the later stage for subacute or chronic sports injuries. Ultrasound is a form of mechanical energy and application of ultrasound to injured tissues will speed the rate of healing. Some tissues absorb ultrasound waves more readily than others. Generally, the tissues with the higher protein content will absorb the ultrasound waves better than those with a low protein content. Blood and fat have a low protein content and therefore ultrasound is not suitable for acute bleeding episodes, whereas cartilage, tendon and bone have a high protein content and absorb more of the ultrasound wave. Therefore, soft-tissue injuries, such as a sprained ankle, are well suited to treatment with ultrasound.

CONCLUSION

The future for children with haemophilia is bright. Recombinant blood products will halt the transmission of human blood-borne viruses which have had such devastating effects on the haemophilic population over the past 15 years. Children will, however, continue to have bleeding episodes, but with early intervention by physiotherapy the consequence of joint arthropathy can be prevented. Children and their parents must utilize the resources available and seek early consultation with their centre physiotherapist. Using the techniques available, physiotherapy has been shown to speed up recovery, reduce pain and prevent contractures. However, the resources available in modern developed countries are not available to over 80% of the world's haemophilic population. The World Federation for Haemophilia has initiated programmes to address this problem, such as Operation Improvement and the Twinning Schemes.

REFERENCES

1 Buzzard BM. Sports and haemophilia: antagonist or protagonist. *Clin Orthop* 1996; **328**: 25–30.

2 Kasper CK. Mild haemophilia is less of a burden than severe haemophilia. Isn't it? Or is it? *Haemophilia World* 1996; **3**: 3.

3 Wynne-Davis R. Acetabular dysplasia and familial joint laxity, two aetiological factors in congenital dislocation of the hip. *J Bone Joint Surg (Br)* 1970; **52B**: 704–8.

4 Buzzard BM, Heim M. A study to evaluate the effectiveness of 'Air-Stirrup' splints as a means of reducing the frequency of ankle haemarthrosis in children with haemophilia A and B. *Haemophilia* 1995; **1**: 133–6.

5 Bachmayer F, Holdredge S. Developmental activities, sports and games. *Haemophilia World* (World Federation of Haemophilia) 1991; **7**: 5–6.

6 Jones PM, Buzzard BM, Heinmen L. *Go for it: Guidelines on Physical Activity and Sports for People with Haemophilia and Related Diseases*. World Federation of Haemophilia: 1998.

7 Boone DC. Management of musculo-skeletal problems of haemophilia. *Phys Ther* 1974; **54**: 123–7.

8 Buzzard BM, Saeed C. The physiotherapy management of sports injuries in haemophilia. In: Heijnen L, ed. *Recent Advances in Rehabilitation in Haemophilia*. Hove, East Sussex: Medical Education Network, 1995: 73–7.

9 Heijnen L, de Klein P. Sport. In: Heijnen L, ed. *Recent Advances in Rehabilitation in Haemophilia*. Hove: Medical Education Network, 1995: 66–72.

10 Onwuzunke N, Warrier I, Lusher JM. Types of bleeding seen during the first 30 months of life in children with severe haemophilia A and B. *Haemophilia* 1996; **2**: 137–40.

11 Janco RL, MacLean WE, Perrin JM, Gortmaker SL. A prospective study of patterns of bleeding in boys with haemophilia. *Haemophilia* 1996; **2**: 202–6.

12 Haemophilia Chartered Physiotherapy Association. *Haemophilia Standards of Care*. London: Chartered Society of Physiotherapy, 1996.

13 Buzzard BM. Physiotherapy for prevention and treatment of chronic haemophilic synovitis. *Clin Orthop* 1997; **343**: 42–6.

14 Nilsson IM, Berntrop E, Löquist E, Pettersson H. Twenty-five years' experience of prophylactic treatment in severe haemophilia A and B. *J Intern Med* 1992; **232**: 25–32.

15 Liesner RJ, Khair K, Haan IM. The impact of prophylactic treatment on children with severe haemophilia. *Br J Haematol* 1996; **92**: 973–8.

16 Kreuz W, Escuriola-Ettinghausen C, Funk M, Schmidt H, Kornhuber B. When should prophylactic treatment in patients with haemophilia A and B start? The German Experience. *Haemophilia* 1998; **4**: 413–17.

17 Ljung R. Second workshop of the European Paediatric Network for haemophilia management. *Haemophilia* 1999; **5**: 286–91.

18 American College of Sports Medicine. *ACSM Guidelines for Exercise Testing and Prescription*. Baltimore: William

and Wilkins, 1995.

19 Miser AN, Miser JS, Newton WA. Intensive factor replacement for management of chronic synovitis in haemophilic children. *Am J Pedriat Hematol Oncol* 1986; **8**: 66–90.

20 Beeton K, Ribbans WJ, Lee CA. Removal of anterior osteophytes in haemophiliac arthropathy of the ankle. *Haemophilia* 1996; **2**: 39.

21 Buzzard BM, Briggs PJ. Functional outcome following removal of distal tibial osteophytes in haemophila. *Proceedings of the 5th Musculoskeletal Congress of World Federation of Haemophilia.* Sydney, Australia, 1999.

22 Buzzard BM. Propioceptive training in haemophilia. *Haemophilia* 1998; **4**: 528–31.

23 Lusher JM. Factor VIII inhibitors etiology, characteristics, natural history and management. *Ann NY Acad Sci* 1987; **509**: 89–102.

24 Brettler DB. Inhibitors of factor VIII and IX. *Haemophilia* 1995; **1** (Suppl. 1): 35–9.

25 Warner I, Baird-Cox K, Lusher JM. Use of central venous catheters in children with haemophilia: one haemophilia treatment centre experience. *Haemophilia* 1997; **3**: 194–8.

26 Kloth LC, Feeder JA. Acceleration of wound healing with high voltage monophasic pulsed current. *Phys Ther* 1988; **68**: 503–8.

27 Haynes C. Pulsed high frequency energy: its place in physiotherapy. *Physiotherapy* 1984; **70**: 459–66.

CHAPTER 25

Physiotherapy for Adult Patients with Haemophilia

K S BEETON

INTRODUCTION

Improvements in the medical management of haemophilia, including early and prompt treatment with factor replacement, have reduced the incidence and severity of bleeding episodes for many children with haemophilia [1,2]. Many adult patients did not have access to such effective treatment programmes in the past. The effects of bleeding into joints and muscles can lead to a life of pain, deformity and loss of function. Within the comprehensive care team, the physiotherapist has an important part to play in the management of the adult patient with haemophilia. This chapter will discuss referral to physiotherapy, the physiotherapy examination and the annual review. The clinical presentation and strategies for the physiotherapy management of an acute haemarthrosis or muscle haematoma, chronic synovitis and arthropathy will be outlined. Finally, the role of the physiotherapist in an inpatient orthopaedic setting will be briefly discussed.

REFERRAL TO PHYSIOTHERAPY

Patients with haemophilia may present with neuromusculoskeletal problems as a consequence of their haemophilia, or they may present with problems commonly seen in the general population, such as spinal pain or sports injuries. Depending on the local arrangements of the haemophilia centre, patients may be referred to physiotherapy by haemophilia centre staff including doctors or nurses, or the patient may self-refer for physiotherapy. All physiotherapy appointments should be made promptly to maximize recovery [3].

Initial examination

For patients referred with specific neuromusculoskeletal problems, the initial examination by the physiotherapist includes both subjective and physical components.

Subjective examination

The aims of the subjective examination are to establish baseline information regarding the patient's haemophilia status, determine the source of the symptoms and identify any factors which may be contributing to the problem. It is important to establish whether there are any precautions or contraindications to the physical examination or treatment, and to determine the history of the specific problem [4]. The patient is asked about their type of bleeding disorder, the level of circulating factor, whether they are on prophylaxis or 'on demand' treatment, or if they have inhibitors. If patients are severely affected, this has implications for physiotherapy management, as they need to be handled carefully in order to avoid causing a bleed. Patients with inhibitors need particular care in management, due to the potential difficulties in controlling bleeding [5,6].

The physiotherapist will ask about the symptoms experienced, the aggravating and easing factors, behaviour of the symptoms over 24 hours and functional limitations in order to try to determine the source and extent of the problem [7]. Other factors which may be contributing to the specific problem, such as inadequate footwear, poor seating at work or stiff knees causing increased strain on the upper limb joints, need to be identified. Failure to address these issues may limit the benefits of any treatment [4]. Psychosocial factors such as depression or anxiety and attitudes to haemophilia may also impact on the response to treatment [4,8].

It is essential to identify any precautions or contraindications to physiotherapy management. Enquiries should be made regarding the patient's general health, weight, drug therapy, results of X-rays and other medical investigations [9]. If the physiotherapist has any concerns that the patient may have a non-musculoskeletal cause of symptoms such as septic arthritis [10] or may have developed inhibitors [11], this should be discussed with the appropriate medical personnel prior to any intervention.

The patient is also asked about the history of the specific problem, whether there was a spontaneous or traumatic onset and the behaviour of the symptoms since onset. The physiotherapist must always be vigilant when managing the patient with haemophilia where an acute bleed has followed a traumatic incident, as the bleed may mask a fracture which can be missed initially. Relevant past history including previous target joints and effects of previous physiotherapy interventions should also be discussed.

Physical examination

The aim of the physical examination is to test structures identified from the subjective examination as causing or contributing to the problem. Examination includes evaluation of posture and functional movements as well as assessment of the articular, muscle and neurological system if indicated.

Examination of the articular system includes assessment of active and passive physiological movements and passive accessory movements [7]. The aim of these tests is to reproduce the patient's symptoms and determine the quality of the movements. If active movements are symptom-free, pressure can be applied with care at the end of range to test the end-feel of the joint [7]. In patients with arthropathy associated with contractures, a soft-tissue end-feel indicates that physiotherapy may be able to improve range of movement. A bony, hard end-feel will be less responsive to manual techniques. Other tests may need to be performed in different joint regions, for example, knee ligaments and menisci may need to be tested, especially if the patient has complained of weakness or giving way. Leg length, balance and proprioception are assessed if indicated.

Muscle testing includes assessment of isometric and isotonic strength and muscle imbalances if indicated. Isometric muscle testing is useful in situations where there may be pain following a bleed or in cases of arthropathy. Marked muscle atrophy may be apparent as a result of pain and inhibition of muscles and disuse over time. This can be estimated by measuring limb circumference with a tape measure. In muscle imbalances, some muscles such as hamstrings or gastrocnemius have a tendency to become short and overactive. These muscles are assessed for appropriate length. Other muscles have a predominantly stabilizing role, for example, gluteals or lower fibres of the trapezius, and often become inhibited in the presence of pain. They are assessed by testing their endurance capacity [12].

Peripheral neuropathies may be associated with bleeds in the neuromusculoskeletal system and can lead to marked motor and sensory changes which need to be carefully monitored using neurological tests. The femoral and ulnar nerves are commonly involved. Specific neural tissue tension tests, for example, straight leg raise or upper limb tension tests [13] can be used with care in haemophilic patients to assess the mobility of the nervous system.

At the conclusion of the physical examination, the physiotherapist must make a judgement based on the assessment whether the patient has a neuromusculoskeletal problem which requires specific intervention with various physiotherapy modalities, whether the patient needs advice and a self-management programme, or whether the patient needs further evaluation either from the orthopaedic surgeon or haemophilia consultant. For patients who require specific physiotherapy treatment, the findings from the examination will provide a baseline which can be used as markers for the assessment of progress.

Annual reviews

The neuromusculoskeletal system of a patient with haemophilia needs to be monitored on a long-term basis. Ideally, an annual review of the patient is undertaken to evaluate any deterioration in joint range or muscle strength so that appropriate intervention can be undertaken if necessary. Johnson and Babbit [14] identified a progressive loss of range of movement over time in the knees, ankles and elbows, depending on the stage of the arthropathy. A standardized assessment form may assist in the collection of data [3]. The classification recommended by the Orthopaedic Advisory Committee of the World Federation of Haemophilia can also be used to assess neuromusculoskeletal function.

MANAGEMENT

When considering possible management strategies and treatment options, clinicians should 'base clinical decisions on the best available scientific evidence' [15]. There has been an enormous drive for evidence-based practice in the healthcare professions over the last few years, however, it is essential that the available evidence is critically appraised in conjunction with clinical experience [16]. The following section provides an overview of the clinical presentation and management of acute bleeds, chronic synovitis and arthropathy based on the evidence and clinical experience.

Clinical presentation of acute joint and muscle bleeds

In countries where there is adequate use of factor replacement, joint or muscle bleeds may occur less often. However, 80% of the world's population with haemophilia do not have adequate access to factor replacement and, even in countries with sufficient supplies, patients still present with acute bleeds. The knee, ankle and elbow are the most common sites of haemarthroses, and the iliopsoas, gastrocnemius and forearm flexors are sites where haematomas often occur. The onset of a joint bleed is often preceded by an 'aura' which is followed by pain, swelling, tenderness and loss of range of movement [11]. The degree of pain and other symptoms experienced will depend on the severity of the bleed and how quickly factor replacement is given. In the absence of adequate factor replacement, bleeding in a joint may continue until a tamponade effect occurs [11].

Muscle and soft-tissue bleeds may be associated with marked bruising as well as pain, swelling and loss of movement, particularly on stretching the muscle. Compartment syndromes may occur following muscle bleeds if there is insufficient room for the expansion of tissues due to bleeding. This may result in muscle necrosis and contractures, for example, anterior tibials or Volkmann's ischaemic contractures [17,18]. Peripheral nerve lesions may also occur in association with muscle bleeds, for example, femoral nerve neuropathy following iliopsoas bleeds. Prompt treatment with factor replacement will reduce complications due to peripheral nerve lesions, whereas delayed treatment can hinder recovery. Recovery from nerve lesions has been demonstrated to be significantly slower in patients with inhibitors compared to those who did not have inhibitors [19]. The authors suggested that this could be due to the greater amount of bleeding and prolonged immobilization. Residual sensory loss was common in all patients [20].

Management of acute joint and muscle bleeds

The joint or muscle should be rested until haemostasis has been achieved through adequate dosage of factor replacement. Treatment should be commenced promptly in order to minimize damage and hasten recovery. Factor concentrates should be continued until the bleed has resolved. Further complications can occur if treatment is discontinued too quickly [20]. Excessive pain or paraesthesia or a failure to respond to factor replacement will require prompt medical opinion [11].

The main aims of physiotherapy are to relieve pain, reduce swelling, prevent recurrence of bleeding and maximize function with restoration of full range of movement of joints and normal strength and length of muscles. Modalities of treatment may include ice packs to reduce pain and swelling, and rest in a functional position. For upper limb bleeds, a sling may be required to provide appropriate support and protection. In the lower limb, crutches or splints may be necessary. Electrotherapy including pulsed short-wave [21] and ultrasound [22] may aid the resolution of joint and muscle bleeds. Transcutaneous nerve stimulation (TNS) with modulation in conjunction with factor replacement has also been shown to be beneficial in reducing the effects of haemarthroses in a small group of haemophilic patients [23].

Once active rehabilitation can be commenced, a graded programme of exercises including non-weight-bearing isometric exercises and closed and open chain exercises can be undertaken. It is important to consider exercises with the knowledge of functional activities that the patient needs to do due to the specificity of training [24]. Carefully monitored progression is recommended rather than vigorous treatment programmes, in order to prevent rebleeding [25]. Modification of activities and avoidance of lifting and undue strain are important factors until the bleed has completely resolved. A home maintenance programme should be part of the strategy to facilitate self-management once recovery has been optimized. Counselling may be necessary from members of the comprehensive care team to minimize recurrence [11].

Clinical presentation of chronic synovitis

If the haemarthrosis becomes recurrent, the so-called 'target' joint, a chronic synovitis will develop with hypertrophied synovium and fragile blood vessels which bleed easily. Roosendaal *et al.* [26] have defined chronic synovitis as chronic swelling of the joint lasting for more than 3 months which does not respond to normal replacement therapy. Muscle atrophy is often a significant feature of this stage of deterioration leading to weakness and instability, although pain is often minimal or absent [27,28]. Hyperaemia of the lower limb epiphyseal plates of the growing child can lead to overgrowth of the bones, causing leg length differences. This may be masked by the development of flexion deformities [29].

Management of chronic synovitis

Heijnen *et al.* [28] have described a protocol for the management of chronic synovitis. Other treatment strategies have also been outlined [27]. Essentially, the aims of physiotherapy treatment are to reduce swelling, increase muscle strength and improve coordination and proprioception. Regular prophylaxis is essential to prevent or minimize bleeding. Electrotherapeutic modalities may help to reduce swelling due to effusion and synovial thickening. Splinting or braces may be required to rest the joint and provide additional support for the limb in the presence of muscle weakness. Crutches may be used to decrease weight-bearing. The use of Air Stirrup braces have been evaluated and shown to be beneficial in reducing the number of ankle bleeds in children [30], but their use in adults has not been established. Visco heels may provide benefits for some patients with ankle synovitis by increasing shock absorption [28].

Once the bleeding is under control, a progressive strengthening programme is commenced, as discussed following an acute bleed, with particular emphasis on joint coordination and proprioception training [31]. Hydrotherapy may be indicated in the early stages. The programme should continue until the patient can return to functional activities and sport [29] and may need to be pursued for several months [28]. The marked muscle atrophy which can occur following chronic synovitis may be very slow to recover [2], and clinical experience suggests that residual differences between sides may be apparent in the long term despite prolonged exercise regimes. If conservative measures fail, then surgery may need to be considered. The results are more likely to be successful in the early stages of arthropathy.

Clinical presentation of arthropathy

If bleeding continues, ultimately the joint will be destroyed. The presence of blood in the joint damages the articular cartilage leading to degenerative changes with loss of joint space, sclerosis and osteophytes evident on radiographs [32]. The patient may complain of pain which can be severe. Characteristic deformities, loss of range of movement, swelling, crepitus, decreased muscle strength and reduced function are often apparent. In end-stage disease, soft-tissue changes may have resolved, leaving a joint with marked bony changes and bony or fibrous ankylosis [33]. Joint contractures are common [34].

Management of arthropathy

Physiotherapy can play an important role in preventing and improving the symptoms which may arise as a result of arthropathy. The main aims of treatment are to relieve pain, increase or maintain range of movement and muscle strength, and maximize function. Modalities of treatment used include manual therapy including mobilization of joints and correction of muscle imbalances, hydrotherapy, electrotherapy including TNS, acupuncture, braces and splints, and advice and education.

Mobilization of joints can be useful in reducing pain and restoring range of movement [7]. Mobilizations consist of passive physiological and passive accessory movements produced by the physiotherapist as rhythmical oscillations and they can be used to treat pain, stiffness or spasm [7]. Manipulation or Grade V techniques are contraindicated at all times [3] and vigorous or forceful techniques should be avoided. The application of tape to the skin in conjunction with mobilizations and exercises can relieve pain and provide a passive stretch to soft-tissue structures such as tight lateral retinaculum [35].

Muscle imbalances may need to be addressed. This involves specific re-education of the endurance capacity of those muscles which provide a predominantly stabilizing function and lengthening procedures for muscles which have a tendency to become overactive and tight [36]. If this aspect of management is not adequately assessed and managed, symptoms may recur.

Hydrotherapy exercises in warm water can also be very beneficial for patients with marked muscle weakness or multiple joint involvement. The water can be used to assist or resist movement and graded exercise programmes can be developed depending on the patient's problem. The warmth of the water facilitates relief of pain and reduction of muscle spasm and promotes relaxation and a feeling of well-being [37].

Electrotherapy also has a place in the management of arthropathy. Clinical experience has demonstrated that TNS can be a useful adjunct to relieve chronic pain due to arthropathy. It is thought to work by stimulating large AB fibres, thus moderating small A delta and C fibre activity which transmit pain. It may also stimulate production of the patient's own pain-relieving endorphins [38].

The use of acupuncture has also been described in patients with hae-mophilia. Koh [39] outlined two case reports of haemophilic patients with arthropathy who had relief of pain following acupuncture. The author emphasized the importance of prophylactic factor replacement prior to acupuncture and outlined the strict precautions which must be heeded.

Other options for the treatment of arthropathy include treating contractures using serial casting, reversed dynamic slings and extension desubluxation hinge devices [34]. An intermittent compression system has also been successful in reducing knee flexion contractures [40].

Splinting and braces may be indicated in some cases, although many patients are reluctant to use supports due to bad experiences in the past when splinting was used to rest joints in the absence of factor replacement. Nowadays, splints can often be worn discreetly under clothes and in shoes, so that the tell-tale signs of disability are not apparent. Improvements in pain and function have been identified in small groups of patients with ankle arthropathy following the use of custom-made insoles [41,42].

Advice and education are an essential part of any treatment. For patients with arthropathy, this includes advice on avoiding and minimizing aggravating factors, and teaching the patient how to look after joints to minimize stress [43]. Patient education may take place on an individual basis or in a group setting, where patients can benefit from sharing their experiences with other patients. It is important that the patient has a programme of exercises to do at home in order to maintain progress and to encourage the patient to take responsibility for the problem. The physiotherapist can also advise on sporting and other activities which would be relevant to the patient.

For patients who present with arthropathy, bony and soft-tissue changes may prevent full recovery. The patient and the physiotherapist need to have realistic expectations of what can be achieved with treatment and set goals accordingly. Exercise programmes, particularly in weight-bearing positions, should be progressed with caution. It is important to treat the patient holistically and consider factors which may be contributing to the persistence of symptoms and address all the problems. The patient may need to consider changing aspects of their life-style in order to preserve joint function. This can be difficult for patients who deny or ignore problems [8].

THE ROLE OF THE PHYSIOTHERAPIST FOLLOWING ORTHOPAEDIC SURGICAL PROCEDURES

If conservative measures fail, various surgical procedures such as synovectomy, soft-tissue releases, osteotomy and total joint arthroplasty may be considered. Physiotherapy will be important in the rehabilitation of patients following surgical procedures and the physiotherapist must work closely with the orthopaedic surgeon. Providing appropriate levels of circulating factor are maintained, management should be similar to that of non-haemophilic patients. Some patients, however, will have a more prolonged recovery from surgical procedures [44] and the outcome, particularly in terms of range of movement, may be less good [45] due to the concomitant involvement of other joints and soft-tissue changes. If the patient is not on continuous infusion of factor replacement, physiotherapy sessions should take place immediately after bolus injections so that the risks of bleeding are minimized. Continuous passive motion (CPM) should be used with care in the early postoperative period [46]. Prolonged or vigorous use following total knee replacements may be associated with bleeding episodes. Used appropriately, CPM can assist in restoring range of movement [47], and may also decrease the length of hospital stay [46]. Once the patient has been discharged, rehabilitation may continue on an outpatient basis until maximum function has been achieved.

CONCLUSION

The key to effective physiotherapy management is a thorough assessment. There is increasing evidence to support the inclusion of various treatment modalities into management programmes and, where available, these should be incorporated into practice. However, there is a need for caution before extrapolating evidence from other patient groups to patients with haemophilia, and there is a continued need for research in this field. This will provide the scientific basis to support the effective and successful clinical physiotherapy practice that undoubtedly occurs in these patients.

REFERENCES

1 Nilsson IM, Berntorp E, Löfqvist T, Pettersson H. Twenty-five years' experience of prophylactic treatment in severe haemophilia A and B. *J Intern Med* 1992, **232**: 25–32.

2 Liesner R, Khair K, Hann I. The impact of prophylactic treatment on children with severe haemophilia. *Br J Haematol* 1996; **92**: 973–8.

3 *Standards for Haemophilia.* Haemophilia Chartered Physiotherapists Association. London: Powage Press, 1996.

4 Jones M. Clinical reasoning process in manipulative therapy. In: Boyling J, Palastanga N, eds. *Grieve's Modern Manual Therapy,* 2nd edn. Edinburgh: Churchill Livingstone, 1994: 471–89.

5 Brettler D. Inhibitors in congenital haemophilia. *Bailliere's Clin Haematol* 1996; **9**: 319–30.

6 Cahill M, Colvin B. Haemophilia. *Postgraduate Med J* 1997; **73**: 201–6.

7 Maitland G. *Peripheral Manipulation.* 3rd edn. London:

Butterworth-Heinemann, 1991.

8 Miller R, Beeton K, Goldman E, Ribbans W. Counselling guidelines for managing musculoskeletal problems in haemophilia in the 1990s. *Haemophilia* 1997; **3**: 9–13.

9 Petty N, Moore A. *Neuromusculoskeletal Examination and Assessment*. Edinburgh: Churchill Livingstone, 1998.

10 Gilbert M, Aledort L, Seremetis S, Needleman B, Oloumi G, Forster A. Long-term evaluation of septic arthritis in hemophilic patients. *Clin Orthop* 1996; **328**: 54–9.

11 Ribbans W, Giangrande P, Beeton K. Conservative treatment of haemarthrosis for prevention of hemophilic synovitis. *Clin Orthop* 1997; **343**: 12–18.

12 Richardson C, Jull G, Hodges P, Hides J. *Therapeutic Exercise for Spinal Segmental Stabilisation in Low Back Pain*. Edinburgh: Churchill Livingstone, 1999.

13 Butler D. *Mobilisation of the Nervous System*. Edinburgh: Churchill Livingstone, 1991.

14 Johnson R, Babbitt D. Five stages of joint disintegration compared with range of motion in hemophilia. *Clin Orthop* 1985; **201**: 36–42.

15 Koes B, Hoving J. The value of the randomised clinical trial in the field of physiotherapy. *Manual Therapy* 1998; **3**: 179–86.

16 Bury T. Evidence-based practice: survival of the fittest. *Physiotherapy* 1996; **82**: 75–6.

17 Lancourt J, Gilbert M, Posner M. Management of bleeding and associated complications of hemophilia in the hand and forearm. *J Bone Joint Surg (Am)* 1977; **59A**: 451–60.

18 Heim M, Horoszowski H, Martinowitz U. The short foot syndrome: an unfortunate consequence of neglected raised intracompartmental pressure in a severe hemophilic child: a case report. *Angiology* 1986; **37**: 128–31.

19 Fernandez-Palazzi F, Hernandez S, De Bosch N, De Saez A. Hematomas within the iliopsoas muscles in hemophilic patients. *Clin Orthop* 1996; **328**: 19–24.

20 Katz S, Nelson I, Atkins R, Duthie R. Peripheral nerve lesions in haemophilia. *J Bone Joint Surg (Am)* 1991; **73A**: 1016–19.

21 Scott S. Short-wave diathermy. In: Kitchen S, Bazin S, eds. *Clayton's Electrotherapy*, 10th edn. London: WB Saunders, 1994: 154–8.

22 Young S. Ultrasound therapy In: Kitchen S, Bazin S, eds. *Clayton's Electrotherapy*, 10th edn. London: WB Saunders, 1994: 243–70.

23 Martinowitz U, Beeton K, Heim M, Tuddenham D, Kernoff P. Transcutaneous electrical stimulation in the treatment of haemarthrosis in haemophilia: a double blind study. *Proceedings of XVII International Congress of the World Federation of Hemophilia,* Milan, 1986: 135.

24 McArdle W, Katch F, Katch V. *Exercise Physiology*, 4th edn. Baltimore: Williams and Wilkins, 1996: 393–415.

25 Heim M, Martinowitz U, Graif M, Ganel A, Horoszowski H. Case study: the treatment of soft tissue hemorrhages in a severe classical hemophiliac with an unusual

antibody to factor VIII. *J Orthop Sports Phys Ther* 1988; **10**: 138–41.

26 Roosendaal G, de Kleijn P, Mauser-Bunschoten E, Heijnen L, van den Berg M. Treatment of chronic synovitis. In: Heijnen L, ed. *Recent Advances in Rehabilitation in Haemophilia*. Hove, East Sussex: Medical Education Network, 1995: 8–16.

27 Buzzard B. Physiotherapy for prevention and treatment of chronic haemophilic synovitis. *Clin Orthop* 1997; **343**: 42–6.

28 Heijnen L, Roosendaal G, Heim M. Orthotics and rehabilitation for chronic hemophilic synovitis of the ankle. *Clin Orthop* 1997; **343**: 68–73.

29 Heim M, Horoszowski H, Martinowitz U. Leg-length inequality in haemophilia. *Clin Pediatr* 1985; **24**: 601–2.

30 Buzzard B, Heim M. A study to evaluate the effectiveness of 'Air-Stirrup' splints as a means of reducing the frequency of ankle haemarthroses in children with haemophilia A and B. *Haemophilia* 1995; **1**: 131–6.

31 Buzzard B. Proprioceptive training in haemophilia. *Haemophilia* 1998; **4**: 528–31.

32 Duthie R. Musculoskeletal problems and their management In: Rizza C, Lowe G, eds. *Haemophilia and Other Inherited Bleeding Disorders*. London: WB Saunders, 1997: 227-74.

33 York J. Musculoskeletal disorders in the haemophilias. *Bailliere's Clin Rheumatol* 1991; **5**: 197–220.

34 Rodriguez-Merchan EC. Therapeutic options in the management of articular contractures in haemophiliacs. *Haemophilia* 1999; **5** (Suppl. 1): 5–9.

35 McConnell J. Management of patello-femoral problems. *Man Ther* 1996; **1**: 60–6.

36 Beeton K, Cornwell J, Alltree J. Muscle rehabilitation in haemophilia. *Haemophilia* 1998; **4**: 532–7.

37 Golland A. Basic hydrotherapy. *Physiotherapy* 1981; **67**: 258–62.

38 Frampton V. Transcutaneous electrical nerve stimulation (TENS) In: Kitchen S, Bazin S, eds. *Clayton's Electrotherapy*, 10th edn. London: WB Saunders, 1994: 287–305.

39 Koh T. Acupuncture therapy in hemophilia. *Am J Acupuncture* 1981; **9**: 269–70.

40 Nelson I, Atkins R, Allen A. The management of knee flexion contractures in haemophilia: brief report. *J Bone Joint Surg (Br)* 1989; **71B**: 327–8.

41 Padkin J, Beeton K, Kriss S, Lee C, Goddard N, Miller R, Alltree J. An evaluation of the use of orthoses in haemophilia patients presenting with ankle pain. *World Federation of Hemophilia 5th Musculoskeletal Congress Proceedings*. Sydney, Australia, 1999.

42 Slattery M. Changes to the range of motion of the ankle and the efficacy of function foot orthotics. *World Federation of Hemophilia 5th Musculoskeletal Congress Proceedings*. Sydney, Australia, 1999.

43 Haemophilia Chartered Physiotherapists Association. *Joint Care and Exercises*. London: The Haemophilia

Society, 1993.

44 Heeg M, Meyer K, Smid W, Van Horn J, Van der Meer J. Total knee and hip arthroplasty in haemophilic patients. *Haemophilia* 1998; **4**: 747–51.

45 Teigland J, Tjonnfjord G, Evensen S, Charania B. Knee arthroplasty in hemophilia. *Acta Orthop Scand* 1993; **64**: 153–6.

46 Johnson R. The effect of continuous passive motion on wound healing and joint mobility after knee arthroplasty. *J Bone Joint Surg (Am)* 1990; **72A**: 421–6.

47 Luck J, Kasper C. Surgical management of advanced hemophilic arthropathy. *Clin Orthop* 1989; **242**: 60–82.

4

Miscellaneous

CHAPTER 26

Orthotic Principles and Practice, and Shoe Adaptations

L HEIJNEN AND M HEIM

INTRODUCTION

Haemarthroses and muscle haemorrhages cause impairments of joint and muscle function. If replacement therapy with appropriate clotting factor is available, normal function of the muskeloskeletal system is usually regained within a short time. If replacement therapy is instituted late or not available at all, joint and muscle impairments may be permanent, leading to disabilities and handicaps. In both the acute phase of haemorrhages and in the chronic or permanent situation orthotic devices and shoe adaptations are helpful.

ORTHOTIC PRINCIPLES AND PRACTICE

Definition

An orthosis is an externally applied device used to modify the structural and functional characteristics of the neuromuscular and skeletal systems.

The primary function of an orthosis is the control of motion of certain body segments and/or support of the body. An ideal orthosis controls only those motions that are abnormal or undesirable and permits motion where normal function can occur [1]. Orthotic design must give equal emphasis to mechanical efficiency and accuracy of fit, since comfort is critical for acceptance. Patients accept orthoses only if they have a well-defined therapeutic purpose or if they provide a function that cannot be accomplished in any other fashion [2]. In addition to a good fit, weight and acceptable cosmetic appearance are also important.

Prescription principles

1 Identification of the primary basic purpose for which the orthosis is to be prescribed.
2 Definition and understanding of the major biomechanical deficits present in the patient, that is, an accurate biomechanical analysis of the patient and a systematic functional appraisal of the impaired limb or body segment.

3 Appreciation of the comparative attributes of available orthotic systems, selection of appropriate components and the creation of an orthotic system from the components selected.

4 Re-evaluation of the patient after application of the prescribed orthosis to ensure its effectiveness and its correct use.

Ideally, an orthosis should be prescribed by an orthotic team consisting of a physician with an active interest in the field of rehabilitation, an orthotist trained in this field, and a physiotherapist.

The team identifies the primary purpose for the orthosis, which may be prevention of deformity, protection of a weakened or painful musculoskeletal segment, improvement of function, or weight deviation from a limb upon weight-bearing.

Orthotic components and systems

In the past, orthopaedic appliances were made out of metal and leather. Complaints of excess bulk, weight, noise and rigidity were common. The history of orthotic usage in haemophilia has been described by Heim and Steinbach [3]. The trend has been one of gradual improvement, and nowadays orthotists assemble orthopaedic appliances from prefabricated mass-produced parts of various metals and more recently use thermoplastics, carbon fibre and titanium.

In general, orthopaedic and sports medicine hybrid systems and 'off-the-shelf' orthoses are used, some of which may be useful in cases of musculoskeletal problems in haemophilia. However, no evidence-based material is available from which hard conclusions can be drawn.

Heijnen *et al.* [4] describe their experience with the use of Visco heels (a shock-absorbing shoe insert) which seem to reduce the bleeding frequency in some patients and also seem to generate a reduction in pain for some. However, the numbers were small and hence not subjected to statistical analysis.

Seuser *et al.* [5] analysed the effects of silicone heel cushioning on the ankle motion of haemophilic patients in different stages of haemarthropathy and concluded that a silicone heel cushion has no influence on ankles in the late stage of haemarthropathy. The authors warn that its use might lead to uncontrolled changes of the ankle joint and that they are not useful for prevention and treatment of chronic haemophilic synovitis and may cause additional deterioration of the joint. These two articles from the same journal show that there is a need for more extensive investigations before definite conclusions can be drawn either from laboratory analysis or from the actual use of orthotic appliances by patients.

APPLICATION OF ORTHOSES IN HAEMOPHILIA

Temporary orthoses during acute haemarthroses and muscle haemorrhages

Rest and immobilization

During the initial phase of rest and immobilization, the affected limb should be rested in the most comfortable position. Ice can be applied every 2 hours for 10–20 minutes (no ice on bare skin); compression can be provided by means of an elastic bandage. Cryocuff (Aircast, Summit EJ) adaptive cuff acts as an orthotic and has proved successful in the initial management of acute haemarthroses [6].

For elbow or shoulder bleeds, if it is not possible to rest the arm in a comfortable position with the help of supportive cushions, a sling can be applied during ambulation.

The knee and/or ankle and foot can be rested by means of a simple back splint made either of plaster of Paris or thermoplastic material. Both should be well padded. The limb and the joint or muscle group in which the haemorrhage is present should be evaluated and the splint adapted to the most favourable position in which the patient is comfortable (aiming for extension at the knee joint and dorsiflexion at the ankle joint). Temporary appliances require frequent alteration, keeping pace with improvement in the condition of the limb.

Mobilization

The second phase, mobilization, should be commenced as soon as the pain subsides and the bleeding has stopped. The splint should be removed, at least for part of the day, to allow active movements and exercises.

Passive mobilization should be undertaken with great care and only within the pain limits of the patient. A continuous passive motion machine (CPM) can be used if the patient is very passive and if it is available, but the range of motion should be well within the pain limits. Assisted active exercises will prepare the patient for active exercises. These are a must to enable the patient to regain range of motion during all functional activities.

Physiotechnical applications such as transcutaneous nerve stimulation (TENS) and electrotherapy are also used to diminish pain and stimulate movement. When analysing the causes of a specific recurrent bleeding problem, an orthosis can be prescribed to prevent recurrent bleeding. Orthotic provision should only be used when active training fails to solve the problem.

Temporary orthoses outside the acute bleeding phase

When no acute joint or muscle bleed is present but full range of motion and/or muscle strength have not been regained (due to chronic synovitis or arthropathy), an orthosis can be used temporarily to protect the joint, muscle groups or limb. Joint instability may be caused by lack of muscle strength and poor coordination combined with a slack joint capsule and ligaments. Prescription of an orthosis should always be combined with active exercises and, if needed, other physiotherapeutic measures.

Dynamic bracing

Strapping with an elastic bandage is the most simple form. The elastic bandage is not capable of stabilizing the joint, but the compression gives some patients a 'safe' feeling and makes them aware of their joint and the proprioceptive signals which should enable them to move properly.

Taping, as used in sports medicine, can be applied too. Advantages are that it is not bulky and can be used in all kinds of footwear. Disadvantages are skin irritation, and that it needs a professional to apply it.

Soft elastic orthoses can be useful, for instance, those made of elastic tubing with the addition of silicone pads (Genu Train, Malleo Train and Epi Train, Bauerfind). The Push brace®, which imitates taping by means of non-elastic and elastic bands, and the Air Stirrup brace are also used in sports medicine and are said to give some protection [7].

Static bracing

Static bracing employs braces with uni- or bilateral metal reinforcements and hinges. Many off-the-shelf braces are nowadays available for the knee [3] and elbow [8], with hinges which can be either locked or limited in range of motion (limiting full extension and/or full flexion). The range of motion can be adjusted by an orthotist, who can also adapt the fitting of several of them.

As soon as the limb has regained its full range of motion and muscle strength and the patient feels confident to perform his normal functional activities, the orthosis should be discarded.

A familiar brace which is advised in case of weakness of the quadriceps muscle is the Los Angeles brace, designed by Boone in 1976 [9]. Quadriceps muscle weakness may have been caused by a muscle problem, haemarthrosis or femoral nerve compression, as seen in iliopsoas bleeds. The brace protects and supports the knee joint and stimulates re-education of the quadriceps action. The splint can be made from a thermoplastic material.

Specific orthoses to treat contractures

If replacement therapy, physiotherapy (both traction and translation, assisted active exercises and active exercises) and/or traction and suspension with weights are not able to reduce contractures, specific orthotic devices can be used.

Serial casting by means of plaster of Paris is cheap but needs a specialist experienced in this technique. In cases where posterior tibial subluxation has occurred, knee extension is problematic. Unless the tibia can be returned to its normal anatomical position, the natural gliding and rotatory knee movements will be compromised. This is impossible with the serial casting technique in which wedges are inserted to extend the plaster cast. Boone designed an orthosis which is said to correct the subluxation of the tibia, using a brace with an extension desubluxation hinge [9].

Several other hinges with either a turnbuckle screw, an excentric joint or a damper (gas spring) are available with which an experienced orthotist can make an individual brace.

Permanent orthoses

Elastic bandages are sometimes continuously used for years on end. Some patients keep them on even while taking a shower. They are convinced that they will get an instant joint bleed the moment they do not wear the bandage. There is no proof that this is the case and also no theoretical explanation, but it is very difficult to convince those patients that they should improve their muscle strength by means of active exercises, so that the muscles may take over the function of the elastic bandage.

For persons with severe deformities, lack of muscle power which has not been restored despite a long period of intensive physiotherapy, and irreparable damage of joints, muscles or nerves, a permanent orthosis is necessary. In these cases, an individually fitted orthosis should be manufactured of material that is locally available and most suitable for the purpose. Increasing numbers of articulated commercial orthotics are available nowadays, especially for the knee [3], but also for ankle and elbow joints [8].

For persons with a painful haemophilic arthropathy of the ankle joint a leather ankle gauntlet brace or total contact thermoplastic device, or one made with carbon fibre and leather, can be used.

SHOE ADAPTATIONS AND SPECIAL SHOES

In a large part of the world shoes are used to protect and support normal feet. In warm climates, people may walk barefoot or use sandals. A lot of well-fitting shoes both for children and adults are commercially manufactured. However, fashion and commerce also influence the quality and fitting of shoes. For children and adults with haemophilia, shoes may help to prevent bleeding problems by protecting the feet, by stabilizing the foot during standing and walking, and by transferring weight-bearing stresses and facilitating a rolling motion during walking (from heel strike until toe off).

Requirements for a good shoe

Shoes should be well-fitting in such a way that there is no excessive pressure either on the toes or on the rest of the foot. The part round the heel should fit snugly and keep the foot in the correct position during standing and walking. The upper of the shoe should close preferably with laces or velcro to prevent the foot from sliding forward in the shoe. The shoe should have some toe-spring to facilitate push-off [10].

Shoes are constructed over lasts. (A shoe last is a wooden, plastic or metal form or mould.) Shoes are measured by width (letters) and length (numbers): for each width (A to B) there is a $\frac{1}{4}$ inch differential in girth and $\frac{1}{12}$ to $\frac{1}{24}$ inch differential in length [11].

Temporary adaptations

When there is limited or no dorsiflexion, or even an equinus foot after a fresh calf bleed, a temporary heel raise can be fitted underneath the ordinary shoe. The contralateral shoe should be raised to prevent the occurrence of a leg length discrepancy. The patient should be monitored once a week or even more frequently to assess whether the heel raise can be diminished. If a heel raise of more than 3 cm is needed it is better to manufacture a temporary shoe which can be easily adapted. A high heel raise underneath a normal shoe will deform the shoe and the foot will slide forward and there will be pressure both on the toes and on the heads of the metatarsals.

A temporary flexion contracture in the knee also may demand a heel raise.

Permanent shoe adaptations

Inlays (removable foot or arch supports) have the advantage that they are interchangeable from shoe to shoe and may be modified without disturbing the shoe. They may incorporate multiple corrections and may be constructed from several materials. Rigid arch supports, originally developed to correct a weak or flat longitudinal arch, are not used any more. There is no evidence that this correction of the foot will prevent haemarthrosis of the ankle in haemophilia.

Individually made inlays can spread pressure and unburden painful areas when there is pathological callus underneath the head of one or more metatarsal bones. This may be the case when there is a transverse flat-foot or talipes cavus (club foot).

When there is a slight leg length discrepancy, this may be corrected with an insole which is thicker under the heel of the shorter leg. For a leg length discrepancy of more than 3.5 cm, an individually made shoe should be prescribed. Permanent limited dorsiflexion of the ankle which limits the unrolling of the step can be facilitated by a heel raise and a sole with a rocker bottom. In cases of instability of the ankle which do not react favourably to active exercises, a high, snugly fitting shoe may prevent recurrent haemarthrosis.

In severe arthropathy of the tibiotalar and/or subtalar joints, fixing the ankle and foot in the least painful position and facilitating walking by the nature of the shoe can be realized using an individually designed orthopaedic shoe with a high upper and a stiff, snugly fitting part around the ankle. The same kind of shoe can be used to correct a drop-foot instead of an ankle–foot orthosis.

DISCUSSION

When considering orthoses and special shoe adaptations, one should also consider the necessity for another form of walking adjunct. Deloading of weight through a supporting orthosis may be necessary either temporarily or permanently. The transfer of that weight via an upper limb may be effected by using a cane, a crutch, crutches or a walker. It is better for a patient to walk correctly biomechanically, using an auxiliary device, than to pound the healthy limb. This is of great importance in persons with coagulopathies, for while hopping or jumping on their healthy limb they may cause a haemorrhage. Chronic use of an auxiliary walking device causes other minor problems. No person should be provided with an orthosis or walking device without medical justification, and because a person's status may change there is an absolute necessity for regular assessment visits. These visits should be weekly in acute cases and when the orthosis is permanent on a 3-monthly basis. The rehabilitation team will assess the quality of the brace/shoe and also its fit and function. All deviations from the normal gait pattern force the patient to exert more energy to ambulate. The orthosis provided should allow the person to carry out activities of daily living (ADL) with relative ease. If the energy demand is of such magnitude that ADL is problematic, then usually the person will be better off in a wheelchair. It is of vital importance to preserve the person's independence.

From this point of view, the local situation and the materials available need to be taken into account. Corrections, adaptations and/or repairs are more quickly and easily achieved when orthoses and walking adjuncts are of local origin. In developing countries, canes and crutches are usually preferable to wheelchairs because of the condition of houses and roads.

CONCLUSION

Worldwide, 80% of persons with haemophilia have no or very limited access to replacement therapy. In those persons with severe haemophilia A and B, haemarthroses and muscle haemorrhages occur frequently, causing joint and muscle impairments leading to disabilities and handicaps. Orthotic devices, special shoe adaptations and walking adjuncts will allow those affected to carry out activities of daily living as independently as possible under the circumstances. An orthosis should be prescribed and manufactured by doctors, paramedics and technicians with knowledge and experience in this field. Orthoses should be made of materials which are locally available in order to make adaptations and repairs possible. When prescribing an orthosis, the main purpose and major biomechanical deficits of each individual patient should be assessed. Follow-up assessments should be made available to the patient and instructions about the purpose and duration of use should be given. Orthoses can be used temporarily in acute bleeding situations, when there is lack of muscle strength or joint instability. Recently sustained contractures may be corrected and temporary shoe adaptations may assist during the conservative correction of an equinus foot. Permanent orthoses and shoe adaptations may be necessary when haemophilic arthropathy causes painful deformities or a muscle bleed has caused nerve damage.

Whether for temporary or permanent use, the orthotic device should always fit accurately, be mechanically efficient, should not be heavy and should have an acceptable cosmetic appearance. When prescribing walking adjuncts, knowledge of sociocultural and local circumstances are a prerequisite.

REFERENCES

1 McCollough NC. Biomechanical analysis system. In: *Atlas of Orthotics. Biomechanical Principles and Applications*. St Louis: CV Mosby, 1975: 169–93.

2 Perry J. Prescription principles. In: *Atlas of Orthotics. Biomechanical Principles and Applications*. St Louis: CV Mosby, 1975: 105–27.

3 Heim M, Steinbach T. Update on the use of orthotics in Hemophilia. *Orthop Rev* 1998, **10**: 975–8.

4 Heijnen L, Roosendaal G, Heim M. Orthotics and rehabilitation for chronic haemophilic synovitis of the ankle. *Clin Orthop* 1997; **343**: 68–73.

5 Seuser A, Wallny T, Klein H *et al*. Gait analysis of the hemophilic ankle with silicone heel cushion. *Clin Orthop* 1997; **343**: 74–80.

6 Heim M, Martinowitz U, Horoszowski H. Orthotic management of the knee in patients with hemophilia.

Clin Orthop 1997; **343**: 54–7.

7 Heim M, Heijnen L. Splints, orthotics and prosthetics. In: Heijnen L, ed. *Recent Advances in Rehabilitation in Haemophilia*. Hove, East Sussex: Medical Education Network, 1995: 44–7.

8 Heim M, Wershavski M, Martinowitz U, Varon D, Checicq A, Azaria M. The role of orthoses in the management of elbow joints in persons with haemophilia. *Haemophilia* 1999; **5** (Suppl. 1): 43–5.

9 Boone DC. *Comprehensive Management of Hemophilia*. Philadephia: FA Davis, 1976.

10 Heijnen L, Heim M, InderMaur H. Manufactured shoes and orthopaedic shoes. In: Heijnen L, ed. *Recent Advances in Rehabilitation in Haemophilia*. Hove, East Sussex: Medical Education Network, 1995: 48–53.

11 Jahss MH. Shoes and shoe modifications. In: *Atlas of Orthotics. Biomechanical Principles and Applications*. St Louis: CV Mosby, 1975: 267–79.

CHAPTER 27

Gait Corrective Devices

F QUEROL-FUENTES, C LOPEZ-CABARCOS AND J A AZNAR-LUCEA

INTRODUCTION

One of the main objectives of orthopaedic surgery and rehabilitation is to establish the characteristics of normal and pathological gaits. In the former case the aim is the patient's comfort and the prevention of lesions, while in the latter the aim is to identify the type of disability and ensure that the corrective device used is the appropriate one. Since each device has to be adapted to the needs of the individual patient, the following points have to be considered.

1 Common features of deformities affecting gait in haemophilic patients.
2 Common features of normal and pathological gait.
3 Orthopaedic diagnosis of the lower limbs to monitor the development of locomotion in haemophilic patients.
4 Common haemophilic injuries affecting the lower limbs.
5 Orthotics to prevent musculoskeletal injury in the lower limbs.
6 Orthopaedic and rehabilitation management and devices for acute injuries.
7 Gait corrective devices for chronic injuries.
These aspects will be discussed in turn.

COMMON FEATURES OF DEFORMITIES AFFECTING GAIT IN HAEMOPHILIC PATIENTS

The first references to disabilities affecting the musculoskeletal system as a result of haemophilia date from the beginning of the nineteenth century [1–4]. The impossibility of staunching haemorrhages at that time ruled out surgical procedures that were in use for other illnesses. Moreover, the average life expectancy for haemophiliacs was put at 16, which virtually restricted therapeutic options to haemotological measures [2,3,5–8]. The typical image of restricted motion caused by haemophilia is that of 'the little boy cradled in his mother's arms' who is unable to walk without assistance [9].

Haemarthrosis is the commonest bleeding complication in haemophilia, and is accepted as the main cause of haemophilic arthropathy.

Muscle and joint bleeds occur in all patients with severe haemophilia before the age of 2 years [10,11]. Haematomas appear in the first months of life, whereas joint bleeds in the lower limbs occur as the child is learning to move by himself, when there is a greater risk of injury [10]. It is at this stage of the child's development that the use of orthopaedic devices to prevent disability must be considered.

Musculoskeletal injuries are the main cause of morbidity and disability in haemophilia [3,6,10,12]. We believe, moreover, that an injury to just one of the six joints of the lower limbs is itself a serious disability which may require corrective devices to aid movement. Fernandez-Palazzi and Battistella [12] studied the frequency of bleeding episodes in 120 patients, identifying osteoarticular haemorrhages in 83.3% of cases. In the 10 699 bleeding episodes studied by Magallon and Martin-Villar [10], 87% were identified as musculoskeletal injuries.

The notion of disability is generally associated with inability to walk. The American Medical Association considers that injuries to the lower limbs which either reduce or impede movement represent up to 80% of cases of permanent impairment [13]. If, for example, a haemophilic patient needs two crutches to walk, his ability to lead a normal life is considered to be reduced by 50%, which illustrates the importance of preventing injuries to the lower limbs and using orthoses that prevent disabling injuries and improve the motion and comfort of the lower limbs.

COMMON FEATURES OF NORMAL AND PATHOLOGICAL GAIT

Normal gait is defined as a form of biped locomotion consisting of alternate movements of the lower limbs without the aid of crutches or any other device, and in which dynamic equilibrium is maintained. The consumption of energy during walking must be minimal. In addition, these factors must be considered: characteristics of the surface on which we walk, step frequency, speed of walking and distance covered [14]. Normal gait takes for granted the use of footwear, even though it is an external device that aids walking over different surfaces, be they flat or inclined, hard or soft, sandy, icy, or of any other consistency [15].

Pathological gait is entailed when external devices are needed to give stability to joints, correct aberrant positions (such as flexed and valgus knee) and aid walking. These external devices can include appliances as simple as the adaptation of footwear to correct deficient balance and the use of a cane to aid walking [16].

In analysing gait, the mechanical anatomy of motion and posture must be taken into account. That is to say, the motion of the upper and lower limbs during walking must be studied, as well as horizontal and vertical movements from the centre of gravity of the body. This study would include characteristics of stride, cadences, walking patterns, speed, and different walking cycles and phases. In addition, all the aspects of the musculoskeletal system involved in walking must be considered, in view of the fact that it can be severely affected in haemophilic patients.

Gait analysis begins with a clinical examination. First, the patient, dressed only in his/her underwear, is asked to stand upright and is viewed from the front and side. If possible, such an evaluation should be carried out on a pedigraph so that the features of the plantar print may be studied for possible axial deformities [17,18]. Next, the patient is asked to walk naturally so that general articular motion during walking may be observed. The clinical examination just described is subjective, but it provides the joint evaluation of haemophilic patients with parameters that measure the gait of such patients on a scale of 0–3, which are: abnormalities such as limping, walking with foot turned out, walking on side of foot, no push-off, walking on toes, uneven strides, no or uneven weight-shifting, abnormal running, and galloping or skipping [11].

Gait analysis can be carried out and objectified with technical aids of varying sophistication such as optoelectronic systems, accelerometers, triaxial goniometers, and the like. In our observations, we applied a protocol of instrumented insoles developed in the Institute for Biomechanics, Valencia, Spain, for the prescription, design and evaluation of foot orthoses [19].

Traditionally, orthopaedic pathologies causing gait disorder have been classified as pain in the hip, knee and/or ankle joints, leg length discrepancies, hip rigidity and/or instability, muscular pain in hip, joint flexion contracture and/or rigidity of extension in the knee, and loss of dorsal and/or plantar flexion and angular deformities in the ankle. All these disorders are still very frequent in haemophilic patients [20–22].

STEP-BY-STEP MONITORING OF AMBULATION IN THE HAEMOPHILIC PATIENT AND GENERAL OBSERVATIONS ON THERAPY

Musculoskeletal examination of the lower limbs

The joints should be examined both statically and dynamically. Examination at rest establishes the presence or absence of swelling in the joint, erythema characterized by the redness of the skin, heat resulting from an increase of temperature in the area, and pain in the muscular insertion or the joint. Examination during movement establishes the existence of joint crepitation, impairment of articular or muscular motion, and evident signs of pain during different stages of active or passive movement.

The hips, knees and ankles are assessed in terms of functionality according to muscular, joint and nervous system. The absence of previous injury suggests normal strength and sensitivity, which in theory should favour complete range of movement in the joint. The haemophilic patient should be examined at least once a year, to evaluate in each joint the degree of range or mobility as percentages in flexion, extension, abduction, adduction, and internal and external rotation. The evaluation of motoricity is carried out by examining muscular function on a scale of 0–5 points. The scores on this scales represent the following [18,23]:

0 absence of muscle contraction
1 possibility of contraction without movement
2 movement favoured by gravity

3 movement against gravity
4 movement against resistance
5 normal state.

Basic examinations according to age of patient

A rough but practical classification of patients according to age is to distinguish between infants (0–2-year-olds), pre-school children (2–7-year-olds), schoolchildren (7–10-year-olds), pre-adolescents (10–14-year-olds) and adolescents (14–18-year-olds). With infants examination is necessarily passive. With pre-school children it is necessary to create an appropriate 'playtime' atmosphere to elicit the right response. While a certain degree of cooperation is possible with schoolchildren, the help of their parents is essential so that the child may understand why it is necessary to have orthoses and learn how to use them. More active co-operation concerning physical exercise and the use of orthoses can be elicited from pre-adolescents. Adolescents need to be persuaded of the importance of gait corrective devices and how they can benefit from their use to prevent the crippling effects of arthropathy [3,18].

With infants the first step is to carry out a pyschomotor examination so that neurological disorders may be ruled out as a cause of the abnormalities they may present. Body posture and muscle tone and strength are assessed, as well as the motor responses in the extremities. Although these are uncommon, the absence of gross deformities such as knock knees should be noted so that they may be discounted. It is also important to assess the articular axes of the knees and the axis, mobility and muscle balance of hips, taking note of the absence of dislocations, osteochondrosis, synovitis or epiphysiolysis, disorders which negatively affect gait and necessitate the use of orthoses [24].

In children it is very common to find small haematomas which require the adoption of preventive measures such as protective headwear, knee and shin pads, and the like. According to the degree of autonomy of movement, there are three courses of protective action which we shall term passive prevention, assisted prevention and active prevention [18].

Passive prevention involves conditioning the infant's environment to forestall the likelihood of its sustaining any injury. For example, injuries sustained from the movements of cradles, chairs and other items of furniture can be prevented by padding the edges and corners with a soft material such as foam. Since at such an early age movement is generally limited to small, low-risk areas, orthoses are not usually necessary as long as furniture is adequately padded.

Assisted prevention becomes necessary as soon as the child is able to move by himself. A child first learns to sit up and crawl on his hands and knees, then he learns to stand, first with the help of an older person and then on his own. Finally, he learns to walk. During these stages, the child has to be provided with protective devices such as special headwear to prevent injury when he bumps his head against any object, knee pads to prevent injuries that may be sustained while crawling on hands and knees, or shin pads to prevent bruising caused by blows to the legs.

Active prevention is to be taken once the child has learned to walk unassisted. At this stage, the child begins to pursue games and activities that involve a great deal of physical exertion, becoming aware of the dangers they entail. For instance, when the child is learning to ride a bicycle, his parents should lay down safety measures such as obliging him to wear a helmet and shin pads. A level-headed and disciplined approach will inculcate appropriate habits in the child, such as choosing the right kit to use for the practice of sports, even non-competitive ones [25].

Diagnosis of deformities affecting gait and requiring corrective devices

The most important deformities that affect gait and require orthopaedic diagnosis are the following [16,20,24,26–9]:
- deformities affecting the foot: cavus, flat, talus, valgus and varus foot
- deviation of the knee axis: flexed, recurvatum, valgus and varus knee, and tibial rotation
- dislocation of the hip, osteochondritis, synovitis, and epiphysiolysis
- lower limb length discrepancy.

Given the frequency of deformities affecting the foot, the description of examinations will be limited to this part of the body, with reference to the haemophilic boy.

In haemophilia, the ankle joint ranks third in the frequency of haemarthrosis. If the child has not suffered bleeding episodes, it is reasonable not to expect to find signs of damage to the joints. However, a thorough examination is still indicated to ascertain the presence or absence of synovitis, synovial hypertrophy, strength, trophism, flexion and equinus contracture, range of movement, crepitus on motion, signs of instability, axial deformities and abnormal gait [11].

The feet are assessed both statically and dynamically. The use of a pedoscope is common practice in such examinations. Another common procedure is to take plantar prints with the aid of a pedograph with a rubber mat. This involves an extremely simple functional barographic examination: the foot is placed on a sheet of rubber with its bottom side steeped in ink so that it leaves a plantar imprint on a sheet of squared paper placed underneath the sheet of rubber. Maximum foot pressure is thereby measured on the sheet of paper by observing the size of the print. The cost is reduced to the price of a sheet of paper, and this type of examination is useful for the diagnosis of deformities such as cavus, flat and talus foot, and the like. More sophisticated methods such as isokinetic apparatus and dynamometric insoles permit more detailed assessments but, although their value for research is obvious, their use and cost-effectiveness in the clinical setting are still under study [28–30].

The assessment of deformities affecting the foot requires a clear-cut approach. Such deformities, even if only perceived, are a source of worry for parents, and these concerns are sometimes transmitted to the paediatrician. A child's foot is extremely malleable, particularly in the first year, and therefore heavy loads and inadequate footwear should be avoided [31]. On the other hand, undue parental fears that confuse normal for pathological situations should be dispelled.

When the child is between the ages of 3 and 5 years, paediatricians are often asked about 'abnormal' gaits concerning bow legs, flat feet, and the like. In 90% of cases, there is no cause for concern, although it should be stressed that pathological deformities of the foot may be related to serious conditions that sometimes pass unnoticed such as malformation of the spine, polymalformation, brain damage affecting the motor regions, or hereditary degenerative illnesses [24].

The assessment of the tibiotalar (flexion–extension), subtalar (pronation and supination) and midtarsal (fore- and hindfoot) joints helps in the diagnosis of cavus, flat, talus, valgus and varus foot, conditions which require a common diagnostic and therapeutic criterion because of their effect on foot biomechanics, particularly in haemophilia [26].

It is important to know how the talo-calcaneal angle of the hindfoot can be affected because this may be an indication of serious orthopaedic problems. The talo-calcaneal angle is defined as the angle between the axes that form the external arc – that is, the axis which goes through the calcaneum, cuboid and second metatarsus – and internal arc, or talus. A lateral perspective of the hindfoot affords a good view of the talo-calcaneal angle, which remains constant regardless of the position of the foot, and whose normal angle is 40°. Severe flat-foot is diagnosed when the talo-calcaneal angle is >40°. When the angle is 0–10°, talus foot is diagnosed [24].

The degree to which deformities of the foot can be corrected should also be evaluated, together with that of the hips and knees, and the position of the foot in relation to the tibial axis. One should never forget that a malformation of the foot may conceal other orthopaedic disorders. Talus foot, for example, is often associated with congenital dislocation of the hip.

Finally, muscle balance should also be analysed. The dorsal flexion of the foot should be performed on a strictly sagittal plane with no lateral deviance whatsoever, indicative of a perfect equilibrium between the muscles tibialis anterior and peroneus tertius.

Since physiological orthopaedic deformities such as valgus and varus knee, externally rotated tibia, flat and valgus foot, and talar deviance disappear with growth, the doctor should distinguish the pathology, because in the haemophilic patient it may be a cause of bleeding episodes, which in turn may bring about arthropathy.

COMMON INJURIES AS A RESULT OF HAEMOPHILIA AFFECTING THE LOWER EXTREMITIES

The injuries to the soft tissue which affect the musculoskeletal system can be classified as extra- and intra-articular. In the former, deep haematomas are of particular interest because their inter- and intramuscular location brings about functional deficit. Intra-articular injuries are haemarthroses and synovitis, which constitute the morphological basis of arthropathy [32].

Deep haematomas

Deep haematomas are defined as severe episodes that can seriously impede gait when located in the lower extremities. They affect muscle tissue and are always the cause of functional disorders which require convalescence and, in addition to replacement of deficient factor, usually call for orthotics that help redistribute load during monopodal stance to prevent fresh bleeds brought on by overloading.

During the acute phase the first urgent problem is compartment syndrome. Sometimes a less severe and more localized haematoma causing compression of the nerve brings on neurapraxia, that is, a temporary blocking of nerve conduction. This in turn causes motor and/or sensory disorders which usually disappear as soon as pressure eases off.

A typical episode for its severity is haematoma affecting the iliopsoas, the muscle which controls flexion of the hip. This requires careful diagnosis, and also differential diagnosis to prevent confusing its symptoms with those of appendicitis. The consequences can be serious as to hinder flexion of the hip or paralyse the extensors of the knee [33]. That is why physiotherapy treating problems affecting the iliopsoas muscle must make use of walking aids to ensure adequate rehabilitation. Deep haematomas require thorough control. The encapsulation of a haematoma and renewed bleeds can bring about haemophilic pseudotumours, which can affect the bone and so seriously hinder therapeutic action.

As regards damage to the joints, haemarthrosis is, as we have already indicated, the most frequent, most typical and best-known injury caused by bleeding episodes brought on by haemophilia. Magallon and Martin-Villar [10], drawing on their broad experience in this area, mention haemarthrosis as representing 69% of all the haemorrhages that a patient with haemophilia may experience. The Orthopaedic Outcomes Study established that haemarthrosis constitutes 65% of all bleeding episodes.

Acute haemarthrosis

Acute haemarthrosis is defined as the presence of blood in the joints following trauma. The intensity of the trauma need not be great for haemarthrosis to occur, since there are cases of haemarthrosis occurring without the patient being aware of having sustained any injury. The distinction between subacute and chronic haemarthrosis is made on the basis of the characteristics of the clinical evolution of each, although chronic haemarthrosis presents synovial hypertrophy and muscular atrophy, with the attendant risks of renewed bleeding. Haemarthrosis in the lower extremities always impedes gait and requires recourse to orthotics to immobilize the joint, as well as crutches to aid movement while resting the affected limb.

Synovitis

Synovitis is inflammation of the synovial membrane covering the joint. As is already known, bleeds into the joint originate in the area of the synovial membrane, which sets off a chain reaction: the reabsorption of blood results in inflammatory hyperplasia in the synovial membrane, and causes easing of intracapsular pressure, which in turn causes the damaged blood vessel to reopen. Recurrent bleeding episodes result in hypertrophy. The first stage, or pigmentary hypertrophy, is characterized by abundant vascularization and the thinness of the newly formed vessels, and favours renewed bleeding. The end stage is arthropathy. Synovitis in the lower extremities affects the strength and range of movement of the joints, impedes gait, and requires orthotics and replacement therapy with deficient coagulant factors, and perhaps synoviorthesis or surgical synovectomy [34–37].

ORTHOTICS USED IN PREVENTION OF MUSCULOSKELETAL INJURIES IN THE LOWER EXTREMITIES

Cushioned pads are recommended for the area around the joints and bones of lower extremities with little muscle protection. They are made of non-slip material such as neoprene and include soft materials such as gel polymer and silicone so that they can be used as a type of tubular bandage providing protection against blows (Fig. 27.1). For this reason they are widely used for sports activities, and in haemophilia they are employed to prevent haematomas or torn muscles caused by too much exercise [21,26,29,38–43].

Splints of various materials may be adjusted to functional positions to prevent haemorrhages caused by involuntary movements. Made of plaster and/or thermoplastic material, these splints are used with high-risk patients and are placed at night so that spontaneous haemarthrosis caused by uncontrolled movements during sleep may be prevented [26,27,38,44,45].

Insoles will absorb and cushion pressure on the heel during the stance phase. Instrumented barographic insoles map out the pressure distribution. These insoles have proved their usefulness in ensuring the wearer's comfort and preventing spontaneous haemarthrosis [46–50].

The aim of load-relieving orthotics is to free, partially or completely, the affected joint from weight-bearing. For the ankle, calipers are used made up of an upper and lower segment joined together by articulated bars. The lower segment is the shoe or boot itself, or a plastic splint

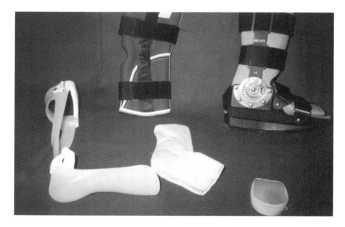

Fig. 27.1 Orthotics used for the prevention of musculoskeletal injuries in the lower limbs.

adjusted to the requirements of the foot; the upper segment is a cuff which encircles the shin to ensure a tight fit. If the characteristics of the appliance allows it, it may be fitted on to the area of the lateral condyle of the tibia. In the light of our experience with haemophilic patients, however, we prefer placing the orthosis on the shin because pressure on bone surfaces usually causes haematomas during gait. This type of appliance is frequently used in the management of injuries caused in the pursuit of sports activities requiring load relief during gait. Studies conducted into their performance show a load decrease of over 40% in full stance, which with the use of crutches offers a safety margin of over 80% in monopodal stance.

The load-relief appliances may consist of calipers that afford protection to all the joints of the lower limb or a support that protects an individual joint. In calipers protecting the knee joint, the two articulated bars end in either a thigh or ischial support, and come equipped with adjustable locked knee joints [51]. If an ischial support is used, load relief of the knee is up to 100%. An ischial support sufficiently cushioned with soft material does not generally cause haematomas, and patients find them comfortable.

Relieving the hip joint of load during gait requires a pelvic corset made of supple material such as leather or plastic that fits on to hip. It can have only one metal shaft, which is fitted to the outer part of the thigh support and pelvic corset. The corset is only able to give partial relief and is generally used to immobilize and limit rotary movements of the hips when this becomes painful as a result of arthrosis.

Shin, knee and elbow pads with joint-stabilizing systems to prevent injury to the ligaments are made of soft materials such as neoprene and reinforced with elastic strips placed in the direction of the ligaments to perform their function. They can also be equipped with lateral metal bars and silicone pads placed over the bony areas to protect them from blows. Some models come equipped with air splints so that they can be placed on the area around the joint more smoothly and increase stability [52–54].

Articularly aligned orthosis

There are many models of this type of orthosis. The most commonly used for the lower extremities in patello-femoral arthropathy are knee pads with an opening that leaves the patella uncovered. Their purpose is to ensure that the patella is stabilized.

Crutches and walking sticks

Crutches and walking sticks improve ambulation because they relieve the joints of the lower limbs of their weight-bearing function, improve balance, provide greater impetus for locomotion, and decrease the amount of energy required.

Ordinary crutches are made up of three main parts: handle, shaft, and pad or cushion, the latter being the part in contact with the ground. The most common are elbow crutches, which have an additional piece containing a brace to support the forearm. One of the main aims of physiotherapy is to help the patient learn to walk with the aid of crutches.

ORTHOPAEDIC AND REHABILITATION MANAGEMENT AND DEVICES FOR ACUTE INJURIES

Besides replacement therapy, acute haemarthrosis in the lower extremities receives two other types of treatment: conservative treatment and arthrocentesis [54–58].

Conservative treatment

Conservative treatment involves the following protocol.

Day 1
Orthotic device. Immobilization with posterior splint in antalgic position, application of ice to the affected joint, and resting the affected limb in a position ensuring unimpaired circulation. Release from loading, prescribing orthotic devices and crutches for locomotion.

Day 2
Medical examination after 24 hours: in the event of satisfactory progress, the orthotic device is adjusted to a functional position, isometric exercises are allowed, and application of ice to and resting of affected joint continued.

Day 3 onwards
Monitoring of progress paying special attention to swelling and mobility, prescription of support of partial load to be stepped up gradually, prescription of orthotic devices such as crutches to aid walking, load-relief footwear for the ankles, knee splints or pelvic corsets, and prescription of active physical exercise to be stepped up gradually.

Arthrocentesis

This treatment involves the following protocol.

Day 1
Orthotic devices include compressive bandage or tubular bandage, and crutches for partial load. Ice is to be applied to the affected joint, and rest to be prescribed.

Day 2 or 3
Orthotic devices: compressive bandage to be taken off, load to be increased gradually, though crutches still needed; stabilizing splints might be used. More strenuous exercise might be prescribed followed by application of ice to the affected joint.

Both conservative treatment and arthrocentesis involve the acquisition of new walking habits by the patient, which may require the use of crutches or other walking aids to control load on the affected joint.

GAIT CORRECTIVE DEVICES FOR CHRONIC INJURIES

Arthropathy of the ankle

The corrective device to be used depends on the degree and severity of the haemarthrosis. However, there are three types of device whose purpose is to prevent ankle and knee haemarthroses and improve comfort: insoles with material to cushion shock in gait phase, insoles to correct deformities, and shin pads with rigid or elastic supports to stabilize the joint, and functional corsets (Fig. 27.2).

Arthropathy of the knee

The devices used for this condition basically consist of ligament-stabilizing knee pads with bars and elastic straps to centralize the patella and correct flexum, recurvatum, valgus and varus knee.

Arthropathy of the hip

The first priority is to prevent the risk of fracture in osteoporosis. In recent years the Hips © device (Hips protection system for flexible use) has been adopted, which consists of a plastic structure with a convex surface used as a shock absorber.

In advanced arthropathy, a total joint arthroplasty is the best solution for the condition [20]. However, in some cases jointed orthoses are preferred as they relieve the hip of weight-bearing by immobilizing it by means of a pelvic belt corset, and ensuring flexion and extension while impeding rotations, the movements which provoke the most intense pain.

CONCLUSIONS

Even today, on the threshold of the twenty-first century, the prevention and treatment of haemophilic arthropathy is still the main goal of prophylaxis with replacement therapy of deficient plasma clotting factors [6,12,58]. Orthoses have proved their usefulness in correcting joint

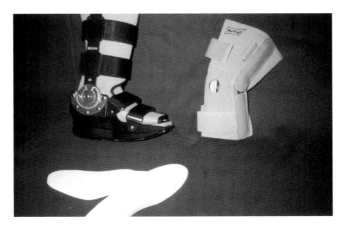

Fig. 27.2 Gait corrective devices used for chronic injuries of the lower limbs.

deformities, surgery and other problems [59–66]. The diagnosis of normal and pathological gait is essential to prevent disability in the haemophilic patient. It also draws attention to the role played by orthopaedic surgery and rehabilitation in haemophilia [67–70] because abnormal gait may cause arthropathy as a result of the joint bearing excessive weight, and because arthropathy of the lower limbs gives rise to abnormal gait, giving rise in turn to a vicious circle which aggravates damage to the joint.

The provision of commercial plasma clotting factor for all haemophiliacs is not yet achievable. As with the population at large, the pursuit of sports activities is recommended to haemophilic patients for the beneficial effects it has on their health [71–76], although one should always bear in mind the risks inherent in such activities, as well as the physical activities of daily life [69,75–78]. Adequate devices should therefore be used to protect the musculoskeletal system.

The description of gait corrective devices is an arduous task in view of the great number of models available, especially when there is not enough space to provide ample illustration. Every year, orthoprosthesists turn out new designs which improve the possibilities of restoring normal gait to disabled patients. On the other hand, the diagnosis of normal and pathological gait requires methodical study so that these corrective devices may be judged on their merits with regard to their use in therapy.

Since the objective of this chapter is to provide a general overview of problems concerning gait and the orthotic devices to remedy them, we believe that the guidelines regarding the care of haemophilic patients should include the following:

1 that orthopaedists and/or specialists in rehabilitation should carry out a precise diagnosis of normal and pathological gait;

2 that target joints should receive protective splinting;

3 that insoles used in footwear should be comfortable in the gait phase and prevent small-scale traumas that cause ankle and knee haemarthrosis;

4 that in acute haemarthroses receiving conservative treatment, the joint should be immobilized first in an antalgic position and, after 24–48 hours, in a functional position, keeping the affected joint at rest and relieving the lower limbs of weight-bearing;

5 that after immobilization in the case of acute haemarthrosis in the lower limbs, the weight which the affected limb may bear should be increased gradually, and that orthotic devices should be used to avoid relapses;

6 that advanced arthropathy benefits from the use of orthotic devices, which control mobility, stability and weight;

7 that surgery performed on the joints of the lower limbs should always make use of gait corrective devices for rehabilitation.

REFERENCES

1 Otto JC. An account of an hemorrhagic disposition existing in certain families. *Review of American Publication in Medicine, Surgery and the Medical Repository* 1803; **6**: 1–4.

2 DiMichele D. Hemophilia 1996: new approach to an old disease. *Pediatr Hematol* 1996; **3**: 709–36.

3 Hilgartner MW. *Hemophilia in the Child and Adult*. New York: Masson, 1982.

4 Kasper CK. An elective orthopaedic surgical repair: a reminiscence. *Haemophilia* 1996; **2**: 120–1.

5 Nilsson MI. *Haemophilia*. Sweden, 1994.

6 Berntorp E. Methods of haemophilia care delivery: regular prophylaxis versus episodic treatment. *Haemophilia* 1995; **1**: 3–7.

7 Boone DC. A perspective on conservative management of musculoskeletal problems: is it time for the next crusade? *Hemophilia World* 1990; **6**: 1–16.

8 Szucs TD, Öffner A, Schramm W. Socioeconomic impact of haemophilia care: results of a pilot study. *Haemophilia* 1996; **2**: 211–17.

9 Kelley LA. *Alexis, El Príncipe que tenía Hemofilia*. Armour Pharmaceutical Company, 1992.

10 Magallon M, Martin-Villar J. Aspectos clínicos, psicológicos y sociales de las hemofilias. In: Universidad de Salamanca, ed. *Enciclopedia Iberoamericana de Hematología*. Salamanca, Spain: Universidad de Salamanca, 1992: 328–39.

11 Manco-Johnson M, Nuss R, Geraghty S, Kilcoyne R, Funk S. A prophylactic program in the United States: experience and issues. In: Berntorp E, ed. *Prophylactic Treatment of Hemophilia A and B: Current and Future Perspectives*. New York: Science & Medicine, 1994: 52–6.

12 Fernandez-Palazzi F, Battistella LR. Ortopedia y rehabilitación en hemofilia. In: Universidad de Salamanca, ed. *Enciclopedia Iberoamericana de Hematología*. Salamanca, Spain: Universidad de Salamanca, 1992: 367–76.

13 American Medical Association (US*). Guias para la evaluación de las deficiencias permanentes*. Department of Preventive Medicine and Public Health (Chicago). Ministerio de Asuntos Sociales (España), 1994.

14 Plas F, Viel E, Blanc Y. *La Marcha Humana*. Barcelona, Spain: Masson, 1984.

15 Ribbans WJ, Phillips M, Stock D, Stibe E. Haemophilic ankle problems: orthopaedic solutions. *Haemophilia* 1995; **1**: 91–6.

16 Viladot R, Cohí O, Clavell S. *Ortesis y Protesis del Aparato Locomotor. Extremidad Inferior*. Barcelona, Spain: Masson, 1989.

17 Pitzen P, Rösller H. *Manual de Ortopedia*. Barcelona, Spain: Doyma, 1993.

18 Querol F, Lorenzo JI, Haya S, Molina R, Aznar JA. Tratamiento rehabilitador de la artropatía inicial en el paciente hemofílico. *Proceedings of the V Simposio Hyland: Artropatía Hemofílica*. Avila, Spain, October 1996: 49–61.

19 Querol F. Rehabilitación en la hemofilia. *Proceedings of the III Congreso Nacional de Hemofilia*; Seville, Spain, November 1995: 60–71.

20 Rodriguez-Merchan EC. Common orthopaedic problems in haemophilia. *Haemophilia* 1999; **5** (Suppl. 1): 53–60.

21 Ribbans WJ, Rees JL. Management of equinus contrac-

tures of the ankle in haemophilia. *Haemophilia* 1999; **5**: 46–52.

22 Fernandez-Palazzi F, Battistella LR. Non-operative treatment of flexion contracture of the knee in haemophilia. *Haemophilia* 1999; **5** (Suppl. 1): 20–4.

23 Gilbert MS. Prophylaxis: musculoskeletal evaluation. *Seminars in Hematology* 1993; **30**: 3–6.

24 Dimeglio A. *Ortopedia Infantil Cotidiana*. Barcelona, Spain: Masson, 1991.

25 Harris NS. *Hemophilia, Sports and Exercise*. New York: National Hemophilia Foundation, 1996.

26 Heijnen L, Roosendaal G, Heim M. Orthotics and rehabilitation for chronic hemophilic synovitis of the ankle. *Clin Orthop* 1997; **343**: 68–73.

27 Dietrich SL, Luck JV, Martinson AM. Problemas musculoesqueléticos. In: Hilgartner MW, ed. *Hemofilia en el Niño y en el Adulto*. Barcelona, Spain: Espaxs, 1984: 117–33.

28 Heim M, Martinowitz U, Horoszowski H. Orthotic management of the knee in patients with hemophilia. *Clini Orthop* 1997; **343**: 54–7.

29 Lopez-Cabarcos C, Martinez-Moreno M: Rehabilitación en la patología del pie hemofílico. *Proceedings of the Congreso Nacional de Hemofilia*. Santander, Spain, 1991: 35–6.

30 Zwart J, Pradas A. La masa ósea a nivel del pie. *Interés biodinámico* 1993; **15**: 75–80.

31 Canelon-Sanchez F. Lesiones del pie en el atleta pediátrico. *Proceedings of the Jornadas de Traumatología Deportiva. XI Curso de doctorado*, Valencia, Spain, May 1998.

32 Roosendaal G. Haemophilic arthropathy compared to osteoarthritis and rheumatoid arthritis. In: *Blood induced cartilage damage in hemophilia*. Doctoral thesis, Utrecht, Holland: Elinnkwijk, 1998: 65–82.

33 Fernandez-Palazzi F, Rivas S, DeBosch NB, DeSaez AR. Hematomas within the iliopsoas muscle in hemophilic patients. *Clin Orthop* 1996; **328**: 19–24.

34 Rodriguez-Merchan EC, Magallon M, Galindo E, Lopez-Cabarcos C. Hamstring release for fixed knee flexion contracture in hemophilia. *Clin Orthop* 1997; **343**: 63–7.

35 Gilbert MS, Radomisli TE. Therapeutic options in the management of hemophilic synovitis. *Clin Orthop* 1997; **343**: 88–92.

36 Lopez-Cabarcos C. Medidas rehabilitadoras en la artropatía hemofílica. *Proceedings of the III Congreso Nacional de Hemofilia*. Seville, Spain, November 1995: 108–11.

37 Ribbans WJ, Giangrande P, Beeton K. Conservative treatment of hemarthrosis for prevention of hemophilic synovitis. *Clin Orthop* 1997; **343**: 12–18.

38 Heijnen L, Haan E, Mauser-Bunschoten EP. The whens and whys of inmobilization. *Proceedings of the XX International Congress of the World Federation of Hemophilia*, Athens, Greece, October 1992.

39 Bachmayer E, Holdredge S. Developmental activities,

sports, and games. *Hemophilia World* 1991; **7**: 5–12.

40 Buzzard BM. Physiotherapy and sports injuries in haemophilia. *Proceedings of the XX International Congress of the World Federation of Hemophilia*, Athens, Greece, October 1992.

41 Gilbert MS, Schorr JB, Holbrook, Tiberio D. *Hemophilia and Sports*. Michigan: National Hemophilia Foundation, 1994.

42 Jones P. *Hemofilia*. Barcelona: Instituto de Hemoderivados Inmuno, 1978.

43 O'Connel D. Los Deportes y su Hijo. *Selecciones de Hemalogia* 1995; **1**: 9–11.

44 Boone DC, Spencer CD. *Terapia fisica en la Hemofilia*. Berkeley, California, USA: Cutter Laboratories, 1977.

45 Lopez-Cabarcos C, Wolanov S. Tratamiento rehabilitador. In: Magallon M, ed. *Hemofilia y Rehabilitación*. Madrid: Real Fundacion Victoria Eugenia, 1996: 21–6.

46 Gilbert MS. Complicaciones musculoesqueléticas de la Hemofilia: Las articulaciones. In: *Guidelines for the Development of a National Programme for Haemophilia*. World Federation of Hemophilia, 1997; **6**: 1–7.

47 Heim M, Horoszowski H, Varon D, Martinowitz U. Podal shock absorption. *Proceedings of the XX International Congress of the World Federation of Hemophilia*, Athens, Greece, October 1992.

48 Querol F, Lorenzo JI, Molina R, Haya S, Aznar JA. Hemartros y actividad física en nuestra población hemofílica de 7 a 18 años. *Proceedings of the III Congreso Nacional de Hemofilia*. Seville, Spain, November 1995: 123.

49 Ribbans WJ, Phillips AM. Hemophilic ankle arthropathy. *Clin Orthop* 1996; **328**: 39–45.

50 Seuser A, Wallny T, Klein H, Ribbans W J, Schumpe G, Brackmann H H. Gait analysis of the hemophilic ankle with silicone heel cushion. *Clin Orthop* 1997; **343**: 74–80.

51 Gilbert MS. *Ortopedia en Hemofilia*. Berkeley, California, USA: Cutter Laboratories, 1981.

52 Janiszewsky DW, Carolyn ZL. Tratamiento de rehabilitación para el enfermo hemofílico. In: Hilgartner MW, ed. *Hemofilia en el Niño y en el Adulto*. Barcelona: Espaxs, 1984: 355–78.

53 Buzzard BM. Twin centre study to evaluate the effectiveness of "Airsplints" as a means of reducing bleeding episodes in the ankle joints of children with haemophilia A and B. *Proceedings of the XXI International Congress of the World Federation of Hemophilia*, Mexico, April 1994: 49.

54 Rodriguez-Merchan EC. Tratamiento ortopédico de las hemartrosis de rodilla en el paciente hemofílico. *Proceedings of the V Simposio Hyland: Artropatía Hemofílica*, Avila, Spain, October 1996: 23–7.

55 Massanet S. Tratamiento del hemartros agudo. *Proceedings of the V Simposio Hyland: Artropatía Hemofílica*, Avila, Spain, October 1996: 34–5.

56 Querol F, Lorenzo JI, Haya S, Molina R, Aznar JA. Tratamiento rehabilitador del hemartros agudo en el paciente hemofílico. *Proceedings of the V Simposio Hyland: Artropatía Hemofílica*, Avila, Spain, October 1996: 38–48.

57 Pettersson C. Orthopedic treatment. In: Nilsson MI, ed. *Hemophilia*. Sweden: Pharmacia Plasma Products, 1994: 76–81.

58 Effenberger W, Weissbach G. Arthropathy in hemophilic adolescents. *Proceedings of the XX International Congress of the World Federation of Hemophilia*, Athens, Greece, October 1992.

59 Horoszowski H, Heim M, Schulman S, Varon D, Martinowitz U. Multiple joint procedures in a single operative session on hemophilic patients. *Clin Orthop* 1996; **328**: 60–4.

60 Lopez-Cabarcos C, Magallon M. La rehabilitación como prevención de las hemorragias en el paciente con hemofilia. *Proceedings of the Seminarios Hyland: Tratamiento Profiláctico de la Hemofilia*. Cuenca, Spain, November 1993: 52–64.

61 Rodriguez-Merchan EC. Therapeutic options in the management of articular contractures in haemophiliacs. *Haemophilia* 1999; **5** (Suppl. 1): 5–9.

62 Rodriguez-Merchan EC. Correction of fixed contractures during total knee arthroplasty in haemophiliacs. *Haemophilia* 1999; **5** (Suppl. 1): 33–8.

63 Gamble JG, Bellah J, Rinsky LA, Glader B. Arthropathy of the ankle in hemophilia. *J Bone Joint Surgery (Am)* 1991; **73A**: 1008–15.

64 Armengol R, Azorin L, Guimera J *et al*. Tratamiento actual de la sinovitis crónica hemofílica. In: Garcia-Talavera J, ed. *Actualidades en Hemofilia*. Barcelona: Espaxs, 1983: 39–48.

65 Brettler DB, Kraus EM, Levine PH. Clinical aspects and therapy for hemophilia A. In: Hoffman R, Benz EJ, Shattil SJ, Cohen HJ, eds. *Hematology: Basic Principles and Practice*. New York: Churchill Livingstone, 1995: 1848–63.

66 Buzzard BM. Physiotherapy for prevention and treatment of chronic hemophilic synovitis. *Clin Orthop* 1997; **343**: 42–6.

67 Greene WB. The role of orthopaedists in the prevention of hemophilic arthropathy (abstract). *Haemophilia* 1996; **2**: 1.

68 Heijnen L. Haemophilia in orthopaedics. *Haemophilia* 1997; **3**: 222–3.

69 Miller R, Beeton K, Goldman E, Ribbans WJ. Counselling guidelines for managing musculoskeletal problems in haemophilia in the 1990s. *Haemophilia* 1997; **3**: 9–13.

70 Iwata N, Hachisuka K, Tanaka S, Naka Y, Ogata H. Measuring activities of daily living among haemophiliacs. *Disabil Rehabil* 1996; **18**: 217–23.

71 Heijnen L, Kleijn P, Van den Berg P. The roles of sports in hemophilia management. Theory and practice. *Proceedings of the XXI International Congress of the World*

Federation of Hemophilia, Mexico, April 1994.

72 Hubert KH, Zauner DA. Rehabilitation at summercamps as an important factor in prevention of haemophilic arthrosis (abstract). *Haemophilia* 1996; **2**: 125.

73 Janco RL, Maclean WE, Perrin JM, Gortmaker SL. A prospective study of patterns of bleeding in boys with haemophilia. *Haemophilia* 1996; **2**: 202–6.

74 Roure E, Vallbona C. Recomendaciones de actividad física desde la atención primaria de salud. *JANO* 1995; **49**: 594–5.

75 Roure E, Vallbona C. Ejercicio físico y enfermedad. *JANO* 1996; **50**: 15.

76 Gonzalez-Iturri JJ, Fernandez J, Commandre F, Ceberio F. Estudio retrospectivo sobre las lesiones de un club de futbol: una temporada deportiva. *Archivos Medicina Deporte* 1994; **11**: 35–40.

77 Gonzalez JC, Guijarro JS, Amigo N. Incidencia y epidemiología de las lesiones ocurridas durante una temporada en un club de futbol. *Archivos Medicina Deporte* 1995; **12**: 189–94.

78 Petrini P, Lindvall N, Egberg N, Blombäck M. Prophylaxis with factor concentrates in preventing hemophilic arthropathy. *Am J Pediatr Hematol Oncol* 1991; **3**: 280–7.

CHAPTER 28

Burnout Syndrome in Haemophilia Staff

P ARRANZ, E C RODRIGUEZ-MERCHAN AND F HERNANDEZ-NAVARRO

INTRODUCTION

Caring for a severely ill person may at times be extremely demanding and distressing, and caring for patients with haemophilia is no exception. In haemophilia almost any organ or system can be affected, leading to the involvement of many professionals from medical, nursing, social work and mental health specialties, as well as voluntary workers. The ability of these health workers to cope with caring for people with haemophilia varies between individuals and within an individual over time. Physicians in Eastern Europe and in underdeveloped countries have to manage with the scarcity of special treatments. They know of their existence and availability in other places but, for a variety of reasons, they have no access to them. This can generate high levels of frustration. The relationship with patients becomes of great importance.

In western countries the problems have a different aspect. There is a large discrepancy between the expectations that professionals may have when they start work in haemophilia and the reality with which they have to cope. There have been many years of steady improvement in the haemophilia community, in which healthcare professionals have been privileged to witness the steady social integration of haemophilic patients. This brought personal satisfaction and professional recognition. However, this has changed in the last few years and has brought increased pressures and demands for reasons that are well-known, which have resulted in tensions and dissatisfaction between healthcare providers and patients with haemophilia. Professionals involved in musculoskeletal related issues also face the professional hazard of burnout. Indeed, members of health and social service groups are often so busy helping others that they neglect their own needs. The definition of burnout and its consequences, risk factors related to musculoskeletal staff and some strategies to cope with the stress associated with this syndrome, are described.

OCCUPATIONAL STRESS AND BURNOUT

Burnout is a term frequently used to describe the experience of health workers dealing with stressful situations, but the term remains imprecise, in spite of the efforts to define and measure it [1]. The concept of burnout is closely related to stress and ways of coping with anxiety. As normal stress increases it can develop into abnormal stress, which is thought to achieve a critical level at some point. This high level of stress can then lead to burnout. Veninga has defined this term as a debilitating psychological condition brought about by the work-related frustrations that result in lower productivity and morale [2]. Burnout can best be described as the process by which a once-committed health professional becomes ineffective in managing the stress of frequent emotional contact with others in the helping context, leading them to experience exhaustion – a feeling of lack of capacity to offer psychological support – and, as a result, disengagement from patients, colleagues and the organization. Burnout also includes a reduced sense of personal accomplishment, involving feelings of dissatisfaction with personal professional competence [3].

Symptoms of burnout occur mainly in four areas of the person's functioning: physical, emotional, behavioural and spiritual. *Physical symptoms* include fatigue, insomnia, lingering minor illness, gastrointestinal disturbances, hypertension, weakness and dizziness, memory problems, headaches or muscle aches. *Emotional symptoms* of burnout include being critical of others, an apathetic attitude, depersonalizing patients, feelings of irritability, low personal accomplishment, frustration with others, hopelessness, depression, poor concentration and feelings of isolation. *Behavioural symptoms* consist of substance abuse, spending less time with patients, rigidity/inflexibility in problem-solving, indecision, absenteeism, impersonal communication or emotional outburst. *Spiritual symptoms* consist of doubt concerning one's value system or beliefs, becoming convinced that a major personal change is necessary such as divorce or a new job, or withdrawing from social contact. Perhaps one of the most striking features of the symptoms described is their severity when taken together [4]. In Table 28.1 we can see the most significant symptoms in detail.

To produce a response to stress, the situation itself is just as important as the subject's perception that he or she can respond effectively to a demand and, therefore, his or her assessment is that of a perception of lack of control, overcoming the healthcare professional's coping capacity. When healthcare professionals lack, or believe themselves to lack, the resources necessary to cope with these demands, and experience feelings of impotence, avoidance behaviour or irritability appear,

Table 28.1 Cognitive, physical and behavioural responses of burnout.

Cognitive	Physical	Behavioural
Recurrent, irrational, intrusive thoughts	Fatigue	Abuse of chemicals
Flashbacks	Insomnia	Avoidance of patients
Sense of insecurity and failure	Headaches and muscular tension	Tardiness and absenteeism
Feelings of low personal accomplishment	Gastrointestinal disturbances	Impersonal communication
Poor concentration	Hypertension	Impulsiveness, irritability
Sadness and boredom		Rigidity in problem-solving
		Propensity to anger and prejudice

and then they are at risk of developing the work-related physical and psychological disorders which constitute burnout syndrome or occupational stress [5]. When professionals can count on sufficient resources the anxiety response disappears and equilibrium is re-established.

STRESSFUL SITUATIONS AT WORK

Despite the fact that surgeons in general are the medical specialty who probably most frequently experience the pleasure of cure, they also have to face a wide range of occupational stressors that fall into a number of categories: personal, organizational and institutional. Musculoskeletal staff carers are no exception. They have to cope with the fear of blood-borne diseases, contagion, overwork, unresolvable uncertainties, over-identification with patients, time pressures, standards, insufficient resources, loneliness in decision-taking, dealing with life and death or difficult issues, demanding chronically ill patients, low recognition or inadequate support personnel, decreased compensation, and an increased threat of litigation, all of which build pressure to practise defensive medicine. Very often there is a lack of time and space to build a real team with a management quality organization. There is a tendency in the work setting to blame people rather than the situation, when the care or service deteriorates and problems appear without solutions. It is important to consider that, for the physician, it is the unanticipated stressors that tend to cause the most problems.

A study of the emotional reactions of haemophilia healthcare providers by Brown *et al.* [6] revealed that the following factors were associated with increased degrees of burnout: greater perceived colleagues' stress, less overall job satisfaction, greater perceived stress in the working environment, fewer team meetings and fewer years of career experience. A minority (7.4% of the 213 respondents) met the criteria for job burnout as assessed by the Maslach and Jackson Burnout Inventory [3]. Some studies have focused on how symptoms of burnout are influenced by staff roles and responsibilities. On a general level, Bates and Moore found that stressors such as role conflict, ambiguity and work overload were more acutely and frequently felt by health professionals who had a high degree of role responsibility [7]. Self-reported stress may not be entirely due to employment or organizational factors, as personal and social factors can also have an influence in the appearance of burnout. Stresses outside work, and pre-existing vulnerability to psychological disorders, may well be of greater relevance in some cases [8]. According to some authors the factors that physicians consider most stressful are: government rules and regulations, insurance or managed care regulations, confronting suffering and death, facing critical decision-making where mistakes have severe consequences, facing increased challenges by patients, fear of being sued for malpractice, and the need to practise defensive medicine. The least stressful factors were time pressures, maintaining clinical competence, maintaining effective relationships with others (teams, patients and families) and facing the realities of medicine that they cannot control.

STRATEGIES TO PREVENT BURNOUT

To face the numerous stressful situations encountered at work, healthcare professionals must adapt continuously and intensely. There have been no systematic reports of intervention to prevent or reduce work-related emotional stress in the haemophilia setting. It is likely that the needs of different professional groups will require different interventions. The emotional stresses faced by junior medical staff involved in caring for patients with chronic medical problems who are able to challenge clinical decisions are likely to be different from those of their more senior colleagues who have been exposed to the continuous demands, accusations or deaths of many of their patients. However, Searle has described active coping styles, stress self-management, self-esteem and expression of feelings in an assertive way, as being the personal qualities that enable staff to deal with work-related difficulties [9].

Besides improving the conditions under which healthcare professionals develop their work, the proposal's approach to management or prevention of burnout implies three levels.

1 Consideration of staff self-evaluation cognitive processes, and the development of strategies that allow them to decrease stressors, avoiding bad experiences or neutralizing the negative consequences of those experiences.

2 Enhancement of training in emotional control and social skills to facilitate adaptive coping resources and strengthening perceptions of self-efficacy and professional competence.

3 Promotion of professional team support.

The final objective is focused on reaching a maximum competence level at a minimal emotional cost. From this perspective, a series of psychological strategies has been proposed to prevent the onset of burnout [10–13].

• It can be hard for physicians to admit negative feelings and recognize their own situation. If the patient is angry or resentful, he or she will probably take it out on the care-giver, who often feels confused, guilty and resentful too. Identifying, admitting and accepting those feelings will help to confront them.

• A high self-esteem and efficiency perception help carers to resist the numerous stressful situations that occur in daily practice. Feeling competent is also a source of motivation at work.

• There is a need to be trained in counselling techniques and in handling emotional reactions. Attention is seldom paid to training doctors in communication skills, despite their enormous importance either in situations of patient conflicts or suffering.

• To make responsible and gratifying use of leisure, to have activities and interests apart from work (sports, hobbies and so on) is also useful as protection against burnout.

• Appreciation and support of the institution they belong to will help the professional to incorporate management initiatives of his/her own, thus increasing motivation towards objectives and shared responsibility.

• There needs to be adequate provision of resources appropriate to the physical and environmental conditions.

• We should discover the art of setting realistic balanced goals, and guiding actions according to them.

• We need to look for adequate training and learn to admit deficiencies, particularly in the communication and handling of emotional skills and how to compensate for shortcomings in these areas. 'Know-how', and when to say 'no'.

• Training in some techniques to reduce anxiety – relaxation, self-hypnosis, yoga, meditation – is very useful. Take a deep breath when beginning to feel anxiety coming on. Dedicating some time to yourself every day is a good way of increasing personal resistance to stress.

• Release tension through enjoyable activities outside work. Engage in the physical exercise of your choice.

• Create well-functioning and coordinated interdisciplinary teams.

• Through attitude and behaviour, foster a team culture. Use agreement and negotiation, instead of imposition, as a better way to resolve conflicts.

• Become an able facilitator inside the team, in a positive atmosphere at work, to be a reinforcer and give support in order to be reinforced and supported. Share delicate decision-taking.

CONCLUSIONS

Healthcare professionals are at risk of developing work-related psychological disorders such as anxiety, low personal accomplishment, boredom, depressive and psychosomatic symptoms, feelings of insecurity and increased irritability. Such mental problems may lead to job dissatisfaction, impaired work performance and a significant number of lost work days. To face the stressful situations encountered at work, physicians should become more aware of the risk of not managing stress related to burnout, incorporate appropriate preventive strategies, starting by understanding the cause of burnout, recognizing where he or she is at risk professionally and personally, reduce the burnout risk and regain emotional control.

The fulfilment obtained through working in the medical and health-care professions occupies a significant part of our real time. It is everyone's task to seek and find the equilibrium that allows them to live, with space and time for creativity and growth, through helping others to improve their quality of life.

REFERENCES

1 Catalan J, Burgess A, Pergami A, Hulme N, Gazzard B, Phillips R. The psychological impact on staff of caring for people with serious diseases: the case of HIV infection and oncology. *J Psychosom Res* 1996; **40**: 425–35.

2 Veninga R. Administrator burnout: causes and cures. *Hosp Progr* 1979; **6**: 45–62.

3 Maslach C, Jackson S. Burnout in health professions: a social psychological analysis. In: Sanders GS, Suls J, eds. *Social Psychology of Illness*. London: Lawrence Erlbaum, 1982.

4 Miller D. Occupational morbidity and burnout: lessons and warnings for HIV/AIDS carers. *Int Rev Psychiat* 1991, **3**: 439–49.

5 Lazarus RS, Folkman S. *Stress, Appraisal and Coping*. New York: Springer, 1984.

6 Brown LK, Stermock AC, Ford HH, Geary M. Emotional reactions of haemophilia health care providers. *Haemophilia* 1999; **5**: 127–31.

7 Bates FM, Moore BN. Stress in hospital personnel. *Med J Austria* 1975; **15**: 751–3.

8 Wilkinson P. Mental health problems at work. *Br Med J* 1993; **306**: 1082–3.
9 Searle E. Knowledge, attitudes and behaviour of heath professionals in relation to AIDS. *Lancet* 1987; **1**: 26–8.
10 Campbell DA Jr. The patient, burnout and the practice of surgery. *Am Surg* 1999; **65**: 601–5.
11 Medical burnout, Inc. webmaster@medicalburnout.com
12 Fields A, Cuerdon T, Brasseux C *et al*. Physician burnout in pediatric critical care medicine. *Crit Care Med* 1995; **23**: 1425–9.
13 Mayou R. Burnout. *Br Med J* 1987; **295**: 284–5.

CHAPTER 29

Some Discussion Essentials for Musculoskeletal Care and Prior to Joint Replacement

R MILLER

INTRODUCTION

The focus of this chapter is on the way that relevant discussion with haemophilic patients and their families about an identified range of issues can contribute to optimal musculoskeletal well-being. Such discussions can be integrated into routine care and specialist orthopaedic clinics by individual haematologists and surgeons in small centres with limited resources, or by members of a multidisciplinary team in highly resourced centres of the world. Some guidelines for identifying and addressing musculoskeletal problems in regular reviews, special orthopaedic clinics [1] and particularly in preparation for joint replacement surgery will be suggested [2].

Achieving optimal musculoskeletal fitness for people with haemophilia is a target for the twenty-first century. Reaching this objective is dependent upon the resources and expertise available for treating bleeding episodes; the skills and techniques of the multidisciplinary specialists; and upon complex psychological and social factors which can impinge upon how patients with haemophilia and their families cope with the condition. Prompt, adequate treatment for bleeds remains the best way to preserve optimal musculoskeletal function [3]. Untreated and under-treated bleeding episodes into muscles and joints can cause pain and deformity and severely limit the functional activities of patients with haemophilia [4,5]. Quality of life is profoundly affected by musculoskeletal problems [6] even in the face of other complicating medical conditions such as HIV and hepatitis C (HCV) infections [7].

Over the last decade HIV and HCV infections have, to some extent, diverted attention away from musculoskeletal problems [8,9]. The improved outlook for patients with HIV on highly active anti-retroviral therapy [10], and the emerging treatments for some patients with HCV, now increases the likelihood of attention focusing on painful, deformed joints.

The orthopaedic surgeon's contribution to haemophilia care through assessment, advice and surgery remains important despite a diminution of joint problems for those patients who have had regular treatment for bleeds. Corrective and palliative surgery for patients with haemophilia has become increasingly possible over the last two decades. There have been advances in more successful surgical interventions, particularly for hips and knees [11–14]. Continuous infusion of concentrates during surgery and the recovery period reduces the risk of bleeding, gives better pain control and can result in shorter admissions [15,16]. Physiotherapy has an important role in maintaining muscle tone and maximum musculoskeletal function generally, and in rehabilitation after major bleeds and following surgery [17].

Haemophilia in 2000

Haemophilia remains a lifelong, potentially life-threatening and often disabling condition. Despite improvements in replacement therapy, bleeds into joints and muscles occur for a variety of reasons which can lead to pain, stiffness and joint deformity.

Home treatment has been a major step forward in improving musculoskeletal care as it enables prompt treatment for bleeding episodes, reducing the worst effects of bleeds and minimizing disruption to daily living activities [18]. Prophylactic treatment, in addition, reduces spontaneous bleeds, thereby giving better protection to joints [19]. However, the potential benefits of treatment can be compromised in some individuals by complex medical, psychological, social and practical factors [1]. Damage to joints, especially ankles, starts early in childhood, even though chronic problems may only occur at a much later age [20].

Concerns about viral infections from factor replacement throughout the 1980s and early 1990s affected attitudes to the management of bleeds [9]. Some patients were hesitant to use blood products and sustained joint damage from untreated bleeds. Some patients who were infected with HIV and HCV are surviving over 15 years with HIV [21], and even longer with HCV [7]. Among these patients there are some with very damaged joints predating adequate treatment. Highly active combination anti-retroviral treatment has improved their health and outlook. This has diverted attention back to their musculoskeletal problems due to the restrictions imposed on their lives from pain and immobility. 'Will I end up in a wheelchair?' is a common concern. Having these infections does not limit interventions that could improve the patient's quality of life, although the stage and prognosis of HIV and liver disease can affect some decisions about orthopaedic surgery. If surgery is feasible, there is no evidence of compromising their immune function and accelerating their disease [22,23], although the risks of sepsis are higher in this group of patients [24,25]. Orthopaedic surgeons have been among the pioneers in gaining experience in operating on HIV-infected patients [26].

Improved availability and effectiveness of replacement factors and prophylactic treatment has fostered a perception of haemophilia being rendered 'normal' among some patients, their families or members of the healthcare team. This attitude can lead to participation in risky activities, such as contact sports, with a reliance on factor replacement if accidents occur. A balance has to be found between enabling patients to partake as fully as possible in 'normal life' activities while educating them about the consequence of taking risks which can lead ultimately to joint damage. Discussion with patients and parents has to focus on helping them make decisions based on the realities of their medical and social situation.

WHY DISCUSSION IS IMPORTANT

An optimum orthopaedic service can be offered if there is a structure within the comprehensive care team for identifying and addressing problems, and specific guidelines for orthopaedic counselling [27].

Targeted discussion with patients and their family helps to use resources well in busy clinics and when costly surgical procedures and replacement therapy are being used. Many patients are reluctant to have joint replacement surgery, and the success of the whole procedure depends on a combination of factors from the patient's and surgeon's perspective [28]. If key issues are explored with patients prior to joint replacement surgery, misunderstandings and unrealistic expectations, preconceptions and beliefs can be identified and addressed. Focused discussion can enhance preoperative understanding and perceptions of both the patient and surgeon. It is often unidentified and unresolved discrepancies that lead to postoperative dissatisfactions and complaints, some of which can lead to litigation. Appropriate discussion can help to avoid such situations which are both time-consuming and stressful for all concerned.

Discussion is especially important when dealing with the 'grey areas' of clinical practice. These are situations where there are no clear answers due to uncertainty of outcome and lack of evidence-based medicine. In such situations, both patient and surgeon may have to take an additional element of risk for the desired 'clinical benefit'. Sometimes surgeons may be ambivalent about how much information should be given to patients. Likewise, patients may be ambivalent about how much they wish to know or not know. It is tempting to avoid difficult discussions when the outlook is unclear, especially if the surgeon considers that the patient's anxiety may be unnecessarily raised due to a lack of certainty.

APPROACH TO COUNSELLING ABOUT ORTHOPAEDIC PROBLEMS

Pertinent medical, practical, psychological and social factors form a background [1,29] to musculoskeletal counselling.

Medical factors

Although the degree of damage to joints usually corresponds to the severity of haemophilia, those with moderate and mild haemophilia can develop significant orthopaedic problems following bleeds. The age and general health of the patient are important considerations, especially if there are other coexistent conditions which might contraindicate surgery, such as cardiovascular or respiratory disease. The stage, current treatment and prognosis for HIV and HCV infections are relevant factors when planning surgery. Obtaining an accurate bleeding history is an integral part of musculoskeletal assessment, including review of the records of bleeding episodes, treatment given, site of the bleed, as well as eliciting the patient's perceptions and beliefs about replacement therapy. Perceptions may differ from the facts, and records may differ from what actually happens. There can be problems with prophylaxis. Some patients get tired of doing it; others have phobias about needles; some have difficulty in gaining venous access and wish to 'preserve' their veins for treating serious bleeding episodes; and yet others treat themselves at a time of day that is not of optimum benefit (at bedtime). Patients on home treatment can develop inappropriate attitudes and habits which must be reviewed and rectified if optimal musculoskeletal care is to be achieved. Although inhibitors to replacement therapy limit surgical interventions, these patients can benefit from specialist orthopaedic and physiotherapy advice about adaptations to daily living and pain reduction. The use of analgesia for the management of chronic and acute pain requires a careful review of daily living activities and propensity to drug dependence [30].

Practical factors

Practical, daily living conditions have an impact on patients' ability to cope adequately with musculoskeletal problems. Quality of life is profoundly affected by mobility. Prolonged walking for those with severe haemophilia can provoke bleeds. Using public transport is very difficult if knees have fixed flexion deformities or are fixed in extension. Adaptations to cars and automatic gears to facilitate ease of driving and protect ankle and knee joints can facilitate participation in daily living activities. Stairs at home, school or work may be difficult to manage and can provoke further bleeding. In some situations consideration must be given, if possible, to installing adaptations, such as rails, stair lifts and downstairs toilets, which may be the only option for those who have inhibitors to replacement therapy and very damaged joints.

Psychological and social factors

These factors can affect how patients cope with haemophilia and subsequently with musculoskeletal complications. Attitudes to haemophilia develop early in life and can be influenced by parents' views. The relationship between parents, the child with haemophilia and unaffected siblings may affect attitudes to and treatment of bleeds. It is difficult for parents to get the correct balance between the reality of haemophilia and allowing children to gain independence. Overprotection is one response. Another is to make life seem as 'normal' as possible by allowing risks to be taken by the child that might subsequently lead to permanently damaged joints. Restricting sport to those activities which have no body contact can be difficult for parents to achieve and the boy to accept. Disclosure of haemophilia to others has always been difficult for those with haemophilia and for their parents for fear of being labelled as disabled. Starting school is often the first time parents have to confront the implications of haemophilia outside the family; with improved treatment many were more willing to talk more openly about haemophilia. Secrecy about the diagnosis of haemophilia emerged again with HIV [31]. Reluctance to tell others about haemophilia can be an obstacle to prompt, adequate treatment. Some patients try to hide the problem at work and in their social lives, but these patients often have considerable walking difficulties, and the tell-tale signs of damaged knee joints are not easy to hide. Some explain deformity and immobility as being due to 'arthritis'.

Against this background regular haemophilia review clinics for those with severe haemophilia A and B, and on a less frequent basis for moderate and mildly affected patients, can be used to ensure that important issues are identified and assessed early. Combined haemophilia–orthopaedic clinics can then focus on the pertinent factors affecting musculoskeletal heath. General advice about joint care and baseline assessment for those whose problems are not yet acute, especially for children, can be offered.

DISCUSSION GUIDELINES

Having clear aims for musculoskeletal counselling facilitates accurate assessment of orthopaedic issues, prepares patients better for orthopaedic surgical intervention and helps to identify and address 'grey areas' of clinical practice. Some guiding principles which help in achieving these aims effectively, include:

• Not making assumptions about patients' concerns, beliefs or wishes.
• Having small, achievable goals for each session with the patient, dealing with the most important concerns first.
• Using words carefully as everything said has an impact, and avoiding the use of technical words and medical jargon to enhance patients' understanding.
• Sharing responsibility with patients about areas of certainty and uncertainty to ensure they are involved in decision-making and resisting the temptation to reassure patients for fear of raising their anxiety.
• Balancing reality (the difficulties of the situation) with hope (for some alleviation of the musculoskeletal difficulty).

Decisions about referral to the orthopaedic surgeon and physiotherapist can be facilitated by using a combination of open and closed questions which identify and address key issues. Eliciting the patient's main concern often leads to identification of a target joint. If the concern is other than orthopaedic, prompting questions can be used, for example: 'You say that your main concern is your falling CD4 count; have you any concerns about your joints?'

Identifying activities or approaches to treatment of bleeding episodes that are not providing optimal protection to joints is part of the bleeding history assessment, for example:

• 'How often do you get a bleed?'
• 'What do you do when you have a bleed'
• 'You say that you are reluctant to treat bleeds; which would you treat and which would you leave?'
• 'What time of day do you usually treat yourself?'
• 'What aspects of treating yourself are easiest? Are there any difficulties?'

Educating young patients, and especially those who continue to take risks, about the effects of bleeds enables them to make more informed decisions for themselves about the degree of risk they are prepared to take, for example:

- 'Do you know what happens when you get a bleed into a joint?'
- 'Each bleed does some damage. Thus early treatment, and avoiding situations that might provoke bleeds, can help preserve your joints. It may not seem a problem now, but how might you view it if your mobility was impaired in 10 years' time?'

At orthopaedic clinics, focus then can be placed on musculoskeletal problems. Differently focused questions from members of the multidisciplinary team (surgeon, haematologist, nurse, physiotherapist, counsellor) provide a comprehensive exploration of the patient's concerns, beliefs and expectations, especially when total joint replacement surgery is being considered. For example:

Surgeon: What would you most want to come out of this consultation?
Patient: For you to tell me that my joints will hold out and I won't land up in a wheelchair.
Surgeon: I cannot guarantee that your joints will not deteriorate as the X-rays show marked damage and you say you have a lot of pain. What would you think about having your knees replaced?
Patient: I don't feel ready for that yet.
Surgeon: What would make you decide that you were ready?

Addressing beliefs about surgery and providing information and advice are important in the process of decision-making and preparation, for example:

- 'If we were to offer you a joint replacement, what do you expect to be able to do that you cannot do now?'
- 'If we replace your knee joint we hope it will improve the pain, but you may not gain a great deal more movement. Would this affect your decision?'
- 'What would have to happen to make the decision about surgery easier to make?'

Helping patients to be specific enables discussion to focus on the main problem joint and clarifies whether the problem is due to bleeding, pain, stiffness, clicking or locking. For example:

- 'Which joint gives you the most problems?'
- 'How often do you get bleeds into that joint?'
- 'What is it about the joint that worries you most?'
- 'Is it pain or stiffness that is the main problem?'
- 'What does the problem stop you doing?'
- 'Is there anything that you do that makes it worse?'
- 'What do you do about the pain?'

Sometimes the views of the patient and surgeon differ about the main problem joint. For example, the patient may complain about an ankle problem, whereas the surgeon may be more concerned about a badly damaged knee joint. The two damaged joints may adversely affect each other. In some cases, it is neither the pain nor the limitations of movement that is the patient's main concern, but the fact that he looks disabled. When contemplating major surgery, it is important that such views are uncovered so that they can be addressed realistically. Surgery may not completely remove outward signs of disability.

If an operation is being suggested, there are a series of questions that help to assess the patient's knowledge, expectations and the optimum time for the procedure to be done.

- 'What would make you decide that you could not go on as you are?'
- 'What do you understand about what a joint replacement might achieve for you?'
- 'What might be your main concern about the operation?'

An assessment of the patient's view about hospitalization and his support system during the rehabilitation period is also important. If the patient has no help, or might place himself in circumstances that could jeopardize the beneficial results of the operation, these need to be identified and addressed. For example:

- 'If you have to be in hospital and away from work for quite some time, what effect will that have on your work situation?'
- 'The rehabilitation after some surgery can be quite prolonged. Are you prepared to do exercises and attend physiotherapy regularly?'

Assessment of unrealistic expectations, such as walking great distances after a knee replacement, is important.

- 'How does the knee problem rank alongside all your other difficulties that you have mentioned?'
- 'What is it that you want to do that you are prevented from doing now?'
- 'What do you hope and expect this operation to achieve?'
- 'How might you cope if the surgery did not achieve exactly what you want?'
- 'If the decision is not to operate at present – how will you manage – what will help – what might make it more difficult?'

Patients also have a series of questions including:

- 'How long will I be in hospital?'
- 'Will you do the two knees at the same time and is this more risky? Will it take twice as long?'
- 'If you operate on my knees, how will my ankles be affected? And what about my bad hip?'
- 'What kind of joint will you use? What is it made of?'
- 'How long will the new joint last? How will I know if it is not holding out? What signs will I get? What can be done if it wears out?'

Some of these questions are easier to answer than others that enter the realms of the 'grey areas' where there is more uncertainty. Skills to open, continue and end difficult conversations with patients are required where there are no clear answers. Information can be given in a way that is understood by the patient, and throughout the conversation it is important to check that the patient's understanding matches with the reality of the situation and those of the surgeon. It is always important to keep careful records about what was discussed, the patient's reactions and the surgeon and other team members' concerns.

CONCLUSIONS

The various members of the multidisciplinary team (physiotherapist, counsellor, nurse, haematologist, surgeon) each have a perspective to add which enhances optimal musculoskeletal care by the comprehensive coverage of issues. Using targeted questions which address key issues helps to gather pertinent information rapidly about patients' wishes, beliefs and expectations. This helps the surgeon to address unrealistic expectations; the patient to gain a better understanding; other team members to address fears, personal and family difficulties, and practical problems. Decision-making is made easier for surgeon and patient and there are less postoperative difficulties [6]. Probing questions help patients to identify issues they might not have otherwise considered and thus to clarify their expectations of joint surgery. Focused discussions bring more clarity to 'grey areas' of total joint replacement and other orthopaedic surgery. Questions can raise anxieties not previously considered, but if dilemmas and uncertainties are identified they can then be addressed. Such an approach can also help surgeons and others who work in busy clinics without the backup of the multidisciplinary team. Questions can be refined over time and adapted to different settings.

Musculoskeletal treatment remains a major component of haemophilia care. Patients can become depressed and isolated due to limitations on daily activities. The development of improved replacement therapy, home treatment and advances in surgical techniques have all contributed to a better musculoskeletal outlook for those with haemophilia. Appropriate, focused discussion will facilitate and enhance musculoskeletal management.

REFERENCES

1 Miller R, Beeton, K, Goldman E, Ribbans WJ. Counselling guidelines for managing musculoskeletal problems in haemophilia in the 1990s. *Haemophilia* 1997; **3**: 9–13

2 Miller R, Beeton K, Madgwick C *et al*. Joint replacements from 1983 to 1998 in patients with haemophilia and HIV infection: medical, psychological and social factors (abstract). 23rd International Congress of the World Federation of Hemophilia, The Hague, 17–21 May 1998. *Haemophilia* 1998; **4**: 320.

3 Petrini P, Lindvall N, Egberg N, Blomback M. Prophylaxis with factor concentrates in preventing hemophilic arthropathy. *Am J Pediatr Hematol Oncol* 1991; **13**: 280–7.

4 Rodriguez-Merchan EC. Effects of hemophilia on articulations of children and adults. *Clin Orthop* 1996; **328**: 7–13.

5 York JR. Musculoskeletal disorders in the haemophilias. *Bailliere's Clin Rheumatol* 1991; **5**: 197–220.

6 Miller R, Beeton K, Miners A, Padkin J, Goddard N. Quality of life issues: patients with haemophilia and joint replacements 1996-99 (abstract). Presented at the *5th Musculoskeletal Congress of the World Federation of Hemophilia*, Sydney, 14–16 April, 1999.

7 Telfer P, Sabin C, Devereux H, Scott F, Dusheiko G, Lee C. The progression of HCV-associated liver disease in a cohort of haemophilic patients. *Br J Haematol* 1994; **87**: 555–61.

8 Kernoff PBA, Miller R. AIDS-related problems in the management of haemophilia. In: Miller D, Weber J, Green J, eds. *The Management of AIDS Patients.* Basingstoke: Macmillan, 1986: 81–91.

9 Lee CA, Miller R, Goldman E. Treatment dilemmas for HIV infected haemophiliacs. *AIDS Care* 1989; **1**: 153–8.

10 BHIVA Guidelines Co-ordinating Committee. British HIV Association guidelines for antiretroviral treatment of HIV seropositive individuals. *Lancet* 1997; **349**: 1086–92.

11 Ribbans WJ, Phillips M, Stock D, Stibe E. Haemophilic ankle problems: orthopaedic solutions. *Haemophilia* 1995; **1**: 91–6.

12 Birch NC, Ribbans WJ, Goldman E, Lee CA. Knee replacement in haemophilia. *J Bone Joint Surg (Br)* 1994; **76B**: 165–6.

13 Heck DA, Robinson RL, Partridge CM, Lubitz RM, Freund DA. Patient outcomes after knee replacement. *Clin Orthop* 1998; **356**: 93–110.

14 Heeg M, Meyer K, Smid WM, Van Horn JR, Van der Meer J. Total knee and hip arthroplasty in haemophilic patients. *Haemophilia* 1998; **4**: 747–51.

15 Hathaway WE, Christian MJ, Clarke SL, Hasiba U. Comparison of continuous and intermittent Factor VIII concentrate therapy in hemophilia A. *Am J Hematol* 1984; **17**: 85–8.

16 Martinowitz U, Schulman S, Gitel S, Horozowski H,

Heim M, Varon D. Adjusted dose continuous infusion of factor VIII in patients with haemophilia A. *Br J Haematol* 1992; **82**: 729–34.

17 Heijnen L. *Recent Advances in Rehabilitation in Haemophilia*. Hove: Medical Education Network, 1995.

18 Le Quesne B, Britten MI, Maragaki C, Dormandy KM. Home treatment for patients with haemophilia. *Lancet* 1974; **2**: 507–9.

19 Nilsson IM, Berntorp K, Löfqvist T, Pettersson H. Twenty-five years' experience of prophylactic treatment in severe haemophilia A and B. *J Intern Med* 1992; **232**: 25–32.

20 Ribbans WJ, Phillips AN. Hemophilic ankle arthropathy. *Clin Orthop* 1996; **328**: 39–45.

21 Phillips AN, Sabin CA, Elford J, Bofill M, Janossy G, Lee CA. Use of CD4 lymphocyte count to predict long-term survival free of AIDS after HIV infection. *Br Med J* 1994; **309**: 309–13.

22 Phillips M, Sabin C, Ribbans WJ. The effect of open joint surgery on CD4 counts of HIV positive haemophilics. 3rd Musculoskeletal Congress of the World Federation of Hemophilia, Herzilya, Israel, June 1995. *Haemophilia*, 1996; **2**: 45–55.

23 Phillips AN, Sabin C, Ribbans WJ, Lee CA. Orthopaedic surgery in hemophilic patients with human immunodeficiency virus. *Clin Orthop* 1997; **343**: 81–7.

24 Ragni MV, Crossett LS, Herndon JH. Postoperative infection following orthopaedic surgery in human immunodeficiency virus-infected hemophiliacs with CD4 counts <200/mm³. *J Arthroplasty* 1995; **10**: 716–21.

25 Greene WB, DeGnore LT, White GC. Orthopaedic procedures and prognosis in haemophilic patients who are seropositive for human immunodeficiency virus. *J Bone Joint Surg (Am)* 1990; **72A**: 2–11.

26 Ribbans W. "Reducing the risk": barrier protection in the orthopaedic operating room. *New World Health* 1997; Jan: 63–4.

27 Bor R, Miller R, Latz, M, Salt, H. *Counselling in Health Care Settings*. London: Cassell, 1998.

28 Miller R, Beeton K, Goddard N: Some discussion essentials prior to joint replacement in patients with haemophilia (abstract). In: *Abstracts of 5th Musculoskeletal Congress of the World Federation of Hemophilia*, Sydney, 14–16 April, 1999.

29 Miller R. *A Framework for Psycho-social Services in Haemophilia Care*. World Federation of Haemophilia, Alpha Therapeutic, 1988.

30 Phillips M, Birch N, Ribbans WJ. Post-operative analgesia requirements in haemophiliacs. 3rd Musculoskeletal Congress of the World Federation of Hemophilia, Herzilya, Israel, 1995. *Haemophilia* 1996; **2**: 45–55.

31 Miller R, Goldman E, Bor R, Kernoff PB. Counselling children and adults about AIDS/HIV: the ripple effect on haemophilia care settings. *Counselling Psychol* 1989; **2**: 65–72.

CHAPTER 30

Anti-Inflammatory Drugs in the Management of Haemophilic Arthropathy: A Rheumatologist's Point of View

J YORK

INTRODUCTION

The role of drug therapy in haemophilic arthropathy is limited. Konig in 1892 initially described the pathology in the haemophilic joint where the synovitis resembles that seen in the synovium in rheumatoid arthritis, while the changes in bone resemble those seen in osteoarthritis [1]. There is compelling evidence that the initiating event is the deposition of iron in the synovium, and more importantly in the chondrocyte complex of articular cartilage [2,3]. Treatment therefore may be directed towards suppression of inflammation and/or the protection of cartilage and bone.

In general rheumatological terms there are five broad pharmacological groups of therapeutic agents (Table 30.1). All may have a part at some stage for some patients with haemophilia, but their precise roles have not been clearly defined. This chapter deals with the use of nonsteroidal anti-inflammatory drugs and corticosteroids, and the limited experience with so-called anti-rheumatic and chondroprotective agents.

Immunosuppressive and cytotoxic therapy has been used in selected cases to lower levels of clotting factor inhibitors, the major experience being in acquired forms of haemophilia [4–6]. Nonsteroidal anti-inflammatory drugs (NSAIDs) are the most commonly used drugs, but their principal disadvantages are the risk of occult or symptomatic gastrointestinal blood loss and their effect on platelet function, which is variable in both extent and duration. In the context of haemophilia their effects can be catastrophic. Ibuprofen, indomethacin and salicylates and the now discredited benoxprofen have all been used in small and most-

Table 30.1 Groups of pharmacological agents.

1	Analgesics
2	Anti-inflammatory agents, including nonsteroidal anti-inflammatory drugs, local intra-articular anti-inflammatory agents and corticosteroids
3	Anti-rheumatic and chondroprotective agents
4	Immunosuppressive and cytotoxic agents
5	General supportive drugs

ly uncontrolled studies [7–10]. Experience at the International Haemophilia Training Centre at the Royal Prince Alfred Hospital has been with the use of sulindac, a so-called pro-drug, said to be less likely to cause gastrointestinal bleeding. It is absorbed as the inactive form, which is attached to a sulphide radical within the liver and excreted in the bile as the active agent which is then reabsorbed and part of which undergoes enteropathic recirculation. However, the circulating active drug may have an effect on gastroprotection, and our studies have also shown that it has a measurable effect on platelet function. The newly released COX-2 selective NSAIDs, for example, celecoxib or rofecoxib, with improved gastrointestinal tolerance and no observable effect on platelet function, will be a welcome addition to the therapeutic options.

Corticosteroid agents, both locally injected intra-articularly after appropriate factor replacement, and as short courses of oral therapy, have been widely used [11–13]. The use of local intra-articular anti-inflammatory agents, such as rifampicin, yttrium-90 or dysprosium, are covered in Chapter 6.

The so-called anti-rheumatic drugs and some of the newly developed chondroprotective agents have not been adequately tried, but a small series of patients with haemophilia have been treated with D-penicillamine [14], and there is interest in the use of the metalloproteinase inhibitors such as tetracycline in the protection of articular cartilage [15,16].

The role of intra-articular hyaluronate has been studied in a small uncontrolled trial in haemophilia, but the need for repeated intra-articular injection limits its practicability [17]. This chapter is an attempt to provide perspective in the use of the available agents.

DRUG THERAPY

In the acute bleeding episode, the essential principles remain early recognition of bleeding, adequate factor replacement, initial immobilization, the use of physical measures, such as ice and so on, and then intensive physiotherapy. The use of prophylactic treatment in all newly diagnosed children is an ideal which can be achieved in developed countries, but is unfortunately well beyond the 80% of the world's haemophilic population who do not have access to treatment.

In the subacute phase, where the hallmark of the condition is a so-called boggy synovitis, again the essential principles of treatment are prophylactic factor replacement, intensive physiotherapy, short-term oral corticosteroid therapy in selected cases [12], or under some circumstances arthroscopic washing out of blood clot and instillation of corticosteroid. At a later stage, the use of either chemical or radioactive synovectomy and where available arthroscopic or open surgical synovectomy may be necessary.

Nonsteroidal anti-inflammatory drugs (NSAIDs) in our hands have had very limited, if any, value at this stage and this is the general experience of most clinicians. The use of D-penicillamine [14] has been reported in one comparatively small series, and our experience of its use in only one or two cases has not given us any grounds for optimism, but there have been no properly conducted controlled trials. The occurrence of thrombocytopenia as a well-recognized side-effect of the drug may temper any therapeutic enthusiasm. At all stages of the disease, there is always the possibility that the acute symptoms may be due to intra-articular infection, and as home treatment is the norm in many developed countries, a high index of suspicion for sepsis must be maintained, and where appropriate, aspiration of the joint and culture of the synovial fluid performed. There is an important role at this stage for the use of splints and shock absorption orthotics in ankle involvement.

It is in the chronic stage of the disease where NSAIDs are of more value. The differentiation of symptoms due to intra-articular bleeding from those due to arthritic disease may be difficult. The treatment of bleeding is replacement therapy, whereas arthritic symptoms may respond to anti-inflammatory agents. NSAIDs have proved valuable for symptom relief, but patients must be warned to be vigilant to detect gastric irritation and especially evidence of gastrointestinal bleeding. The choice of agent is an individual preference but aspirin, in view of its prolonged and irreversible effect on platelet function, should be avoided.

Local corticosteroid injections

Intra-articular and soft-tissue injections are of value to deal with a target joint in both the subacute and chronic stages of the arthropathy. The knee, elbow, ankle and shoulder joints are most frequently injected, and soft-tissue and intrabursal infiltration may be necessary.

Given the high prevalence of viral infections in many older haemophilic patients, protective clothing (gloves, face masks, goggles) should be worn by the physician. After appropriate factor replacement, the skin should be prepared with iodine or a similar antiseptic and the joint injected using standard techniques [18]. In badly deformed joints, the use of an image intensifier or ultrasonic guidance should be used to ensure accurate placement of the corticosteroid, which is often given mixed with local anaesthetic. If there is any doubt about joint sepsis, the synovial fluid aspirated should be cultured and the procedure deferred. The presence of any local skin sepsis adjacent to the joint contraindicates corticosteroid injection.

GENERAL MEASURES

The use of non-pharmacological methods of pain control may be helpful, such as relaxation and pain control techniques, the use of forms of electrical pain relief, such as transcutaneous nerve stimulation, antidepressant therapy, and above all else compassionate supportive counselling. Unfortunately, many patients with end-stage joint disease ultimately require surgical procedures.

REFERENCES

1 Konig F. Die Gelenkerkrankungen bei Blutern mit besonderer Berücksichtigung der Diagnose. *Klin Vorträge* 1892; **36**: 233–40. [Translation in *Clin Orthop* 1967; **52**: 5–11.]

2 Rosendaal G, Vianen M, van Rinsom A *et al*. Iron deposits and catabolic properties of synovial tissue in haemophilic arthropathy (abstract). *Br J Rheumatol*

1997; **36** (suppl. 1): 86.

3 Roosendaal G. *Blood-induced Cartilage Damage in Haemophilia*. Monograph. Utrecht: Elinwijk, 1998.

4 Green D, Schuette PT, Wallace WH. Factor VIII antibodies in rheumatoid arthritis: effect of cyclophosphamide. *Arch Intern Med* 1980; **140**: 1232–5.

5 Herbst KD, Rapaport SI, Kenoyer DG *et al*. Syndrome of an acquired inhibitor of factor VIII responsive to cyclophosphamide and prednisone. *Ann Intern Med* 1981; **95**: 575–8.

6 Lafferty TE, Smith J Bruce, Schuster J, De Heratius RJ. Treatment of acquired factor VIII inhibitor using intravenous immunoglobulin in two patients with systemic lupus erythematosus. *Arthritis Rheum* 1997; **40**: 775–8.

7 Hasiba U, Scranton P, Lewis J *et al*. Efficacy and safety of ibuprofen for hemophilic arthropathy. *Arch Intern Med* 1980; **140**: 1583–5.

8 Inwood MJ, Killackey B, Startup J. The use and safety of ibuprofen in the hemophiliac. *Blood* 1983; **61**: 709–11.

9 Steven MM, Small M, Pinkerton L *et al*. Non-steroidal anti-inflammatory drugs in haemophilic arthritis – a clinical and laboratory study. *Haemostasis* 1985; **15**: 204–9.

10 Thomas P, Hepburn B, Kim H *et al*. Nonsteroidal anti-inflammatory drugs in the treatment of hemophilic arthropathy. *Am J Hematol* 1982; **12**: 131–7.

11 Stefanini M. Effect of long-term treatment of haemophiliacs with flavenoids or glucocorticoids: preliminary communication. *Lancet* 1962; **1**: 194–5.

12 Kisker CT, Burke C. Double-blind studies on the use of corticosteroids in the treatment of acute hemarthrosis in patients with hemophilia. *N Engl J Med* 1970; **282**: 639–42.

13 Shupak R, Teital J, Garvey M *et al*. Intra-articular methyl prednisolone therapy in hemophilic arthropathy. *Am J Haematol* 1998; **27**: 26–9.

14 Corrigan J, Kolbac S, Gall E *et al*. Treatment of hemophilic arthritis with D-penicillamine. a preliminary report. *Am J Haematol* 1985; **19**: 255–64.

15 Howell D, Altman R, Pelletier J *et al*. Disease-modifying antirheumatic drugs: current status of their application in animal models of osteoarthritis. In: Kuettner K, Goldberg V, eds. *Osteoarthritic Disorders*. Rosemont, IL: American Academy of Orthopaedic Surgeons 1995: 365–77.

16 Brandt K. Modification by oral doxycycline administration of articular cartilage breakdown in osteoarthritis. *J Rheumatol* 1995; **22** (Suppl. 43): 149–51.

17 Wallny T, Brachmann H, Semper H *et al*. Hyaluronic acid and hemophilic arthropathy of the knee. In: *Proceedings of 5th World Federation of Haemophilia Musculoskeletal Congress*. Sydney, April 1999.

18 Canoso J. Aspiration and injection of joints and periarticular tissues. In: Klippel J, Dieppe P, eds. *Rheumatology*, 2nd edn. London: Mosby, 1998: 2.12.1–2.12.11.

Index